## Blood Pressure (BP) Levels for Girls by Age and Height Percentile

| AGE (yr) | BP PERCENTILE | SYSTOLIC BP (mm Hg) PERCENTILE OF HEIGHT | | | | | | | DIASTOLIC BP (mm Hg) PERCENTILE OF HEIGHT | | | | | | |
|---|---|---|---|---|---|---|---|---|---|---|---|---|---|---|---|
| | | 5th | 10th | 25th | 50th | 75th | 90th | 95th | 5th | 10th | 25th | 50th | 75th | 90th | 95th |
| 1 | 50th | 83 | 84 | 85 | 86 | 88 | 89 | 90 | 38 | 39 | 39 | 40 | 41 | 41 | 42 |
| | 90th | 97 | 97 | 98 | 100 | 101 | 102 | 103 | 52 | 53 | 53 | 54 | 55 | 55 | 56 |
| | 95th | 100 | 101 | 102 | 104 | 105 | 106 | 107 | 56 | 57 | 57 | 58 | 59 | 59 | 60 |
| | 99th | 108 | 108 | 109 | 111 | 112 | 113 | 114 | 64 | 64 | 65 | 65 | 66 | 67 | 67 |
| 2 | 50th | 85 | 85 | 87 | 88 | 89 | 91 | 91 | 43 | 44 | 44 | 45 | 46 | 46 | 47 |
| | 90th | 98 | 99 | 100 | 101 | 103 | 104 | 105 | 57 | 58 | 58 | 59 | 60 | 61 | 61 |
| | 95th | 102 | 103 | 104 | 105 | 107 | 108 | 109 | 61 | 62 | 62 | 63 | 64 | 65 | 65 |
| | 99th | 109 | 110 | 111 | 112 | 114 | 115 | 116 | 69 | 69 | 70 | 70 | 71 | 72 | 72 |
| 3 | 50th | 86 | 87 | 88 | 89 | 91 | 92 | 93 | 47 | 48 | 48 | 49 | 50 | 50 | 51 |
| | 90th | 100 | 100 | 102 | 103 | 104 | 106 | 106 | 61 | 62 | 62 | 63 | 64 | 64 | 65 |
| | 95th | 104 | 104 | 105 | 107 | 108 | 109 | 110 | 65 | 66 | 66 | 67 | 68 | 68 | 69 |
| | 99th | 111 | 111 | 113 | 114 | 115 | 116 | 117 | 73 | 73 | 74 | 74 | 75 | 76 | 76 |
| 4 | 50th | 88 | 88 | 90 | 91 | 92 | 94 | 94 | 50 | 50 | 51 | 52 | 52 | 53 | 54 |
| | 90th | 101 | 102 | 103 | 104 | 106 | 107 | 108 | 64 | 64 | 65 | 66 | 67 | 67 | 68 |
| | 95th | 105 | 106 | 107 | 108 | 110 | 111 | 112 | 68 | 68 | 69 | 70 | 71 | 71 | 72 |
| | 99th | 112 | 113 | 114 | 115 | 117 | 118 | 119 | 76 | 76 | 76 | 77 | 78 | 79 | 79 |
| 5 | 50th | 89 | 90 | 91 | 93 | 94 | 95 | 96 | 52 | 53 | 53 | 54 | 55 | 55 | 56 |
| | 90th | 103 | 103 | 105 | 106 | 107 | 109 | 109 | 66 | 67 | 67 | 68 | 69 | 69 | 70 |
| | 95th | 107 | 107 | 108 | 110 | 111 | 112 | 113 | 70 | 71 | 71 | 72 | 73 | 73 | 74 |
| | 99th | 114 | 114 | 116 | 117 | 118 | 120 | 120 | 78 | 78 | 79 | 79 | 80 | 81 | 81 |
| 6 | 50th | 91 | 92 | 93 | 94 | 96 | 97 | 98 | 54 | 54 | 55 | 56 | 56 | 57 | 58 |
| | 90th | 104 | 105 | 106 | 108 | 109 | 110 | 111 | 68 | 68 | 69 | 70 | 70 | 71 | 72 |
| | 95th | 108 | 109 | 110 | 111 | 113 | 114 | 115 | 72 | 72 | 73 | 74 | 74 | 75 | 76 |
| | 99th | 115 | 116 | 117 | 119 | 120 | 121 | 122 | 80 | 80 | 80 | 81 | 82 | 83 | 83 |
| 7 | 50th | 93 | 93 | 95 | 96 | 97 | 99 | 99 | 55 | 56 | 56 | 57 | 58 | 58 | 59 |
| | 90th | 106 | 107 | 108 | 109 | 111 | 112 | 113 | 69 | 70 | 70 | 71 | 72 | 72 | 73 |
| | 95th | 110 | 111 | 112 | 113 | 115 | 116 | 116 | 73 | 74 | 74 | 75 | 76 | 76 | 77 |
| | 99th | 117 | 118 | 119 | 120 | 122 | 123 | 124 | 81 | 81 | 82 | 82 | 83 | 84 | 84 |
| 8 | 50th | 95 | 95 | 96 | 98 | 99 | 100 | 101 | 57 | 57 | 57 | 58 | 59 | 60 | 60 |
| | 90th | 108 | 109 | 110 | 111 | 113 | 114 | 114 | 71 | 71 | 71 | 72 | 73 | 74 | 74 |
| | 95th | 112 | 112 | 114 | 115 | 116 | 118 | 118 | 75 | 75 | 75 | 76 | 77 | 78 | 78 |
| | 99th | 119 | 120 | 121 | 122 | 123 | 125 | 125 | 82 | 82 | 83 | 83 | 84 | 85 | 86 |
| 9 | 50th | 96 | 97 | 98 | 100 | 101 | 102 | 103 | 58 | 58 | 58 | 59 | 60 | 61 | 61 |
| | 90th | 110 | 110 | 112 | 113 | 114 | 116 | 116 | 72 | 72 | 72 | 73 | 74 | 75 | 75 |
| | 95th | 114 | 114 | 115 | 117 | 118 | 119 | 120 | 76 | 76 | 76 | 77 | 78 | 79 | 79 |
| | 99th | 121 | 121 | 123 | 124 | 125 | 127 | 127 | 83 | 83 | 84 | 84 | 85 | 86 | 87 |
| 10 | 50th | 98 | 99 | 100 | 102 | 103 | 104 | 105 | 59 | 59 | 59 | 60 | 61 | 62 | 62 |
| | 90th | 112 | 112 | 114 | 115 | 116 | 118 | 118 | 73 | 73 | 73 | 74 | 75 | 76 | 76 |
| | 95th | 116 | 116 | 117 | 119 | 120 | 121 | 122 | 77 | 77 | 77 | 78 | 79 | 80 | 80 |
| | 99th | 123 | 123 | 125 | 126 | 127 | 129 | 129 | 84 | 84 | 85 | 86 | 86 | 87 | 88 |
| 11 | 50th | 100 | 101 | 102 | 103 | 105 | 106 | 107 | 60 | 60 | 60 | 61 | 62 | 63 | 63 |
| | 90th | 114 | 114 | 116 | 117 | 118 | 119 | 120 | 74 | 74 | 74 | 75 | 76 | 77 | 77 |
| | 95th | 118 | 118 | 119 | 121 | 122 | 123 | 124 | 78 | 78 | 78 | 79 | 80 | 81 | 81 |
| | 99th | 125 | 125 | 126 | 128 | 129 | 130 | 131 | 85 | 85 | 86 | 87 | 87 | 88 | 89 |
| 12 | 50th | 102 | 103 | 104 | 105 | 107 | 108 | 109 | 61 | 61 | 61 | 62 | 63 | 64 | 64 |
| | 90th | 116 | 116 | 117 | 119 | 120 | 121 | 122 | 75 | 75 | 75 | 76 | 77 | 78 | 78 |
| | 95th | 119 | 120 | 121 | 123 | 124 | 125 | 126 | 79 | 79 | 79 | 80 | 81 | 82 | 82 |
| | 99th | 127 | 127 | 128 | 130 | 131 | 132 | 133 | 86 | 86 | 87 | 88 | 88 | 89 | 90 |
| 13 | 50th | 104 | 105 | 106 | 107 | 109 | 110 | 110 | 62 | 62 | 62 | 63 | 64 | 65 | 65 |
| | 90th | 117 | 118 | 119 | 121 | 122 | 123 | 124 | 76 | 76 | 76 | 77 | 78 | 79 | 79 |
| | 95th | 121 | 122 | 123 | 124 | 126 | 127 | 128 | 80 | 80 | 80 | 81 | 82 | 83 | 83 |
| | 99th | 128 | 129 | 130 | 132 | 133 | 134 | 135 | 87 | 87 | 88 | 89 | 89 | 90 | 91 |
| 14 | 50th | 106 | 106 | 107 | 109 | 110 | 111 | 112 | 63 | 63 | 63 | 64 | 65 | 66 | 66 |
| | 90th | 119 | 120 | 121 | 122 | 124 | 125 | 125 | 77 | 77 | 77 | 78 | 79 | 80 | 80 |
| | 95th | 123 | 123 | 125 | 126 | 127 | 129 | 129 | 81 | 81 | 81 | 82 | 83 | 84 | 84 |
| | 99th | 130 | 131 | 132 | 133 | 135 | 136 | 136 | 88 | 88 | 89 | 90 | 90 | 91 | 92 |
| 15 | 50th | 107 | 108 | 109 | 110 | 111 | 113 | 113 | 64 | 64 | 64 | 65 | 66 | 67 | 67 |
| | 90th | 120 | 121 | 122 | 123 | 125 | 126 | 127 | 78 | 78 | 78 | 79 | 80 | 81 | 81 |
| | 95th | 124 | 125 | 126 | 127 | 129 | 130 | 131 | 82 | 82 | 82 | 83 | 84 | 85 | 85 |
| | 99th | 131 | 132 | 133 | 134 | 136 | 137 | 138 | 89 | 89 | 90 | 91 | 91 | 92 | 93 |
| 16 | 50th | 108 | 108 | 110 | 111 | 112 | 114 | 114 | 64 | 64 | 65 | 66 | 66 | 67 | 68 |
| | 90th | 121 | 122 | 123 | 124 | 126 | 127 | 128 | 78 | 78 | 79 | 80 | 81 | 81 | 82 |
| | 95th | 125 | 126 | 127 | 128 | 130 | 131 | 132 | 82 | 82 | 83 | 84 | 85 | 85 | 86 |
| | 99th | 132 | 133 | 134 | 135 | 137 | 138 | 139 | 90 | 90 | 90 | 91 | 92 | 93 | 93 |
| 17 | 50th | 108 | 109 | 110 | 111 | 113 | 114 | 115 | 64 | 65 | 65 | 66 | 67 | 67 | 68 |
| | 90th | 122 | 122 | 123 | 125 | 126 | 127 | 128 | 78 | 79 | 79 | 80 | 81 | 81 | 82 |
| | 95th | 125 | 126 | 127 | 129 | 130 | 131 | 132 | 82 | 83 | 83 | 84 | 85 | 85 | 86 |
| | 99th | 133 | 133 | 134 | 136 | 137 | 138 | 139 | 90 | 90 | 91 | 91 | 92 | 93 | 93 |

## Centigrade to Fahrenheit Temperature Conversions

| °C | °F | °C | °F | °C | °F |
|---|---|---|---|---|---|
| 35.0 | 95.0 | 37.0 | 98.6 | 39.0 | 102.2 |
| 35.2 | 95.4 | 37.2 | 99.0 | 39.2 | 102.6 |
| 35.4 | 95.7 | 37.4 | 99.3 | 39.4 | 102.9 |
| 35.6 | 96.1 | 37.6 | 99.7 | 39.6 | 103.3 |
| 35.8 | 96.4 | 37.8 | 100.0 | 39.8 | 103.6 |
| **36.0** | **96.8** | **38.0** | **100.4** | **40.0** | **104.0** |
| 36.2 | 97.2 | 38.2 | 100.8 | 40.2 | 104.4 |
| 36.4 | 97.5 | 38.4 | 101.1 | 40.4 | 104.7 |
| 36.6 | 97.9 | 38.6 | 101.5 | 40.6 | 105.1 |
| 36.8 | 98.2 | 38.8 | 101.8 | 40.8 | 105.4 |
| | | | | **41.0** | **105.8** |

*Conversion formulas:*
$°F = (°C \times \frac{9}{5}) + 32$ or $(°C \times 1.8) + 32$
$°C = (°F - 32) + \frac{5}{9}$ or $(°F - 32) + 0.55$

## Normal Temperatures in Children

| AGE | TEMPERATURE | |
|---|---|---|
| | °F | °C |
| 3 months | 99.4 | 37.5 |
| 6 months | 99.5 | 37.5 |
| 1 year | 99.7 | 37.7 |
| 3 years | 99.0 | 37.2 |
| 5 years | 98.6 | 37.0 |
| 7 years | 98.3 | 36.8 |
| 9 years | 98.1 | 36.7 |
| 11 years | 98.0 | 36.7 |
| 13 years | 97.8 | 36.6 |

Modified from Lowrey GH: *Growth and development of children,* ed 8, St Louis, 1986, Mosby.

## Normal Heart Rates for Infants and Children

| Age | RATE (beats/min) | | |
|---|---|---|---|
| | Resting (Awake) | Resting (Sleeping) | Exercise (Fever) |
| Newborn | 100-180 | 80-160 | Up to 220 |
| 1 week to 3 months | 100-220 | 80-200 | Up to 220 |
| 3 months to 2 years | 80-150 | 70-120 | Up to 200 |
| 2 years to 10 years | 70-110 | 60-90 | Up to 200 |
| 10 years to adult | 55-90 | 50-90 | Up to 200 |

From Gillette PC: Dysrhythmias. In Adams FH, Emmanoulides GC, Riemenschneider TA, editors: *Moss' heart disease in infants, children, and adolescents,* ed 4, Baltimore, 1989, Williams & Wilkins.

## Normal Respiratory Rates for Children

| AGE | RATE (breaths/min) |
|---|---|
| Newborn | 35 |
| 1 to 11 months | 30 |
| 2 years | 25 |
| 4 years | 23 |
| 6 years | 21 |
| 8 years | 20 |
| 10 years | 19 |
| 12 years | 19 |
| 14 years | 18 |
| 16 years | 17 |
| 18 years | 16-18 |

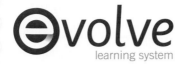
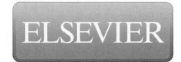
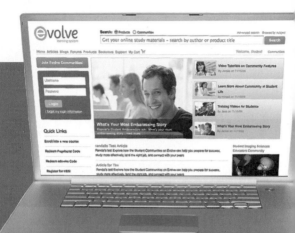

EIGHTH EDITION

## WONG'S

# CLINICAL MANUAL OF

# Pediatric Nursing

**David Wilson, MS, RNC**
Staff, Children's Hospital, Saint Francis Hospital;
Faculty, Langston University School of Nursing
Tulsa, Oklahoma

**Marilyn J. Hockenberry, PhD, RN, PNP-BC, FAAN**
Director of Nurse Practitioners, Texas Children's Cancer Center;
Professor, Department of Pediatrics, Baylor College of Medicine;
Houston, Texas
Consulting Professor
Duke School of Nursing
Durham, North Carolina

**ELSEVIER**
MOSBY

# ELSEVIER
## MOSBY

3251 Riverport Lane
St. Louis, Missouri 63043

---

### Notices

Knowledge and best practice in this field are constantly changing. As new research and experience broaden our understanding, changes in research methods, professional practices, or medical treatment may become necessary.

Practitioners and researchers must always rely on their own experience and knowledge in evaluating and using any information, methods, compounds, or experiments described herein. In using such information or methods, they should be mindful of their own safety and the safety of others, including parties for whom they have a professional responsibility.

With respect to any drug or pharmaceutical products identified, readers are advised to check the most current information provided (i) on procedures featured or (ii) by the manufacturer of each product to be administered, to verify the recommended dose or formula, the method and duration of administration, and contraindications. It is the responsibility of practitioners, relying on their own experience and knowledge of their patients, to make diagnoses, to determine dosages and the best treatment for each individual patient, and to take all appropriate safety precautions.

To the fullest extent of the law, neither the Publisher nor the authors, contributors, or editors assume any liability for any injury and/or damage to persons or property as a matter of products liability, negligence, or otherwise, or from any use or operation of any methods, products, instructions, or ideas contained in the material herein.

---

Library of Congress Cataloging-in-Publication Data
Wilson, David, 1950 Aug. 25-
    Wong's clinical manual of pediatric nursing.—8th ed. / David Wilson, Marilyn J. Hockenberry.
       p. ; cm.
    Clinical manual of pediatric nursing
    Includes bibliographical references and index.
    ISBN 978-0-323-07781-1
    1. Pediatric nursing—Handbooks, manuals, etc.   I. Hockenberry, Marilyn J.   II. Wong, Donna L., 1948-2008. Clinical manual of pediatric nursing.   III. Title.   IV. Title: Clinical manual of pediatric nursing.
    [DNLM:   1. Pediatric Nursing—methods.   WY 159]
    RJ245.H59 2012
    618.92'00231—dc22

                                                                            2011005669

*Managing Editor:* Michele D. Hayden
*Developmental Editor:* Heather Bays
*Publishing Services Manager:* Jeff Patterson
*Senior Project Manager:* Anne Konopka
*Design Direction:* Margaret Reid

Printed in the United States of America

Last digit is the print number:   9   8   7   6   5   4   3

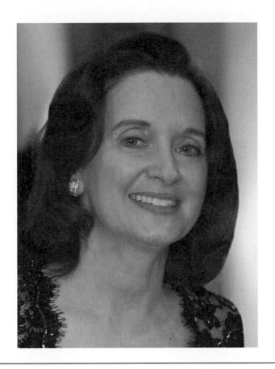

We dedicate this edition of *Wong's Clinical Manual of Pediatric Nursing* to Donna Lee Wong, PhD, RN, PNP, CPN, FAAN, who passed away on May 4, 2008, following complications of leukemia. Donna was the original coauthor of this book. Among her numerous publications, she is best known as the author of *Wong's Nursing Care of Infants and Children, Wong's Essentials of Pediatric Nursing, Wong's Nursing Care of Infants and Children,* and the *Pediatric Quick Reference.* She codeveloped the Wong-Baker FACES Pain Rating Scale, a tool used worldwide to assess pain in children and adults and which has been used in extensive research on pain. She was a fellow in the American Academy of Nursing (FAAN) and is listed in *Who's Who in American Nursing* and *The World's Who's Who of Women.* She was awarded many honors and was the first recipient of the Audrey Hepburn/Sigma Theta Tau International (Honorary Nursing Society) Award for Contributions to the Health and Welfare of Children, Rutger's University Outstanding Alumni,

and the Society of Pediatric Nursing Barbara Larson Humanitarian Award.

For those of us who had the honor of knowing this remarkable individual, she is most remembered for her outstanding generosity and concern for others. Her commitment to pediatric nursing is reflected in her never-ending pursuit of excellence. Her belief that no child should experience pain when interventions are possible led to the development of the concept of "atraumatic care." Donna taught us that nursing is about providing the best care possible and that our patients will be the better for it. She led by example, always looking for ways to improve care for pediatric patients. Donna Wong was an example for all of us who strive for excellence in our nursing profession. We hold her dear to our hearts and will continue to work to carry on her outstanding legacy. She will never be forgotten.

*Chris Humphrey, Photographer*

# Contributors and Reviewers

## Contributing Editor

**Terri L. Brown, MSN, RN, CPN**
Faculty, Evidence-Based Practice Specialist
Center for Research and Evidence-Based Practice
Texas Children's Hospital
Houston, Texas

## Contributors

**Melissa Parker, BS, CCLS**
Child Life Coordinator
Saint John Medical Center
Tulsa, Oklahoma

**Carol Reece, DNP, RN, CPNP**
Dwight Schar College of Nursing
Ashland University
Mansfield, Ohio

## Reviewers

**William T. Campbell, EdD, RN**
Assistant Professor
RN Coordinator
Department of Nursing
Salisbury University
Salisbury, Maryland

**Karyn Casey, RN, CPNP, PhD**
Assistant Professor
University of Tennessee College of Nursing
Knoxville, Tennessee

**Erica Fooshee, MSN, RN, CNE, CPN**
Nursing Student Mentor
Western Governors University
Salt Lake City, Utah

**Kathleen M. McLane, MSN, RN, CPNP, CWCN, COCN**
Pediatric Nurse Practitioner/WOC Nurse
Texas Children's Hospital, Houston
Houston, Texas

**Carol Reece, DNP, RN, CPNP**
Assistant Professor
Ashland University
Dwight Shar College of Nursing
Mansfield, Ohio

**Rebecca Shabo, RN, PNP-BC, PhD**
Associate Professor
Kennesaw State University
Kennesaw, Georgia

**Teresa Smiley, PhD, RN**
Assistant Professor
University of Oklahoma College of Nursing
Okalahoma City, Oklahoma

**Linda Wofford, RN, CPNP, DNP**
Associate Professor, Nursing
Belmont University, College of Health Science and Nursing
Nashville, Tennessee

# Preface

The eighth edition of *Wong's Clinical Manual of Pediatric Nursing,* like its previous editions, serves a unique function in the study and practice of pediatric nursing. This work benefits from the addition of several contributors whose expertise in pediatric nursing is reflected in this new edition. The *Manual* is a practical guide for practicing nurses and students engaged in the care of children and their families—a compendious collection of clinical information, resources, and data packaged for convenient use and easy access. For the practicing nurse, the book is a ready resource of material that is otherwise available only in a wide array of journal articles, texts, federal publications, professional association recommendations, and brochures. Examples of current "cutting-edge" information are recommendations from the American Academy of Pediatrics, Agency for Healthcare Research and Quality, American Pain Society, National Center for Health Statistics, and Centers for Disease Control and Prevention. For the student, it is an indispensable guide to the care of children and their families.

As an adjunct to clinical practice, the *Manual* assumes the thorough preparation and basic theoretical knowledge only a textbook can provide. Although it is not designed to accompany any particular textbook, it serves as a valuable addition to *Wong's Nursing Care of Infants and Children* and *Wong's Essentials of Pediatric Nursing.*

The *Manual* is authoritative and up-to-date. An **evidence-based practice** approach is used to present existing knowledge relevant to nursing care. Its content reflects the latest research and current clinical practice. This edition of the *Manual* has been extensively revised to include a unit on evidence-based practice nursing care of the pediatric patient and family. This unit provides Evidence-Based Practice boxes, which provide the latest research information on issues such as appropriate needle length for intramuscular injections and reduction of minor procedural pain in infants. The Evidence-Based Practice features enhance the practicing nurse's role in the provision of quality pediatric patient care. The Patient and Family Guidelines have been incorporated into this unit in an effort to streamline the book and still provide instructions for certain nursing care procedures.

In an attempt to further streamline this manual the nursing care plans have been moved to the Evolve website. The existing nursing care plans have been revised and include the current North American Nursing Diagnosis Association (NANDA), Nursing Interventions Classification (NIC), and Nursing Outcomes Classification (NOC) nomenclature. The care plans provided serve as a guide and must be individualized according to the patient's and family's unique needs. Users will appreciate access to the latest information on childhood immunizations; end-of-life care interventions; asthma management; central line care; arterial blood gas interpretation; management of the patient requiring mechanical ventilation; neonatal and child pain assessment and management;

blood pressure guidelines based on age, height, and gender; and a resource of standard laboratory values. The *Manual* is designed to ensure that specific information can be located quickly and easily when it is needed. Color tabs printed on the cover facilitate quick access to each of the six units, which have coordinating black thumbtabs. In addition to a detailed table of contents in the front of the book, a unit outline with page references is included at the beginning of each unit. A list of related topics found elsewhere in the book is included in most units. Vital reference data appear inside the front and back covers, where they can be located at a moment's notice.

As in past editions, material designed to be distributed to families is clearly identified. Permission is given to photocopy this material and provide it to caregivers to ensure that they have access to accurate, current information; to improve the quality of care; and to facilitate the nurse's teaching responsibilities.

Greater attention is given to **critical thinking** by emphasizing essential nursing observations and interventions in **Safety Alert** and Drug Alert boxes. These call the reader's attention to considerations which, if ignored, could lead to a deteriorating or emergency situation. Key assessment data, risk factors, and danger signs are among the kinds of information in this feature. The concept of **atraumatic care**—the provision of therapeutic care in settings by personnel and through the use of interventions that eliminate or minimize the psychologic and physical distress experienced by children and their families in the health care system—is incorporated throughout the text and highlighted as boxed material.

**Unit 1** focuses on the **assessment of the child and family**. It includes history taking; assessment of present and past physical health; and a summary of developmental achievements, both general and age specific. New information to this unit includes the addition of a cultural assessment tool, a revised discussion of temperature measurement, and history taking regarding alternative therapies.

**Unit 2** emphasizes **health promotion** in the areas of preventive care, infant and childhood nutrition, immunization, safety and injury prevention, parental guidance, and play. The material on childhood immunizations and on current car restraint guidelines is completely revised to reflect current recommendations.

A unique feature in this new edition is the development of a new chapter devoted to critical assessment and management of pain in children. **Unit 3** now incorporates neonatal, child, and adolescent pain assessment and management into one section for easy ready access. Although the literature on pain assessment and management in children has grown considerably, this knowledge has not been widely applied in practice. Unit 3 has been added to address this concern by presenting detailed pain assessment and management strategies, including discussion of common pain states in children. This unit is a resource for all nurses caring for children in pain.

**Unit 4** outlines **basic nursing procedures** adapted for the child. This section has been extensively revised and provides **Evidence-Based Practice** summaries on numerous nursing interventions. Unit 4 includes an extensive collection of skills and procedures including preparation for procedures, collection of specimens, administration of medicine, venous access devices, invasive and noninvasive oxygen monitoring, and cardiopulmonary resuscitation. The Patient and Family education guidelines have been incorporated into the skills and procedure sections of this unit. These guidelines have been revised for use by nurses as well as families in the care of a child in the acute care or home setting. New sections have been added on end-of-life care interventions, skin and wound care, mechanical ventilation, arterial blood gas interpretation, blood product administration, and chest tube management. The latest American Heart Association recommendations for performing cardiopulmonary resuscitation on an infant or child and for caring for a choking infant or child are included.

Unit 5 has been revised to reflect current educational and clinical practice. This unit has been revised to include more online care plans that the student may access and individualize according to the patient's unique needs. Each nursing care plan consists of assessment guidelines specific to the condition, relevant nursing diagnoses, patient/family goals, interventions, and expected patient/family outcomes. The nursing diagnoses conform to the most recent nomenclature accepted by NANDA, and they are prioritized within the care plans. The nursing diagnoses include Defining Characteristics and Subjective and Objective Data, which assist the student in the validation of assumptions that lead to selected relevant nursing diagnoses. In addition, NOC and NIC nomenclature has been added to further standardize and validate nursing care. The revised nursing care plans have been written to provide the student with a general guideline for critical thinking to encourage further problem solving and meet the patient's individualized care needs. The student may use the care plans as a springboard for developing outcomes and interventions that are applicable to the individual pediatric patient. The

Nursing Care Plan on pain can be used to meet The Joint Commission's current pain standards. The health problems were selected to avoid repetition while including a variety of pediatric disorders.

Unit 6 includes basic resource information for interpretation of **laboratory data,** including values in International Units.

Although the information in the *Manual* is carefully researched, references are included only when citations are required to appropriately credit the work. The reader is directed to the current editions of *Wong's Nursing Care of Infants and Children* and *Wong's Essentials of Pediatric Nursing* for additional references and discussion of material, especially for growth and development, interviewing, and health problems.

This edition of the *Manual* also includes a new section of color photos of common pediatric dermatology conditions. This feature enhances the overall quality of the *Manual* as a reference source for the practicing clinician and student.

Every effort has been made to ensure that the information is accurate and up-to-date at the time of publication. However, as new research and experience broaden our practice, standards of care change accordingly. Therefore, the reader may find some differences in local and regional practices.

A number of people have contributed time and expertise to this edition. We are grateful to Patrick Barrera and Terri Brown, whose contributions to the Wong nursing textbooks greatly benefit the *Manual.* Numerous reviewers and contributors have provided invaluable expertise for updating the material in this *Manual.* Melissa Parker provided valuable input from the perspective of a child life specialist. These outstanding experts have helped us achieve our goal of presenting data that are both current and accurate. And finally, we are so fortunate to have an outstanding Elsevier team— Shelly Hayden, Anne Konopka, and Heather Bays—who make the book a reality.

David Wilson
Marilyn J. Hockenberry

# Contents

# Assessment

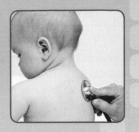

## evolve WEBSITE

**http://evolve.elsevier.com/Wong/clinical**

**Emergency Treatment**
- Fracture
- Hypoglycemia

**Nursing Care Plans**
- The Child in Shock
- The Child Who Is Maltreated
- The Child with a Fracture
- The Child with Acute Diarrhea (Gastroenteritis)
- The Child with Acute Renal Dysfunction
- The Child with Acute Respiratory Infection
- The Child with Appendicitis

- The Child with Asthma
- The Child with Attention Deficit Hyperactivity Disorder (ADHD)
- The Child with Bacterial Meningitis
- The Child with Burns
- The Child with Congestive Heart Failure (CHF)
- The Child with Diabetes Mellitus
- The Child with Fluid and Electrolyte Disturbances
- The Child with Impaired Cognitive Function

- The Child with Nephrotic Syndrome
- The Child with Seizure Disorder
- The Child with Toxic Ingestion or Inhalation
- The Unconscious Child

**Patient and Family Education—Spanish Translations**
- Caring for Your Child's Teeth (Cuidado de la Dentadura de su Niño)
- Measuring Your Child's Temperature (Medición de la Temperatura de su Niño)

# Health History

One of the most significant aspects of a health assessment is the health history. To take a thorough history, the nurse must be well versed in communication and interviewing principles. An overview of the process is presented in terms of general guidelines for communication and interviewing, with additional specific guidelines for children. Because of the frequent need for interpreters with non–English speaking families, guidelines for using interpreters are included.

The history furnishes information about the child's physical health since birth, details the events of the present problem, and includes social and family history facts that are essential for providing comprehensive care. The objective of each assessment area is the identification of nursing diagnoses.

The summary is primarily intended for the recording of data, not the acquisition of information from the informant. Therefore it is not meant to be used as a questionnaire. The column titled "Comments" is intended to enhance and detail sections of the history, as well as to emphasize areas of possible intervention. For a more comprehensive discussion of approaches to taking a history, see *Wong's Nursing Care of Infants and Children* or *Wong's Essentials of Pediatric Nursing.**

---

*Hockenberry M, Wilson D: *Wong's nursing care of infants and children,* ed 9, St Louis, 2011, Mosby; Hockenberry M, Wilson D: *Wong's essentials of pediatric nursing,* ed 8, St Louis, 2009, Mosby.

# General Guidelines for Communication and Interviewing

Assess ability to speak and understand English.

Conduct the interview in a private, quiet area.

Begin the interview with appropriate introductions.
- Address each person by name.

Clarify the purpose of the interview.

Inform the interviewees of the confidential limits of the interview.

Demonstrate interest in the interview by sitting at eye level and close to interviewees (not across a desk), leaning slightly forward, and speaking in a calm, steady voice.

Begin with general conversation to put the interviewees at ease.
- Use comments such as, "How have things been since we talked last?" or (to the child) "What do you think is going to happen today?" to let the family express the main concern.

Include all parties in the interview.
- Direct age-appropriate questions to children (e.g., "What grade are you in at school?" or "What do you like to eat?").
- Be sensitive to instances in which family members, such as adolescents, may wish to be interviewed separately.
- Recognize and respect cultural patterns of communication, e.g., avoiding direct eye contact (American Indian) or nodding for courtesy rather than to express actual agreement or understanding (many Asian cultures).
- Use open-ended questions or statements that begin with "What," "How," "Tell me about," or "You were saying," and reflect back key words or phrases to encourage discussion.
- Encourage continued discussion with nodding and eye contact, saying "Uh-huh," "I see," or "Yes."
- Use focused questions (questions that ask for a specific response, e.g., "What did you try next?") and closed-ended questions (questions that ask for a single answer, e.g., "Did you call the doctor?") to direct the focus of the interview.
- Ensure mutual understanding by frequently clarifying and summarizing information.
- Use active listening to attend to the verbal and nonverbal aspects of the communication.
- Verbal cues to important issues include the following techniques:
  - Frequent reference to a topic
  - Repetition of key words
  - Special reference to an event or person
- Nonverbal cues to important issues include the following:
  - Changes in body position (e.g., looking away or leaning forward)
  - Changes in pitch, rate, intonation, and volume of speech (e.g., speaking rapidly, frequent pauses, whispering, or shouting)
- Use silence to allow persons to do the following:
  - Sort out thoughts and feelings
  - Search for responses to questions
  - Share feelings expressed by another
- Break silence constructively with statements such as, "Is there anything else you wish to say?", "I see you find it difficult to continue; how may I help?", or "I don't know what this silence means. Perhaps there is something you would like to put into words but find difficult to say."
- Convey empathy by attending to the verbal and nonverbal language of the interviewee and reflecting back the feeling of the communication (e.g., "I can see how upsetting that must have been for you").
- Provide reassurance to acknowledge concerns and any positive efforts used to deal with problems.
- Avoid the following blocks to communication:
  - Socializing
  - Giving unrestricted and sometimes unasked-for advice
  - Offering premature or inappropriate reassurance
  - Giving overready encouragement
  - Defending a situation or opinion
  - Using stereotyped comments or clichés
  - Limiting expression of emotion by asking directed, close-ended questions
  - Interrupting and finishing the person's sentence
  - Talking more than the interviewee
  - Forming prejudged conclusions
  - Deliberately changing the focus
- Watch for the following signs of information overload:
  - Long periods of silence
  - Wide eyes and fixed facial expression
  - Constant fidgeting or attempting to move away
  - Nervous habits (e.g., tapping, playing with hair)
  - Sudden disruptions (e.g., asking to go to the bathroom)
  - Looking around
  - Yawning, eyes drooping
  - Frequently looking at a watch or clock
  - Attempting to change the topic of discussion

Close the interview with an opportunity for others to bring up overlooked or sensitive concerns with a statement such as, "Have we covered everything?"

Summarize the interview, especially if problems were identified or interventions were planned.

Discuss the need for follow-up, and schedule a time.

Express appreciation for each person's participation.

# Specific Guidelines for Communicating with Children

Allow children time to feel comfortable.

Avoid sudden or rapid advances, broad smiles, extended eye contact, or other gestures that may be seen as threatening.

Talk to the parent if the child is initially shy.

Communicate through transition objects such as dolls, puppets, or stuffed animals before questioning a young child directly.

Give older children the opportunity to talk without the parents present.

Assume a position that is at eye level with the child.

Speak in a quiet, unhurried, and confident voice.

Speak clearly, be specific, and use simple words and short sentences.

State directions and suggestions positively.

Offer a choice only when one exists.

Be honest with children.

Allow children to express their concerns and fears.

Use a variety of communication techniques.

# Creative Communication Techniques with Children

## Verbal Techniques

### "I" Messages

Relate a feeling about a behavior in terms of "I."

Describe the effect the behavior had on the person.

Avoid use of "you."

- "You" messages are judgmental and provoke defensiveness.
  - Example: "You" message—"You are being very uncooperative about doing your treatments."
  - Example: "I" message—"I am concerned about how the treatments are going because I want to see you get better."

### Third-Person Technique

Involves expressing a feeling in terms of a third person ("he," "she," "they")

Is less threatening than directly asking children how they feel, because it gives them an opportunity to agree or disagree without being defensive

- Example: "Sometimes when a person is sick a lot, he feels angry and sad because he cannot do what others can." Either wait silently for a response, or encourage a reply with a statement such as, "Did you ever feel that way?"

Approach allows children three choices: (1) to agree and, hopefully, express how they feel; (2) to disagree; or (3) to remain silent, in which case they probably have such feelings but are unable to express them at this time.

### Facilitative Responding

Involves careful listening and reflecting back to patients the feelings and content of their statements.

Responses are empathic and nonjudgmental and legitimize the person's feelings.

Formula for facilitative responses: "You feel _____ because _____."

- Example: If child states, "I hate coming to the hospital and getting needles," a facilitative response is, "You feel unhappy because of all the things that are done to you."

### Storytelling

Uses the language of children to probe into areas of their thinking while bypassing conscious inhibitions or fears

Simplest technique is asking children to relate a story about an event, such as being in the hospital.

Other approaches:

- Show children a picture of a particular event, such as a child in a hospital with other people in the room, and ask them to describe the scene.
- Cut out comic strips, remove words, and have child add statements for scenes.

### Mutual Storytelling

Reveals child's thinking and attempts to change child's perceptions or fears by retelling a somewhat different story (more therapeutic approach than storytelling)

Begins by asking child to tell a story about something, followed by another story told by the nurse that is similar to child's tale but with differences that help child in problem areas

- Example: Child's story is about going to the hospital and never seeing his or her parents again. Nurse's story is also about a child (using different names but similar circumstances) in a hospital whose parents visit every day, but in the evening after work, until the child is better and goes home with them.

### Bibliotherapy

Uses books in a therapeutic and supportive process

Provides children with an opportunity to explore an event that is similar to their own but sufficiently different to allow them to distance themselves from it and remain in control

General guidelines for using bibliotherapy are as follows:

- Assess child's emotional and cognitive development in terms of readiness to understand the book's message.
- Be familiar with the book's content (intended message or purpose) and the age for which it is written.
- Read the book to the child if child is unable to read.

- Explore the meaning of the book with the child by having child do the following:
  - ○ Retell the story.
  - ○ Read a special section with the nurse or parent.
  - ○ Draw a picture related to the story and discuss the drawing.
  - ○ Talk about the characters.
  - ○ Summarize the moral or meaning of the story.

### Dreams
Often reveal unconscious and repressed thoughts and feelings
- Ask child to talk about a dream or nightmare.
- Explore with child what meaning the dream could have.

### "What If?" Questions
Encourage child to explore potential situations and to consider different problem-solving options.
- ○ Example: "What if you got sick and had to go to the hospital?" Children's responses reveal what they know already and what they are curious about and provide an opportunity for helping children learn coping skills, especially in potentially dangerous situations.

### Three Wishes
Involves asking, "If you could have any three things in the world, what would they be?"
If child answers, "That all my wishes come true," ask child for specific wishes.

### Rating Game
Uses some type of rating scale (numbers, sad to happy faces) to rate an event or feeling
- Example: Instead of asking children how they feel, ask how their day has been "on a scale of 1 to 10, with 10 being the best."

### Word Association Game
Involves stating key words and asking children to say the first word they think of when they hear each word
- Start with neutral words, and then introduce more anxiety-producing words, such as "illness," "needles," hospitals," and "operation."
- Select key words that relate to some relevant event in child's life.

### Sentence Completion
Involves presenting a partial statement and having child complete it
Some sample statements are as follows:
- The thing I like best (least) about school is _____ _____.
- The best (worst) age to be is _____ _____.
- The most (least) fun thing I ever did was _____ _____.
- The thing I like most (least) about my parents is ____ _____.

- The one thing I would change about my family is ____ _____.
- If I could be anything I wanted, I would be _____ _____.
- The thing I like most (least) about myself is _____ _____.

### Pros and Cons
Involves selecting a topic, such as being in the hospital, and having child list five good things and five bad things about it
Is an exceptionally valuable technique when applied to relationships, such as things family members like and dislike about each other

## Nonverbal Techniques
### Writing
Is an alternative communication approach for older children and adults
Specific suggestions include the following:
- Keep a journal or diary.
- Write down feelings or thoughts that are difficult to express.
- Write letters that are never mailed (a variation is making up a pen pal to write to).
- Keep an account of child's progress from both a physical and an emotional viewpoint.

### Drawing
One of the most valuable forms of communication, it provides both nonverbal (from looking at the drawing) and verbal (from child's story of the picture) information.
Children's drawings tell a great deal about them because they are projections of their inner selves.
Spontaneous drawing involves giving child a variety of art supplies and providing the opportunity to draw.
Directed drawing involves a more specific direction, such as "draw a person" or the "three themes" approach (state three things about child and ask child to choose one and draw a picture).

#### Guidelines for Evaluating Drawings
Use spontaneous drawings, and evaluate more than one drawing whenever possible.
Interpret drawings in light of other available information about child and family.
Interpret drawings as a whole rather than concentrating on specific details of the drawing.
Consider the following individual elements of the drawing that may be significant:
- **Gender of figure drawn first**—Usually relates to child's perception of own gender role
- **Size of individual figures**—Expresses importance, power, or authority
- **Order in which figures are drawn**—Expresses priority in terms of importance
- **Child's position in relation to other family members**—Expresses feelings of status or alliance

- **Exclusion of a member**—May denote feeling of not belonging or desire to eliminate
- **Accentuated parts**—Usually express concern for areas of special importance (e.g., large hands may be a sign of aggression)
- **Absence of or rudimentary arms and hands**—Suggests timidity, passivity, or intellectual immaturity; tiny, unstable feet may be an expression of insecurity, and hidden hands may mean guilt feelings
- **Placement of drawing on the page and type of stroke**—Free use of paper and firm, continuous strokes express security, whereas drawings restricted to a small area and lightly drawn in broken or wavering lines may be a sign of insecurity
- **Erasures, shading, or cross-hatching**—Expresses ambivalence, concern, or anxiety with a particular area

### Magic

Uses simple magic tricks to help establish rapport with child, encourage compliance with health interventions, and provide effective distraction during painful procedures

Although "magician" talks, no verbal response from child is required.

### Play

Is universal language and "work" of children

Tells a great deal about children because they project their inner selves through the activity

Spontaneous play involves giving child a variety of play materials and providing the opportunity to play.

Directed play involves a more specific direction, such as providing medical equipment, a doll, or a dollhouse for focused reasons, such as exploring child's fear of injections or exploring family relationships.

## Guidelines for Using an Interpreter

Explain to interpreter the reason for the interview and the type of questions that will be asked.

Clarify whether a detailed or brief answer is required and whether the translated response can be general or literal.

Introduce interpreter to family, and allow some time before the actual interview so that they can become acquainted.

Give reassurance that interpreter will maintain confidentiality.

Communicate directly with family members when asking questions to reinforce interest in them and to observe nonverbal expressions, but do not ignore interpreter.

Pose questions to elicit only one answer at a time, such as "Do you have pain?" rather than "Do you have any pain, tiredness, or loss of appetite?"

Refrain from interrupting family members and interpreter while they are conversing.

Avoid commenting to interpreter about family members, since they may understand some English.

Be aware that some medical words, such as "allergy," may have no similar word in another language; avoid medical jargon whenever possible.

Respect cultural differences; it is often best to pose questions about sex, marriage, or pregnancy indirectly—ask about "child's father" rather than "mother's husband."

Allow time after the interview for interpreter to share something that he or she felt could not be said earlier; ask about interpreter's impression of nonverbal clues to communication and family members' reliability or ease in revealing information.

Arrange for family to speak with same interpreter on subsequent visits whenever possible.

## Outline of a Health History

**A. Identifying information**
  1. Name
  2. Address
  3. Telephone number
  4. Age and birth date
  5. Birth place
  6. Race or ethnic group
  7. Gender
  8. Religion
  9. Nationality
  10. Date of interview
  11. Informant
**B. Chief complaint**
**C. Present illness**
  1. Onset
  2. Characteristics
  3. Course since onset

**D. Past history**
  1. Pregnancy (maternal)
  2. Labor and delivery
  3. Perinatal period
  4. Previous illnesses, operations, or injuries
  5. Allergies
  6. Current medications
  7. Cultural remedies
  8. Pain
  9. Immunizations
  10. Growth and development
  11. Habits
**E. Review of systems**
  1. General
  2. Integument
  3. Head
  4. Eyes

5. Nose
6. Ears
7. Mouth
8. Throat
9. Neck
10. Chest
11. Respiratory
12. Cardiovascular
13. Gastrointestinal
14. Genitourinary
15. Gynecologic
16. Musculoskeletal
17. Neurologic
18. Endocrine
19. Lymphatic

**F. Nutrition history***
  1. Patterns of eating
  2. Dietary intake

**G. Family medical history**
  1. Family pedigree
  2. Familial diseases
  3. Family members with congenital anomalies
  4. Family habits
  5. Geographic location

**H. Alternative therapies**

**I. Family personal and social history***
  1. Family structure
  2. Family function
  3. Daycare

**J. Sexual history**
  1. Sexual concerns and activity of child
  2. Sexual concerns and activity of adults if warranted

**K. Patient profile (summary)**
  1. Health status
  2. Psychologic status
  3. Socioeconomic status

## Summary of a Health History

| Information | Comments |
|---|---|
| **Identifying Information** | |
| 1. Name<br>2. Address<br>3. Telephone number<br>4. Age<br>5. Birth date<br>6. Race or ethnic group<br>7. Gender<br>8. Religion or spiritual beliefs<br>9. Nationality<br>10. Date of interview<br>11. Informant | Additional information appropriate to older adolescent may include occupation, marital status, and temporary and permanent addresses.<br>Under "informant," include subjective impression of reliability, general attitude, willingness to communicate, overall accuracy of data, and any special circumstances, such as use of an interpreter.<br>Informants should include parent and child, as well as others who may be primary caregivers, such as a grandparent. |
| **Chief Complaint (CC)** | |
| To establish the major specific reason for the individual's seeking professional health attention | Record in patient's own words; include duration of symptoms.<br>If informant has difficulty isolating one problem, ask which problem or symptom led person to seek help now.<br>In case of routine physical examination, state CC as reason for visit. |
| **Present Illness (PI)** | |
| To obtain all details related to the chief complaint<br>1. Onset<br>  a. Date of onset<br>  b. Manner of onset (gradual or sudden)<br>  c. Precipitating and predisposing factors related to onset (emotional disturbance, physical exertion, fatigue, bodily function, pregnancy, environment, injury, infection, toxins and allergens, therapeutic agents) | In its broadest sense, illness denotes any problem of a physical, emotional, or psychosocial nature.<br>Present information in chronologic order; may be referenced according to one point in time, such as prior to admission (PTA).<br>Concentrate on reason for seeking help now, especially if problem has existed for some time. |

*Continued*

---

*Because of the importance of the nutrition history and family personal and social history, separate sections devoted to assessment of these two topics are on pp. 112 and 110, respectively.

## Summary of a Health History—cont'd

| Information | Comments |
|---|---|

### Present Illness (PI)—cont'd

2. Characteristics
   a. Character (quality, quantity, consistency, or other)
   b. Location and radiation (e.g., pain)
   c. Intensity or severity
   d. Timing (continuous or intermittent, duration of each, temporal relationship to other events)
   e. Aggravating and relieving factors
   f. Associated symptoms
3. Course since onset
   a. Incidence
      Single acute attack
      Recurrent acute attacks
      Daily occurrences
      Periodic occurrences
      Continuous chronic episode
   b. Progress (better, worse, unchanged)
   c. Effect of therapy

### Past History (PH)

To elicit a profile of the individual's previous illnesses, injuries, or operations
1. Pregnancy (maternal)
   a. Number (gravida)
      Dates of delivery
   b. Outcome (parity)
      Gestation (full-term, preterm, postterm)
      Stillbirths, abortions
   c. Health during pregnancy
   d. Medications taken
2. Labor and delivery
   a. Duration of labor
   b. Type of delivery
   c. Place of delivery
   d. Medications
3. Perinatal period
   a. Weight and length at birth
   b. Time of regaining birth weight
   c. Condition of health immediately after birth
   d. Apgar score
   e. Presence of problems including congenital anomalies
   f. Date of discharge from nursery
4. Previous illnesses, operations, or injuries
   a. Onset, symptoms, course, termination
   b. Occurrence of complications
   c. Incidence of disease in other family members or in community
   d. Emotional response to previous hospitalization
   e. Circumstances and nature of injuries
5. Allergies
   a. Hay fever, asthma, or eczema
   b. Unusual reactions to foods, drugs, animals, plants, latex products, or household products

*Comments:*

Importance of perinatal history depends on child's age; the younger the child, the more important the perinatal history.
Explain relevance of obstetric history in revealing important factors relating to the child's health.
Assess parents' emotional attitudes toward the pregnancy and birth.

Assess parents' feelings regarding delivery; investigate factors that may affect bonding, such as separation from infant.

If birth problems are reported, inquire about treatment, such as use of oxygen, phototherapy, and surgery, and parents' emotional response to the event.

Ask about diphtheria, scarlet fever, measles, rubella, chickenpox, mumps, tonsillitis, strep throat, pertussis, allergies, and common illnesses such as colds and earaches.
Elicit a description of disease to verify the diagnosis.
Be alert to areas of injury prevention.

Have parent describe the type of allergic reaction and its severity.

## Summary of a Health History—cont'd

| Information | Comments |
|---|---|

### Past History (PH)—cont'd

**Information**

6. Current medications
   a. Name, dose, schedule, duration, and reason for administration
7. Cultural remedies*
   a. Herbs, natural products, special foods, drinks
8. Pain
   a. Previous experiences
   b. Reactions
   c. Effective management
   d. Cultural influences
9. Immunizations
   a. Name, number of doses, age when given
   b. Occurrence of reaction
   c. Administration of horse or other foreign serum, gamma-globulin, or blood transfusion

**Comments**

Assess parents' knowledge of correct dosage of common drugs, such as acetaminophen; note underuse or overuse.

Ask about names of the products used, frequency given, and dosages.

When age-appropriate, elicit information from child as well as parent.

Does the child tend to be stoic or expressive with pain?

What is the family's attitude about taking pain medications?

Parents may refer to immunizations as "baby shots."

Whenever possible, confirm information by checking medical or school records.

> **! SAFETY ALERT**
> Inquire about previous administration of any horse or other foreign serum, recent administration of gamma globulin or blood transfusion, and anaphylactic reactions to neomycin or chicken eggs.

**Information**

10. Growth and development
    a. Weight at birth, 6 months, 1 year, and present
    b. Dentition
       Age of eruption/shedding
       Number
       Problems with teething
    c. Age of head control, sitting unsupported, walking, first words
    d. Present grade in school, scholastic achievement
    e. Interaction with peers and adults
    f. Participation in organized activities, such as Scouting, sports
11. Habits
    a. Behavior patterns
       Nail biting
       Thumb sucking
       Pica

       Rituals, such as use of security blanket
       Unusual movements (head banging, rocking)
       Temper tantrums
    b. Activities of daily living
       Hour of sleep and arising
       Duration of nighttime sleep or naps
       Age of toilet training
       Pattern of stools and urination; occurrence of enuresis or encopresis

**Comments**

Compare parents' responses with own observations of child's achievement and results from objective tests, such as Denver II (see p. 121).

School and social history can be more thoroughly explored under Family Assessment.

Assess parents' attitudes toward habits and any remedies used to curtail them, such as punishment for bed-wetting.

Pica, the habitual ingestion of nonfood items, may be risk factor for lead poisoning.

Record child's usual terms for defecation and urination.

---

*From American Academy of Pediatrics, Committee on Children with Disabilities: Counseling families who choose complementary and alternative medicine for their child with chronic illness or disability, *Pediatrics* 107(3):598-601, 2001.

*Continued*

## Summary of a Health History—cont'd

| Information | Comments |
|---|---|

### Type of Exercise

c. Use or abuse of drugs, alcohol, coffee (caffeine), tobacco, vitamins and supplements, or alternative therapies.
d. Usual disposition; response to frustration

With adolescents, ask about quantity and frequency of chemicals used.

### Review of Systems (ROS)

To elicit information concerning any potential health problem (Box 1-1)

Explain relevance of questioning to parents (similar to pregnancy section) in composing total health history of child.

Make positive statements about each system (e.g., "Mother denies headaches, bumping into objects, squinting, or excessive rubbing of eyes").

Use terms parents are likely to understand, such as "bruises" for ecchymoses.

---

**BOX 1-1 | Review of Systems**

**General**—Overall state of health, fatigue, recent and/or unexplained weight gain or loss (period of time for either), contributing factors (change of diet, illness, altered appetite), exercise tolerance, fevers (time of day), chills, night sweats (unrelated to climatic conditions), frequent infections, general ability to carry out activities of daily living

**Integument**—Pruritus, pigment or other color changes, acne, moles, discoloration, eruptions, rashes (location), tendency toward bruising, petechiae, excessive dryness, general texture, disorders or deformities of nails, hair growth or loss, hair color change (for adolescent, use of hair dyes or other potentially toxic substances such as hair straighteners)

**Head**—Headaches, dizziness, injury (specific details)

**Eyes**—Visual problems (ask about behaviors indicative of blurred vision, such as bumping into objects, clumsiness, sitting very close to the television, holding a book close to the face, writing with head near desk, squinting, rubbing the eyes, bending the head in an awkward position), cross-eye (strabismus), eye infections, edema of lids, excessive tearing, use of glasses or contact lenses, date of last optic examination

**Nose**—Nosebleeds (epistaxis), constant or frequent running or stuffy nose, nasal obstruction (difficulty breathing), alteration or loss of sense of smell

**Ears**—Earaches, discharge, evidence of hearing loss (ask about behaviors such as need to repeat requests, loud speech, inattentive behavior), results of any previous auditory testing, pulling or rubbing ear

**Mouth**—Mouth breathing, gum bleeding, toothaches, toothbrushing, use of fluoride, difficulty with teething (symptoms), last visit to dentist (especially if temporary dentition is complete), response to dentist

**Throat**—Sore throats, difficulty in swallowing, choking (especially when chewing food—may be from poor chewing habits), hoarseness or other voice irregularities

**Neck**—Pain, limitation of movement, stiffness, difficulty in holding head straight (torticollis), thyroid enlargement, enlarged nodes or other masses

**Chest**—Breast enlargement, discharge, masses, enlarged axillary nodes (for adolescent female, ask about breast self-examination)

**Respiratory**—Chronic cough, frequent colds (number per year), wheezing, shortness of breath at rest or on exertion, difficulty in breathing, sputum production, infections (pneumonia, tuberculosis), date of last chest x-ray examination, and skin reaction from tuberculin testing

**Cardiovascular**—Cyanosis or fatigue on exertion, history of heart murmur or rheumatic fever, anemia, date of last blood count, blood type, recent transfusion

**Gastrointestinal**—Nausea, vomiting (not associated with eating, may be indicative of brain tumor or increased intracranial pressure), jaundice or yellowing skin or sclera, belching, flatulence, recent change in bowel habits (blood in stools, change in color, diarrhea, and constipation)

**Genitourinary**—Pain on urination, frequency, hesitancy, urgency, hematuria, nocturia, polyuria, unpleasant odor to urine, force of stream, discharge, change in size of scrotum, date of last urinalysis (for adolescent, sexually transmitted disease, type of treatment; for male adolescent, ask about testicular self-examination)

**Gynecologic**—Menarche, date of last menstrual period, regularity or problems with menstruation, vaginal discharge, pruritus, date and result of last Pap smear (include obstetric history as discussed under birth history when applicable); if sexually active, type of contraception

**Musculoskeletal**—Weakness, clumsiness, lack of coordination, unusual movements, back or joint stiffness, muscle pains or cramps, abnormal gait, deformity, fractures, serious sprains, activity level, redness, swelling, tenderness

**Neurologic**—Seizures, tremors, dizziness, loss of memory, general affect, fears, nightmares, speech problems, any unusual habit

**Endocrine**—Intolerance to weather changes, excessive thirst and urination, excessive sweating, salty taste to skin, signs of early puberty

**Lymphatic**—History of frequent infections, enlarged lymph nodes in any region, swelling, tenderness, red streaks

## Summary of a Health History—cont'd

| **Information** | **Comments** |
|---|---|

### Nutrition History

To elicit information about adequacy of child's dietary intake and eating patterns (see p. 112)

### Family Medical History

| | |
|---|---|
| To identify the presence of genetic traits or diseases that have familial tendencies; to assess family habits and exposure to a communicable disease that may affect family members | Choose terms wisely when asking about child's parentage: for example, inquire about paternal history by referring to the child's "father" rather than mother's husband; use the term "partner" rather than "spouse." |
| 1. Family pedigree and guidelines for construction | A pedigree is a pictorial representation or diagram of a family tree to visualize patterns of disease transmission. |
| 2. Familial diseases such as heart disease, hypertension, cancer, diabetes mellitus, obesity, congenital anomalies, allergy, asthma, tuberculosis, seizures, sickle cell disease, depression, mental retardation, mental illness or other emotional problems, syphilis, or rheumatic fever; indicate symptoms, treatment, and sequelae | |
| 3. Family members with congenital anomalies | |
| 4. Family habits, such as smoking or chemical use | |
| 5. Geographic location, including birth place, present location, and travel or contact with foreign visitors | Important for identification of endemic disease |

### Alternative Therapies*

| | |
|---|---|
| The American Academy of Pediatrics (2001) has the following recommendations when discussing alternative, complementary, and unproven therapies: | These recommendations should be used by nurses when discussing CAM with families. Remember, introducing the subject of CAM requires tactful communication skills. An approach such as, "I am very interested in how nontraditional or alternative therapies can be used to help children. What things have you tried?" is a positive and nonthreatening entrée to a discussion with the family. When families are using an unfamiliar intervention, ask for their sources of information and review them before giving advice. In general, if a therapy produces no adverse effect, including significant financial burden, do not discourage its use. Maintaining a trusting, supportive relationship with the family generally outweighs any benefit from trying to disprove the value of nonconventional therapy. |
| 1. Obtain information for yourself, and be prepared to share it with families. | |
| 2. Evaluate the scientific merits of specific therapeutic approaches. | |
| 3. Identify risks or potential harmful effects. | |
| 4. Provide families with information on treatment options. | |
| 5. Educate families to evaluate information and treatment options. | |
| 6. Avoid dismissal of complementary and alternative therapies (CAM) in ways that indicate a lack of sensitivity or concern. | |
| 7. Recognize feeling threatened, and guard against becoming defensive. | |
| 8. If the CAM approach is endorsed, offer to provide monitoring and evaluate the response. | |
| 9. Actively listen to the family and child with a chronic illness or disability. | |

### Family Personal and Social History

To gain an understanding of the family's structure and function (see p. 110)

*From American Academy of Pediatrics, Committee on Children with Disabilities: Counseling families who choose complementary and alternative medicine for their child with chronic illness or disability, *Pediatrics* 107(3):598-601, 2001.

*Continued*

## Summary of a Health History—cont'd

| Information | Comments |
|---|---|
| **Sexual History** | |
| To elicit information concerning young person's concerns and/or activities and any pertinent data regarding adult's sexual activity that influence child | Sexual history is an essential component of preadolescents' and adolescents' health assessments. |
| 1. Sexual concerns and activity of child | Degree of investigation into parents' sexual history depends on its relevance to the child's health. It may be limited to family planning concerns, or it may be more detailed if overt sexual activity or abuse is suspected. |
| 2. Sexual concerns and activity of adults if warranted | Investigate toward end of history when rapport is greatest. |
| | Respect sensitive and complex nature of questioning. |
| | Give parents and child the option of discussing sexual matters alone with nurse. |
| | Ensure confidentiality. |
| | Clarify terms such as "sexually active" or "having sex." |
| | Refer to sexual contacts as "partners" not "girlfriends" or "boyfriends" to avoid biasing discussion of homosexual activity. |
| | Discussion may flow easily after review of genitourinary tract, such as asking female about menstruation or male about urinary problems. |
| | Suggestions for beginning discussion include the following: |
| | "Tell me about your social life." |
| | "Who are your closest friends?" |
| | "Is there one very special friend?" |
| | "Some teenagers have decided to have sex. What do you think about that?" |
| | Take detailed history of all contacts if sexually transmitted disease is suspected or diagnosed. |
| **Patient Profile (Summary)** | |
| To summarize the interviewer's overall impression of the child's and family's physical, psychologic, and socioeconomic background | A comprehensive summary often identifies nursing diagnoses based on subjective and objective findings. |
| 1. Health status | |
| 2. Psychologic status | |
| 3. Socioeconomic status | |

## Habits to Assess During a Health Interview*

Behavior patterns such as nail biting, thumb sucking, pica (habitual ingestion of nonfood substances), rituals ("security" blanket or toy), and unusual movements (head banging, rocking, overt masturbation, and walking on toes)

Activities of daily living, such as hour of sleep and arising, duration of nighttime sleep and naps, type and duration of exercise, regularity of stools and urination, age of toilet training, and occurrences of daytime or nighttime bed-wetting

Unusual disposition, as well as response to frustration

Use or abuse of alcohol, drugs, coffee, or tobacco

## Taking an Allergy History*

Has your child ever taken any drugs or tablets that have disagreed with him or her or caused an allergic reaction (Guidelines box)? If yes, can you remember the name(s) of these drugs?

Can you describe the reaction?

Was the drug taken by mouth (as a tablet or medicine), or was it an injection?

How soon after starting the drug did the reaction happen?

*Modified from Cantrill JA, Cottrell WN: Accuracy of drug allergy documentation, *Am J Health Syst Pharm* 54(14):1627-1629, 1997.

## GUIDELINES
### Identifying Allergy

Does the child have any symptoms (e.g., sneezing, coughing, rashes, wheezing) when handling rubber products (balloons, tennis or Koosh balls, adhesive bandage strips) or when in contact with rubber hospital products, such as gloves and catheters?

Has your child ever had an allergic reaction during surgery?

Does the child have a history of rashes, asthma, or allergic reactions to medication or foods, especially milk, kiwi fruit, bananas, or chestnuts?

How would you identify or recognize an allergic reaction in your child?

What would you do if an allergic reaction occurred?

Has anyone ever discussed latex or rubber allergy or sensitivity with you?

Has the child had any allergy testing?

When did the child last come in contact with any type of rubber product? Were you present?

How long ago did this happen?

Did anyone tell you it was an allergic reaction, or did you decide for yourself?

Has your child ever taken this drug, or a similar one, again? If yes, did your child experience the same problems?

Have you told the doctors or nurses about your child's reaction or allergy?

## Adolescent Health Issues

For teenagers, a psychosocial review of systems is at least as important as the physical exam.

The popular and effective HEADSS* method of interviewing has been expanded to

HEEADSSS, and focuses on assessment of the Home environment, Education and employment,

Eating, peer-related Activities, Drugs, Sexuality, Suicide/depression, and Safety from injury and violence.

# Cultural Assessment

Cultural assessment helps identify the family's understanding of the health-related problem in relation to how their culture may affect the plan of care. The cultural assessment identifies the family beliefs, values, and practices that may facilitate or interfere with health care. Careful assessment can assist the nurse in better understanding the patient and family.

## Strategies for Gathering Cultural Information

Listen to the patient and family's understanding of the health problem.

Use cultural resources to promote understanding of different ethnic and religious cultures.

Assess cultural influences throughout the comprehensive nursing assessment.

### Culturally Sensitive Interactions
#### Nonverbal Strategies

Invite family members to choose where they would like to sit or stand, allowing them to select a comfortable distance.

Observe interactions with others to determine which body gestures (e.g., shaking hands) are acceptable and appropriate. Ask when in doubt. Know when physical contact is prohibited.

Avoid appearing rushed.

Be an active listener.

Observe for cues regarding appropriate eye contact.

Avoiding eye contact may be a sign of respect.

Learn appropriate use of pauses or interruptions for different cultures.

Ask for clarification if nonverbal meaning is unclear.

Learn if smiling indicates friendliness.

### Verbal Strategies

Learn proper terms of address.

Use a positive tone of voice to convey interest.

Speak slowly and carefully, not loudly, when families have poor language comprehension.

Encourage questions.

Learn basic words and sentences of family's language, if possible.

Avoid professional terms.

When asking questions, tell family why the questions are being asked, the way in which the information they provide will be used, and how it might benefit their child.

Repeat important information more than once.

Always give the reason or purpose for a treatment or prescription.

Use information written in the family's language.

Arrange for the services of an interpreter when necessary.

Learn from families and representatives of their culture methods of communicating information without creating discomfort.

Address intergenerational needs (e.g., family's need to consult with others).

Be sincere, open, and honest, and, when appropriate, share personal experiences, beliefs, and practices to establish rapport and trust.

## Cultural Assessment Outline

### Communication

What language is spoken at home?

How does the family demonstrate respect or disrespect?

How well does the family understand English (spoken and written)?

Is an interpreter needed?

### Health Beliefs

How are health and illness defined by the family?

How are feelings expressed regarding illness or death?

What are the attitudes toward sickness?

Who makes the decisions regarding health practices in the family?

Are there cultural practices that would restrict the type of care needed?

Is a health professional of the same gender or ethnic background an issue for the family?

### Religious Practices and Rituals

What is the family's religious preference?

Who does the family turn to for support and counseling?

Are there special practices or rituals that may affect care?

Are there special rituals or ceremonies when a patient is ill or dying?

Are special rituals or ceremonies attached to birth, baptism, puberty, or death?

### Dietary Practices

Are some foods restricted by the family's culture?

Are there cultural practices in observance of certain occasions or events?

How is food prepared?

Who is responsible for food preparation?

Do certain foods have special meaning to the family or child?

Are special foods believed to cause or cure an illness or disease?

Are there times of required food fasting?

How are the periods of fasting defined, and who fasts in the family?

### Family Characteristics

Who makes the decisions in the family?

How many generations are considered to be a single family?

Which relatives compose the family unit?

When are children disciplined or punished?

How is affection demonstrated in the family?

How are emotions exhibited in the family?

What is the attitude toward children?

### Sources of Support

To what ethnic or cultural organizations does the family belong?

How do the organizations influence the family's approach to health care?

Who is most responsible for influencing the family's health beliefs?

Is there a specific cultural group with which the family identifies?

Is the specific cultural group identified by where the child was born and has lived?

### Resources for Cultural Information

Giger & Davidhizar. (2004). Transcultural Nursing: Assessment and Intervention.

Leininger & McFarland. (2002). Transcultural Nursing: Concepts, Theories and Practice.

Lipson, & Dibble. (2005). Culture & Clinical Care.

Purnell & Paulanka. (2003). Transcultural Health Care: A Culturally Competent Approach

Spector. (2003). Cultural Diversity in Health and Illness.

http://ethnomed.org

*www.ggalanti.com/cultural_profiles*

*www.tcns.org*

## Cultural Characteristics Related to Health Care of Children and Families

| Health Beliefs | Health Practices | Family Relationships | Communication |
|---|---|---|---|
| **African-American** | | | |
| Illness classified as:<br>*Natural*—affected by forces of nature without adequate protection (e.g., cold air, pollution, food, and water)<br>*Unnatural*—God's punishment for improper behavior<br>May see illness as "will of God" | Self-care and folk medicine prevalent<br>Folk therapies usually religious in origin<br>Folk therapies often not shared with medical provider<br>Prayer is common means for prevention and treatment | Strong kinship bonds in extended family, with members coming to aid of others in crisis<br>Less likely to view illness as a burden<br>Place strong emphasis on work and ambition<br>Older adults cared for and respected | Alert to any evidence of discrimination<br>Place importance on nonverbal behavior<br>Affection shown by touching and hugging<br>Silence may indicate lack of trust<br>Eye contact important to establish trust<br>Best to use direct, but caring approach |

Data from Lipson JG, Dibble SL, Minarik PA: *Culture and nursing care: a pocket guide,* San Francisco, 1998, UCSF Nursing Press; Spector RE: *Cultural diversity in health and illness,* Upper Saddle River, NJ, 2000, Prentice Hall.

## Cultural Characteristics Related to Health Care of Children and Families—cont'd

| Health Beliefs | Health Practices | Family Relationships | Communication |
|---|---|---|---|
| **Chinese** | | | |
| View healthy body as gift from parents and ancestors that must be cared for | Goal of therapy: to restore balance of yin and yang | Extended family pattern common | Open expression of emotions unacceptable |
| Health one result of balance between the forces of yin (cold) and yang (hot)—energy forces that rule world | Acupuncture: needles applied to appropriate meridians identified in terms of yin and yang | Strong concept of loyalty of young to old | Often smile when they do not comprehend |
| Illness caused by imbalance | Acupressure and t'ai chi replacing acupuncture in some areas | Respect for elders taught at early age—acceptance without questioning or talking back | |
| | | Children's behavior a reflection on family | |
| Believe blood is source of life and is not regenerated | Moxibustion: application of heat to skin over specific meridians | Family and individual honor and "face" important | |
| Chi is innate energy | Wide use of medicinal herbs procured and applied in prescribed ways | Self-reliance and self-esteem highly valued; self-expression repressed | |
| | Meals sometimes planned to balance "hot" and "cold" | | |
| **Filipino** | | | |
| Health a result of balance | May not respond to illness until it is advanced | Family highly valued, with strong family ties | Immigrants and older persons may not be able to speak or understand English |
| Illness a result of imbalance | May use herbal medicine | Multigenerational family structure common, often including collateral members | Sensitive to tone and manner of speaker |
| To be healthy again is to correct an evil deed | Eating appropriate amounts, not necessarily eating right, promotes good health | Avoid behavior that would bring shame on family | Limited direct eye contact |
| | Physical ailment possibly caused by the supernatural | | |
| **Haitian** | | | |
| Illness a punishment | Health seen as personal responsibility | Maintenance of family reputation paramount | Recent immigrants and older persons may speak only Haitian Creole |
| Natural cause (*maladi bone die*—disease of the Lord) caused by environmental factors, movement of blood within body, changes between "hot" and "cold," and bone displacement | Foods have properties of "hot"/"cold" and "light"/"heavy" and must be in harmony with one's life cycle and bodily states | Lineal authority supreme; children in subordinate position in family hierarchy | Often smile and nod in agreement when do not understand |
| Supernatural (*loa*—spirits' anger) | Natural illnesses treated by home and folk remedies first | Children valued for parental social security in old age and expected to contribute to family welfare at early age | Quiet and gentle communication style and lack of assertiveness, leading health care providers to falsely believe they comprehend health teaching and are compliant |
| Good health: maintenance of equilibrium | May use religious medallions, rosary beads, or figure of saint to pray with | | May not ask questions if health care provider is busy or rushed |
| Prayer and good spiritual habits important | | | |

*Continued*

## Cultural Characteristics Related to Health Care of Children and Families—cont'd

| Health Beliefs | Health Practices | Family Relationships | Communication |
|---|---|---|---|
| **Hmong** | | | |
| Health a balance between social, natural, and supernatural forces<br>There is a belief that in the chest there is a pool of blood that was vital to life. If a person lost this pool of blood, he or she would die | Shamans, soul callers, herbalists, massage therapists, and magic healers are used<br>Often seek traditional healers before seeking Western medicine help.<br>Shaman ceremonies are not only a component of the traditional healing system but also a symbol of cultural identity and caring within the family<br>Shaman ceremonies reaffirm ethnic identity and are perceived by many Hmong elders as being essential to their culture | Hmong people are patriarchal and organized into clans<br>Members of the same clan consider each other to be *kwv tij* "brothers" or "siblings." Clan members are expected to offer one another mutual support<br>The Hmong person's primary identity is not as an individual but as a member of the family and clan. Important decisions are likely to affect all family members, so the individual does not have the right to make decisions independently for himself or herself | Most Hmong households speak a language other than English in the home<br>Husband is seen as the head of the house and announces decisions<br>Women seek advice and approval from their husband and head of the clan when facing health decisions |
| **Japanese** | | | |
| Shinto religious influence<br>Humans inherently good<br>Evil caused by outside spirits<br>Illness caused by contact with polluting agents (e.g., blood, corpses, skin diseases)<br>Health achieved through harmony and balance between self and society<br>Disease caused by disharmony with society and not caring for body | Energy restored by means of acupuncture, acupressure, massage, and moxibustion along affected meridians<br>Kampõ medicine—use of natural herbs<br>Believe in removal of diseased parts<br>Trend to use both Western and Asian healing methods<br>Care for disabled viewed as family's responsibility<br>Take pride in child's good health<br>Seek preventive care, medical care for illness | Close intergenerational relationships<br>Generational categories:<br>Issei—first generation to live in United States<br>Nisei—second generation<br>Sansei—third generation<br>Yonsei—fourth generation<br>Family tendency to keep problems to self<br>Value self-control and self-sufficiency<br>Concept of haji (shame) imposes strong control; unacceptable behavior of children reflects on family | Issei—born in Japan; usually speak Japanese only<br>Nisei, Sansei, *and* Yonsei have few language difficulties<br>Make significant use of nonverbal communication with subtle gestures and facial expression<br>Tend to suppress emotions<br>Will often wait silently |
| **Mexican-American** | | | |
| Health controlled by environment, fate, and will of God<br>Certain illnesses considered "hot" and "cold" states and are treated with food that complements those states<br>Disease based on imbalance between individual and environment | Seek help from curandero or curandera, especially in rural areas<br>Curandero(a) receives position by birth, apprenticeship, or "calling" via dream or vision<br>Treatments with herbs, rituals, and religious artifacts<br>For severe illness, make promises, visit shrines, offer medals and candles, offer prayers<br>Adhere to "hot" and "cold" food prescriptions and prohibitions for prevention and treatment of illness | Strong kinship ties; extended families include compadres (godparents) established by ritual kinship<br>Children valued highly and desired, taken everywhere with family<br>Elderly treated with respect | Spanish speaking or bilingual<br>May have strong preference for native language and revert to it in times of stress<br>May shake hands or engage in introductory embrace<br>Interpret prolonged eye contact as disrespectful<br>Relaxed concept of time—may be late to appointments |

## Cultural Characteristics Related to Health Care of Children and Families—cont'd

| Health Beliefs | Health Practices | Family Relationships | Communication |
|---|---|---|---|
| **Middle Eastern** | | | |
| Illness often associated with bad luck or poverty, health with good luck and wealth<br>Illness may be sent by God as punishment—each person's fate is sealed at the time their soul is created. | Preventive care is not practice in the Middle East, and medication is heavily used<br>May fear hospital admission because they are considered places of misfortune<br>Muslims may be concerned that the body may not be treated correctly according to religious customs | Need for affiliation, thrive on a large repertoire of relationships;<br>Affiliation needs often intensified during illness; patient often accompanied by family members who expect to be present during the examination and often speak for the patient<br>Children often live with their parents until they marry and maintain close contact with family after marriage | Ritual courtesy toward strangers<br>The one with the most authority makes the decisions<br>Include the family spokesperson in the discussion<br>Often communicate negative information in stages |
| **Puerto Rican** | | | |
| Subscribe to "hot-cold" theory of causation of illness<br>Believe some illness caused by evil forces<br>Destiny (*Si Dios quiere*—if God wants) in control of health | Infrequent use of health care system<br>Seek folk healers (*espiritistas*)—use of herbs, rituals<br>Treatment classified as "hot" or "cold"<br>Many varieties of herbal teas used to treat illness and promote healing | Family usually large and home centered—core of existence<br>Father has authority in family<br>Great respect for elders<br>Children valued—seen as gift from God<br>Children taught to obey and respect parents | Spanish speaking or bilingual<br>Strong sense of family privacy—may view questions regarding family as impudent |
| **Vietnamese** | | | |
| Good health considered balance between yin and yang<br>Concept of health based on harmony and balance<br>Many use rituals to prevent illness | Family uses all means possible before using outside agencies for health care<br>Regard health as family responsibility; outside aid sought when resources run out<br>Use herbal medicine, spiritual practices, and acupuncture<br>May use cupping, coin rubbing, or pinching skin<br>May inhale aromatic oils, drink herbal teas, or wear strings tied on body | Family revered institution and chief social network<br>Multigenerational families<br>Children highly valued<br>Individual needs and interests subordinate to those of family group<br>Father main decision maker<br>Women taught submission to men<br>Parents expect respect and obedience from children | Many immigrants not proficient in speaking and understanding English<br>May hesitate to ask questions<br>Questioning authority seen as a sign of disrespect; asking questions considered impolite<br>May avoid eye contact with health professionals as sign of respect |

# Physical Assessment

Physical assessment is a continuous process that begins during the interview, primarily by using inspection or observation. During the more formal examination, the tools of percussion, palpation, and auscultation are added to enhance and refine the assessment of body systems. Like the health history, the objective of the physical assessment is to formulate nursing diagnoses and evaluate the effectiveness of therapeutic interventions.

Because of important differences in physical assessment of the child and newborn, separate guidelines and summaries for conducting the physical examination of each age group are presented.

The summary of the physical assessment of the newborn is also presented according to the area to be assessed, usual findings, common variations and minor abnormalities, and potential signs of distress or major abnormalities. Common variations and minor abnormalities should be recorded but generally do not require further evaluation. Potential signs of distress or major abnormalities are recorded and need to be reported for further evaluation. The procedures for assessment are not presented here but in the summary of physical assessment of the child. In addition to the newborn summary, assessment of clinical gestational age is also described.

The summary of the physical assessment of the child is presented according to the area to be assessed, the procedure for assessment, usual findings, and comments. The comments column includes findings that deviate from the normal and should be reported, special significance of certain findings, and areas for nursing intervention. This section includes detailed instructions for various assessment procedures.

For a more comprehensive discussion of performing a physical assessment, see *Wong's Nursing Care of Infants and Children* or *Wong's Essentials of Pediatric Nursing.*

## General Guidelines for Physical Examination of the Newborn

Provide a comfortably warm and nonstimulating examination area.
- To prevent heat loss, undress only the body area to be examined unless the newborn is already under a heat source, such as a radiant warmer.

Proceed in an orderly sequence (usually head to toe) with the following exceptions:
- Perform first all procedures that require quiet observation (position, attitude, skin color); then proceed with quiet procedures, such as auscultating the lungs, heart, and abdomen.
- Perform disturbing procedures, such as testing reflexes, last.

- Measure head and length at same time to compare results.

Proceed quickly to avoid stressing the infant.
- Check that equipment and supplies are working properly and are accessible.

Comfort the infant during and after the examination if upset.
- Talk softly.
- Hold infant's hands against his or her chest.
- Swaddle and hold.
- Provide nonnutritive sucking.

## Summary of Physical Assessment of the Newborn

| Usual Findings | Common Variations and Minor Abnormalities | Potential Signs of Distress or Major Abnormalities |
| --- | --- | --- |
| **General Measurements** | | |
| *Head circumference*—33-35 cm (13-14 inches); about 2-3 cm (1 inch) larger than chest circumference | Molding after birth may decrease head circumference. | Head circumference <10th or >90th percentile |
| *Chest circumference*—30.5-33 cm (12-13 inches). | Head and chest circumference may be equal for first 1-2 days after birth. | |
| *Crown-to-rump length*—31-35 cm (12.5-14 inches); approximately equal to head circumference | | |
| *Head-to-heel length*—48-53 cm (19-21 inches) | | |
| Birth weight—2700-4000 g (6-9 pounds) | Loss of 10% of birth weight in first week; regained in 10-14 days | Birth weight <10th or >90th percentile |

## Summary of Physical Assessment of the Newborn—cont'd

| Usual Findings | Common Variations and Minor Abnormalities | Potential Signs of Distress or Major Abnormalities |
|---|---|---|
| **Vital Signs** | | |
|  *Temperature (axillary)*—36.5°-37° C (97.9°-98° F) | Crying may increase body temperature slightly.<br>Radiant warmer may falsely increase axillary temperature. | Hypothermia<br>Hyperthermia |
| *Heart rate (apical)*—120-140 beats/min | Crying will increase heart rate; sleep will decrease heart rate.<br>During first period of reactivity (6-8 hours), rate can reach 180 beats/min. | Bradycardia—Resting rate below 80-100 beats/min<br>Tachycardia—Rate above 180 beats/min<br>Irregular rhythm |
| *Respirations*—30-60 breaths/min | Crying will increase respiratory rate; sleep will decrease respiratory rate.<br>During first period of reactivity (6-8 hours), rate can reach 80 breaths/min. | Irregular rhythm<br>Apnea >15 seconds |
| *Blood pressure (oscillometric)*—65/41 mm Hg in arm and calf | Crying and activity will increase blood pressure.<br>Placing cuff on thigh may agitate infant; thigh blood pressure may be higher than arm or calf blood pressure by 4-8 mm Hg and is least preferred method.<br>See Guidelines box. | Oscillometric systolic pressure in calf 6-9 mm Hg less than in upper extremity (possible sign of coarctation of aorta—correlate extremity pulses and pulse oximeter readings as well). Recommend taking blood pressure in same limb each time for consistent comparisons. Blood pressure in preterm infants may vary according to age and illness factors. |
| **General Appearance** | | |
| *Posture*—Flexion of head and extremities, which rest on chest and abdomen | *Frank breech*—Extended legs, abducted and fully rotated thighs, flattened occiput, extended neck | Limp posture, extension of extremities |

*Continued*

---

### GUIDELINES

#### Using the Blood Pressure Tables

1. Use the standard height charts to determine the height percentile.
2. Measure and record the child's systolic blood pressure (SBP) and diastolic blood pressure (DBP).
3. Use the correct gender table for SBP and DBP.
4. Find the child's age on the left side of the table. Follow the age row horizontally across the table to the intersection of the line for the height percentile (vertical column).
5. There, find the 50th, 90th, 95th, and 99th percentiles for SBP in the left columns and for DBP in the right columns.
   - BP <90th percentile is normal.
   - BP between the 90th and 95th percentile is prehypertension. In adolescents, BP ≥120/80 mm Hg is prehypertension, even if this figure is <90th percentile.
   - BP >95th percentile may be hypertension.
6. If the BP is >90th percentile, the BP should be repeated twice at the same office visit, and an average SBP and DBP should be used.
7. If the BP is >95th percentile, BP should be staged. If stage 1 (95th percentile to 99th percentile plus 5 mm Hg), BP measurements should be repeated on two more occasions. If hypertension is confirmed, evaluation should proceed. If BP is stage 2 (>99th percentile plus 5 mm Hg), prompt referral should be made for evaluation and therapy. If the patient is symptomatic, immediate referral and treatment are indicated.

From National High Blood Pressure Education Program Working Group on High Blood Pressure in Children and Adolescents: The fourth report on the diagnosis, evaluation, and treatment of high blood pressure in children and adolescents, *Pediatrics* 114(2 Suppl 4th Report):555-576, 2004.

## Summary of Physical Assessment of the Newborn—cont'd

| Usual Findings | Common Variations and Minor Abnormalities | Potential Signs of Distress or Major Abnormalities |
|---|---|---|
| **Skin** | | |
| At birth, bright red, puffy, smooth<br>Second to third day, pink, flaky, dry<br>Vernix caseosa<br>Lanugo<br>Edema around eyes, face, legs, dorsa of hands, feet, and scrotum or labia<br>*Acrocyanosis*—Cyanosis of hands and feet<br>*Cutis marmorata*—Transient mottling when infant is exposed to stress, decreased temperature, or overstimulation | Neonatal jaundice after first 24 hours<br>Ecchymoses or petechiae caused by birth trauma<br>*Milia*—Distended sebaceous glands that appear as tiny white papules on cheeks, chin, and nose<br>*Miliaria* or *sudamina*—Distended sweat (eccrine) glands that appear as minute vesicles, especially on face<br>*Erythema toxicum*—Pink papular rash with vesicles superimposed on thorax, back, buttocks, and abdomen; may appear in 24-48 hours and resolve after several days<br>*Harlequin color change*—Clearly outlined color change as infant lies on side; lower half of body becomes pink or red, and upper half is pale<br>*Mongolian spots*—Irregular areas of deep blue pigmentation, usually in sacral and gluteal regions; seen predominantly in newborns of African, Native American, Asian, or Hispanic descent<br>*Telangiectatic nevi* ("stork bites")—Flat, deep pink, localized areas usually seen on back of neck | Progressive jaundice, especially in first 24 hours<br>Cracked or peeling skin<br>Generalized cyanosis<br>Cyanosis of one extremity that persists<br>Pallor<br>Mottling<br>Grayness<br>Plethora<br>Hemorrhage, ecchymoses, or petechiae that persist<br>*Sclerema*—Hard and stiff skin<br>Poor skin turgor<br>Rashes, pustules, or blisters<br>*Café-au-lait spots*—Light brown spots<br>*Nevus flammeus*—Port-wine marks<br>Lacerations or abrasions |
| **Head** | | |
| *Anterior fontanel*—Diamond shaped, 2.5-4 cm (1-1.75 inches) (Figure 1-1) | Molding following vaginal delivery<br>Third sagittal (parietal) fontanel<br>Bulging fontanel because of crying | Fused sutures<br>Bulging or depressed fontanels when quiet<br>Widened sutures and fontanels.<br>Occipital or generalized scalp edema associated with vacuum delivery |
| *Posterior fontanel*—Triangular, 0.5-1 cm (0.2-0.4 inch)<br>Fontanels should be flat and firm.<br>Widest part of fontanel measured from bone to bone, not suture to suture | *Caput succedaneum*—Edema of soft scalp tissue<br>*Cephalhematoma (uncomplicated)*—Hematoma between periosteum and skull bone | *Craniotabes*—Snapping sensation along lambdoidal suture that resembles indentation of Ping-Pong ball |

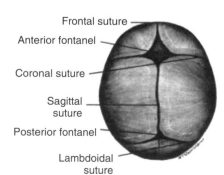

Frontal suture

Anterior fontanel

Coronal suture

Sagittal suture

Posterior fontanel

Lambdoidal suture

FIGURE **1-1**   Locations of sutures and fontanels.

## Summary of Physical Assessment of the Newborn—cont'd

| Usual Findings | Common Variations and Minor Abnormalities | Potential Signs of Distress or Major Abnormalities |
|---|---|---|
| **Eyes** | | |
| Lids usually edematous | Epicanthal folds in Asian infants | Pink color of iris |
| Iris color—Slate gray, dark blue, brown | Searching nystagmus or strabismus | Purulent discharge |
| Absence of tears | *Subconjunctival (scleral) hemorrhages*—Ruptured capillaries, usually at limbus | Upward slant in non-Asians |
| | | Hypertelorism (3 cm or greater) |
| Presence of red reflex | | Hypotelorism |
| Corneal reflex in response to touch | | *Congenital cataracts*—unilateral or bilateral |
| Pupillary reflex in response to light | | Constricted or dilated fixed pupil |
| | | Absence of red reflex |
| Blink reflex in response to light or touch | | Absence of pupillary or corneal reflex |
| Rudimentary fixation on objects and ability to follow to midline | | Inability to follow object or bright light to midline |
| | | Blue sclera |
| | | Yellow sclera |
| **Ears** | | |
| Position—Top of pinna on horizontal line with outer canthus of eye | Inability to visualize tympanic membrane because of filled aural canals | Low placement of ears |
| | Pinna flat against head | Absence of startle reflex in response to loud, sudden noise |
| Startle reflex elicited by a loud, sudden noise | Irregular shape or size | Minor abnormalities may be signs of various syndromes, especially renal |
| Pinna flexible, cartilage present | Pits or skin tags | |
| **Nose** | | |
| Nasal patency | Flattened and bruised | *Nonpatent canals*—Inability to pass nasogastric tube |
| | | Transient cyanosis and apnea with nonpatent canal may be sign of coanal atresia |
| Nasal discharge—Thin, white mucus | | Thick, bloody nasal discharge |
| Sneezing | | Flaring of nares (*alae nasi*) |
| Milia | | Copious nasal secretions or stuffiness (may be minor) |
| **Mouth and Throat** | | |
| Intact, high-arched palate | *Natal teeth*—Teeth present at birth; benign but may be associated with congenital defects | Cleft lip |
| Uvula in midline | | Cleft palate |
| Frenulum of tongue | | Large, protruding tongue or posterior displacement of tongue |
| Frenulum of upper lip | *Epstein pearls*—Small, white epithelial cysts along midline of hard palate | Profuse salivation or drooling |
| Sucking reflex—Strong and coordinated | Lingual frenulum extends to tip of tongue limiting tongue movement | *Candidiasis (thrush)*—White, adherent patches on tongue, palate, and buccal surfaces |
| Rooting reflex | | |
| Gag reflex | | |
| Extrusion reflex | | Inability to pass orogastric tube |
| Absent or minimal salivation | | Hoarse, high-pitched, weak, absent, or other abnormal cry |
| Vigorous cry | | |
| **Neck** | | |
| Short, thick, usually surrounded by skinfolds | *Torticollis (wry neck)*—Head held to one side with chin pointing to opposite side | Excessive skinfolds |
| | | Resistance to flexion |
| Tonic neck reflex | Fractured clavicle | Absence of tonic neck reflex |

*Continued*

## Summary of Physical Assessment of the Newborn—cont'd

| Usual Findings | Common Variations and Minor Abnormalities | Potential Signs of Distress or Major Abnormalities |
|---|---|---|
| **Chest** | | |
| Anteroposterior and lateral diameters equal | Funnel chest (pectus excavatum) | Depressed sternum |
| Slight sternal retractions evident during inspiration | Pigeon chest (pectus carinatum) | Marked retractions of chest and intercostal spaces during respiration |
| Xiphoid process evident | Supernumerary nipples | Asymmetric chest expansion |
| Breast enlargement | Secretion of milky substance from breasts ("witch's milk") | Redness and firmness around nipples |
| | | Wide-spaced nipples |
| **Lungs** | | |
| Respirations chiefly abdominal | Rate and depth of respirations may be irregular; periodic breathing. | Inspiratory stridor |
| Cough reflex absent at birth, present by 1-2 days | Crackles shortly after birth | Expiratory grunt |
| Bilateral, equal bronchial breath sounds | | Retractions |
| | | Persistent irregular breathing |
| | | Periodic breathing with repeated apneic spells (>20 seconds) |
| | | Seesaw respirations (paradoxic) |
| | | Unequal breath sounds |
| | | Persistent fine crackles |
| | | Wheezing |
| | | Diminished breath sounds |
| | | Peristaltic sounds on one side with diminished breath sounds on same side |
| **Heart** | | |
| *Apex*—Fourth to fifth intercostal space, lateral to left sternal border | *Sinus arrhythmia*—Heart rate increases with inspiration and decreases with expiration. | *Dextrocardia*—Heart on right side |
| S2 slightly sharper and higher in pitch than S1 | Transient cyanosis on crying or straining | Displacement of apex, muffled |
| | | Cardiomegaly |
| | | Abdominal bruit |
| | | Murmurs |
| | | Thrills |
| | | Persistent cyanosis |
| | | Hyperactive precordium |
| | | Unequal peripheral pulses |
| **Abdomen** | | |
| Rounded shape | Umbilical hernia | Abdominal distention |
| Bowel sounds present in all four quadrants | *Diastasis recti*—Midline gap between recti muscles | Localized bulging |
| *Liver*—Palpable 2-3 cm below right costal margin | *Wharton's jelly*   Unusually thick umbilical cord | Distended veins |
| *Spleen*—Tip palpable at end of first week of age | | Absent bowel sounds |
| *Kidneys*—Palpable 1-2 cm above umbilicus | | Enlarged liver and spleen |
| *Umbilical cord*—Bluish white at birth with two arteries and one vein | | Ascites |
| *Femoral pulses*—Equal bilaterally | | Visible peristaltic waves |
| | | Scaphoid or concave abdomen |
| | | Green umbilical cord |
| | | Presence of only one artery in cord |
| | | Urine or stool leaking from cord |
| | | Palpable bladder distention following scanty voiding |
| | | Absent femoral pulses |

## Summary of Physical Assessment of the Newborn—cont'd

| Usual Findings | Common Variations and Minor Abnormalities | Potential Signs of Distress or Major Abnormalities |
|---|---|---|
| **Abdomen—cont'd** | | |
| | | Cord bleeding, hematoma, or mass contained within cord (possible omphalocele) |
| | | *Bladder exstrophy*—externalization of bladder (possibly with epispadias) with widely separated symphysis pubis |
| **Female Genitalia** | | |
| Labia and clitoris usually edematous | *Pseudomenstruation*—Blood-tinged or mucoid discharge | Enlarged clitoris with urethral meatus at tip |
| Urethral meatus behind clitoris | Hymenal tag | Fused labia |
| Vernix caseosa between labia | Edema, petechiae, bruising from breech presentation (or delivery) | Absence of vaginal opening |
| Urination within 24 hours | | Meconium from vaginal opening, urethral opening, or perineum |
| | | No urination within 24 hours |
| | | Masses in labia |
| | | Ambiguous genitalia |
| **Male Genitalia** | | |
| Urethral opening at tip of glans penis | Urethral opening covered by prepuce | *Hypospadias*—Urethral opening on ventral surface of penis |
| Testes palpable in each scrotum | Inability to retract foreskin | *Epispadias*—Urethral opening on dorsal surface of penis |
| Scrotum usually large, edematous, pendulous, and covered with rugae; usually deeply pigmented in dark-skinned ethnic groups | *Epithelial pearls*—Small, firm, white lesions at tip of prepuce | *Chordee*—Ventral curvature of penis |
| | Erection or priapism | |
| | Testes palpable in inguinal canal | Testes not palpable in scrotum or inguinal canal |
| Smegma | Scrotum small | Micropenis (two standard deviations below the mean of length and width for age) |
| Urination within 24 hours | Edema, ecchymoses, bruising with breech presentation (or delivery) | No urination within 24 hours |
| | | Inguinal hernia |
| | | Hypoplastic or absent scrotum |
| | | *Hydrocele*—Fluid in scrotum |
| | | Masses in scrotum |
| | | Meconium from scrotum, raphe, or perineum |
| | | Discoloration of testes—(bluish-red) possible testicular torsion |
| | | Ambiguous genitalia |
| **Back and Rectum** | | |
| Spine intact; no openings, masses, or prominent curves | Green liquid stools in infant under phototherapy | Anal fissures or fistulas |
| Trunk incurvation reflex | Delayed passage of meconium in very low–birth-weight or sick neonates | Imperforate anus |
| Anal reflex | | Absence of anal reflex |
| Patent anal opening | | No meconium within 36 hours |
| Passage of meconium within 48 hours | | Pilonidal cyst or sinus |
| | | Tuft of hair along spine |
| | | Spina bifida (any degree) |

*Continued*

## Summary of Physical Assessment of the Newborn—cont'd

| Usual Findings | Common Variations and Minor Abnormalities | Potential Signs of Distress or Major Abnormalities |
|---|---|---|
| **Extremities** | | |
| Ten fingers and 10 toes | Partial syndactyly between second and third toes | *Polydactyly*—Extra digits |
| Full range of motion | Second toe overlapping into third toe | *Syndactyly*—Fused or webbed digits |
| Nail beds pink, with transient cyanosis immediately after birth | Wide gap between first (hallux) and second toes | *Phocomelia*—Hands or feet attached close to trunk |
| Creases on anterior two thirds of sole | Deep crease on plantar surface of foot between first and second toes | *Hemimelia*—Absence of distal part of extremity |
| Sole usually flat | Asymmetric length of toes | Hyperflexibility of joints |
| Symmetry of extremities | Dorsiflexion and shortness of hallux | Persistent cyanosis of nail beds |
| Equal muscle tone bilaterally, especially resistance to opposing flexion | | Yellowing of nail beds |
| Equal bilateral brachial and femoral pulses | | Transverse palmar (simian) crease |
| | | Fractures, abrasions, bruises |
| | | Decreased or absent range of motion (ROM) |
| | | Dislocated or subluxated hip |
| | | Limitation in hip abduction |
| | | Unequal gluteal or leg folds |
| | | Unequal knee height (Galeazzi sign) |
| | | Audible clunk on abduction (Ortolani sign) |
| | | Asymmetry of extremities |
| | | Unequal muscle tone or ROM |
| **Neuromuscular System** | | |
| Extremities usually maintain some degree of flexion. | Quivering or momentary tremors | *Hypotonia*—Floppy, poor head control, extremities limp |
| Extension of an extremity followed by previous position of flexion | | *Hypertonia*—Jittery, arms and hands tightly flexed, legs stiffly extended, startles easily |
| Head lag while sitting, but momentary ability to hold head erect | | Asymmetric posturing (except tonic neck reflex) |
| Able to turn head from side to side when prone | | *Opisthotonic posturing*—Arched back |
| Able to hold head in horizontal line with back when held prone | | Signs of paralysis |
| | | Tremors, twitches, and myoclonic jerks |
| | | Marked head lag in all positions |

## Assessment of Reflexes

| Reflexes | Expected Behavioral Responses |
|---|---|
| **Localized** | |
| *Eyes* | |
| Blinking or corneal reflex | Infant blinks at sudden appearance of a bright light or at approach of an object toward cornea; persists throughout life. |
| Pupillary | Pupil constricts when a bright light shines toward it; persists throughout life. |
| Doll's eye | As head is moved slowly to right or left, eyes lag behind and do not immediately adjust to new position of head; disappears as fixation develops; if persists, indicates neurologic damage. |
| *Nose* | |
| Sneeze | Spontaneous response of nasal passages to irritation or obstruction; persists throughout life. |
| Glabellar | Tapping briskly on glabella (bridge of nose) causes eyes to close tightly. |

## Assessment of Reflexes—cont'd

| Reflexes | Expected Behavioral Responses |
|---|---|
| **Mouth and Throat** | |
| Sucking | Infant begins strong sucking movements of circumoral area in response to stimulation; persists throughout infancy, even without stimulation, such as during sleep. |
| Gag | Stimulation of posterior pharynx by food, suction, or passage of a tube causes infant to gag; persists throughout life. |
| Rooting | Touching or stroking the cheek along side of mouth causes infant to turn head toward that side and begin to suck; should disappear at about age 3-4 months but may persist for up to 12 months. |
| Extrusion | When tongue is touched or depressed, infant responds by forcing it outward; disappears by age 4 months. |
| Yawn | Spontaneous response to decreased oxygen by increasing amount of inspired air; persists throughout life. |
| Cough | Irritation of mucous membranes of larynx or tracheobronchial tree causes coughing; persists throughout life; usually present 1 day after birth. |
| **Extremities** | |
| Grasp | Touching palms of hands or soles of feet near base of digits causes flexion of hands and toes; palmar grasp lessens after age 3 months, to be replaced by voluntary movement; plantar grasp lessens by 8 months of age. |
| Babinski | Stroking outer sole of foot upward from heel and across ball of foot causes toes to hyperextend and hallux to dorsiflex; disappears after age 1 year. |
| Ankle clonus | Briskly dorsiflexing foot while supporting knee in partially flexed position results in one or two oscillating movements ("beats"); eventually no beats should be felt. |
| **Mass (Body)** | |
| Moro* | Sudden jarring or change in equilibrium causes sudden extension and abduction of extremities and fanning of fingers, with index finger and thumb forming a *C* shape, followed by flexion and adduction of extremities; legs may weakly flex; infant may cry; disappears after age 3-4 months, usually strongest during first 2 months. |
| Startle* | A sudden loud noise causes abduction of the arms with flexion of elbows; hands remain clenched; disappears by age 4 months. |
| Perez | While infant is prone on a firm surface, thumb is pressed along spine from sacrum to neck; infant responds by crying, flexing extremities, and elevating pelvis and head; lordosis of the spine, as well as defecation and urination, may occur; disappears by age 4-6 months. |
| Asymmetric tonic neck | When infant's head is turned to one side, arm and leg extend on that side, and opposite arm and leg flex; disappears by age 3-4 months, to be replaced by symmetric positioning of both sides of body. |
| Trunk incurvation (Galant) | Stroking infant's back alongside spine causes hips to move toward stimulated side; reflex disappears by age 4 weeks. |
| Dance or step | If infant is held so that sole of foot touches a hard surface, there is a reciprocal flexion and extension of the leg, simulating walking; disappears after age 3-4 weeks, to be replaced by deliberate movement. |
| Crawl | When placed on abdomen, infant makes crawling movements with arms and legs; disappears at about age 6 weeks. |
| Placing | When infant is held upright under arms and dorsal side of foot is briskly placed against hard object, such as table, leg lifts as if foot is stepping on table; age of disappearance varies. |

*Some authorities consider Moro and startle reflexes to be the same response.

# Assessment of Gestational Age

Assessment of gestational age is an important criterion because perinatal morbidity and mortality are related to gestational age and birth weight. One of the most frequently used methods of determining gestational age is based on physical and neurologic findings. The scale in Figure 1-2, A assesses six external physical and six neuromuscular signs. Each sign has a number score, and the cumulative score correlates with a maturity rating from 20 to 44 weeks (see maturity rating box on scale).

The new **Ballard Scale**, a revision of the original scale, can be used with newborns as young as 20 weeks of gestation. The tool has the same physical and neuromuscular sections but includes −1 and −2 scores that reflect signs of extremely premature infants, such as fused eyelids; imperceptible breast tissue; sticky, friable, transparent skin; no lanugo; and square-window (flexion of wrist) angle of greater than 90 degrees. The examination of infants with a gestational age of 20 weeks or less should be performed at a postnatal age of less than 12 hours. For infants with a gestational age of at least 26 weeks, the examination can be performed up to 96 hours after birth, although shortly after birth, preferably within 2 to 8 hours, is suggested. The scale overestimates gestational age by 2 to 4 days in infants less than 37 weeks of gestation, especially between 32 and 37 weeks of gestation. Neurologic maturity may require retesting once the infant's condition has stabilized. The new Ballard gestational age scale has greater validity when performed before 96 hours of age in preterm infants. It is also important to note that the infant's state and period of reactivity will affect the neuromuscular rating. An infant in the second stage of the first period of reactivity may not have an accurate neuromuscular score. (After the initial stage of alertness and activity [may last the first 6 to 8 hours of life], the infant enters the second stage of the first reactive period, which generally lasts 2 to 4 hours. Heart and respiratory rates decrease, temperature continues to fall, mucus production decreases, and urine or stool is usually not passed. The infant is in a state of sleep and relative calm. Any attempt at stimulation usually elicits a minimal response.)

Classification of infants at birth by both weight and gestational age provides a more satisfactory method for predicting mortality risks and providing guidelines for management of the neonate. The infant's birth weight, length, and head circumference are plotted on standardized graphs that identify normal values for gestational age. The infant whose weight is appropriate for gestational age (AGA) (between the 10th and 90th percentiles) can be presumed to have grown at a normal rate regardless of the length of gestation—preterm, term, or postterm. The infant who is large for gestational age (LGA) (above the 90th percentile) can be presumed to have grown at an accelerated rate during fetal life; the small-for-gestational-age (SGA) infant (below the 10th percentile) can be presumed to have grown at a restricted rate during intrauterine life. When gestational age is determined according to the Ballard scale, the newborn will fall into one of the following nine possible categories for birth weight and gestational age: AGA—term, preterm, postterm; SGA—term, preterm, postterm; or LGA—term, preterm, postterm. Figure 1-2, B is a classification of newborns based on intrauterine growth.

To facilitate the use of Figure 1-2, A, the following tests and observations are described:

| Test | Assessment or Description |
|---|---|
| Posture | With the infant quiet and in a supine position, observe the degree of flexion in the arms and legs. Muscle tone and degree of flexion increase with maturity. Full flexion of the arms and legs = 4. |
| Square window | With the thumb supporting the back of the arm below the wrist, apply gentle pressure with index and third fingers on dorsum of hand without rotating the infant's wrist. Measure the angle between the base of the thumb and forearm. Full flexion (hand lies flat on ventral surface of forearm) = 4. |
| Arm recoil | With the infant supine, fully flex both forearms on upper arms, hold for 5 seconds; pull down on hands to fully extend and rapidly release arms. Observe the rapidity and intensity of recoil to a state of flexion. A brisk return to full flexion = 4. |
| Popliteal angle | With the infant supine and the pelvis flat on a firm surface, flex lower leg on thigh, then flex thigh on abdomen. While holding knee with thumb and index finger, extend lower leg with index finger of other hand. Measure the degree of the angle behind the knee (popliteal angle). An angle <90 degrees = 5. |
| Scarf sign | With the infant supine, support the head in the midline with one hand; use other hand to pull infant's arm across the shoulder so that infant's hand touches the opposite shoulder. Determine location of elbow in relation to midline. Elbow does not reach midline = 4. |
| Heel to ear | With the infant supine and the pelvis flat on a firm surface, pull the foot as far as possible up toward the ear on the same side. Measure the distance of the foot from the ear and degree of knee flexion (same as popliteal angle). Knees flexed with a popliteal angle <90 degrees = 4. |

# Estimation of Gestational Age by Maturity Rating

## NEUROMUSCULAR MATURITY

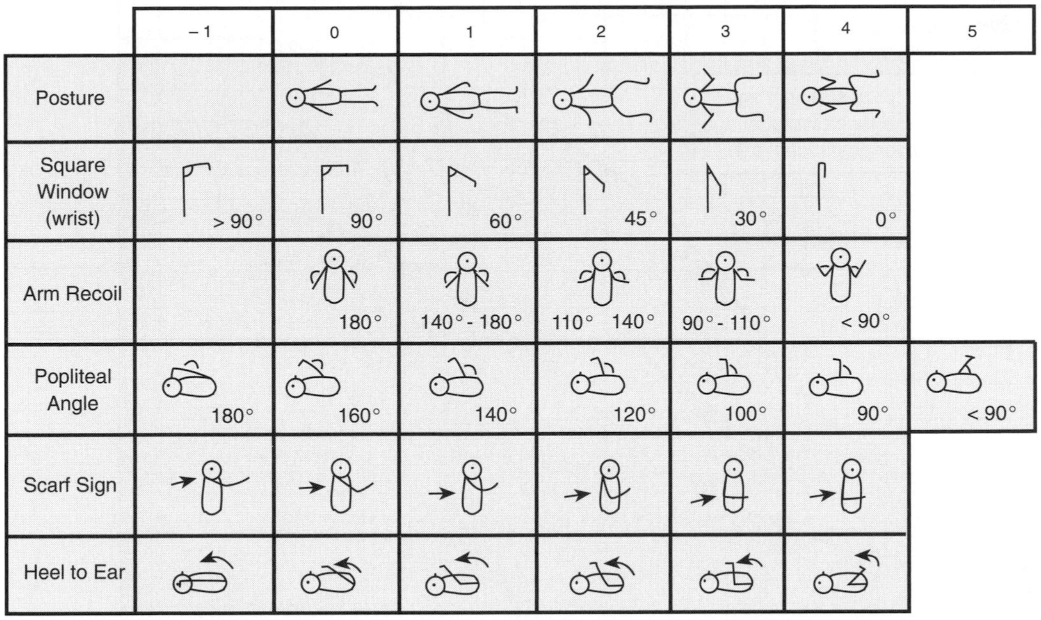

| | −1 | 0 | 1 | 2 | 3 | 4 | 5 |
|---|---|---|---|---|---|---|---|
| Posture | | | | | | | |
| Square Window (wrist) | > 90° | 90° | 60° | 45° | 30° | 0° | |
| Arm Recoil | | 180° | 140° - 180° | 110° 140° | 90° - 110° | < 90° | |
| Popliteal Angle | 180° | 160° | 140° | 120° | 100° | 90° | < 90° |
| Scarf Sign | | | | | | | |
| Heel to Ear | | | | | | | |

## PHYSICAL MATURITY

| | | | | | | | |
|---|---|---|---|---|---|---|---|
| Skin | sticky friable transparent | gelatinous red, translucent | smooth pink, visible veins | superficial peeling &/or rash, few veins | cracking pale areas rare veins | parchment deep cracking no vessels | leathery cracked wrinkled |
| Lanugo | none | sparse | abundant | thinning | bald areas | mostly bald | |
| Plantar Surface | heel-toe 40-50 mm: -1 <40 mm: -2 | >50 mm no crease | faint red marks | anterior transverse crease only | creases ant. 2/3 | creases over entire sole | |
| Breast | imperceptible | barely perceptible | flat areola no bud | stippled areola 1-2 mm bud | raised areola 3-4 mm bud | full areola 5-10 mm bud | |
| Eye/Ear | lids fused loosely: -1 tightly: -2 | lids open pinna flat stays folded | sl. curved pinna; soft; slow recoil | well-curved pinna; soft but ready recoil | formed & firm instant recoil | thick cartilage ear stiff | |
| Genitals (male) | scrotum flat, smooth | scrotum empty faint rugae | testes in upper canal rare rugae | testes descending few rugae | testes down good rugae | testes pendulous deep rugae | |
| Genitals (female) | clitoris prominent labia flat | prominent clitoris small labia minora | prominent clitoris enlarging minora | majora & minora equally prominent | majora large minora small | majora cover clitoris & minora | |

## MATURITY RATING

| score | weeks |
|---|---|
| -10 | 20 |
| -5 | 22 |
| 0 | 24 |
| 5 | 26 |
| 10 | 28 |
| 15 | 30 |
| 20 | 32 |
| 25 | 34 |
| 30 | 36 |
| 35 | 38 |
| 40 | 40 |
| 45 | 42 |
| 50 | 44 |

A

FIGURE **1-2**   A, New Ballard Scale for newborn maturity rating. Expanded scale includes extremely premature infants and has been refined to improve accuracy in more mature infants.

*Continued*

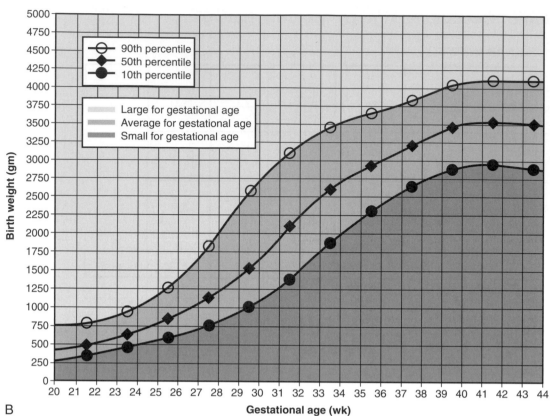

B

FIGURE **1-2, cont'd**   B, Intrauterine growth: birth weight percentiles based on live single births at gestational ages 20 to 44 weeks. (Data from Alexander GR and others: A United States national reference for fetal growth, *Obstet Gynecol* 87(2):163-168, 1996.)

## Assessment of Newborn Bilirubin

Hour-specific serum bilirubin levels to predict newborns at risk for rapidly rising levels may be used as a screening tool before discharge from the hospital. Using a nomogram (Figure 1-3) with three designated risk levels (high, intermediate, and low risk) for hour-specific total serum bilirubin values assists in the determination of which newborns might need further evaluation before and after discharge.

## General Guidelines for Physical Examination During Childhood

Perform examination in pleasant, nonthreatening area.
- Have room well lit and decorated.
- Have room temperature comfortably warm.
- Place all strange and potentially frightening equipment out of sight.
- Have some toys, dolls, stuffed animals, and games available for the child.
- If possible, have rooms decorated and equipped for different-age children.
- Provide privacy, especially for school-age children and adolescents.
- Check that equipment and supplies are working properly and are accessible to avoid disruption.

Provide time for play and becoming acquainted.
- Talking to the nurse
- Making eye contact
- Accepting the offered equipment
- Allowing physical touching
- Choosing to sit on examining table rather than parent's lap

If signs of readiness are not observed, use the following techniques:
- Talk to the parent while essentially "ignoring" the child; gradually focus on the child or a favorite object, such as a doll.
- Make complimentary remarks about the child, for instance, about his or her appearance, dress, or a favorite object.
- Tell a funny story, or perform a simple magic trick.
- Have a nonthreatening "friend," such as a hand puppet or finger puppet, available to "talk" to the child for the nurse.

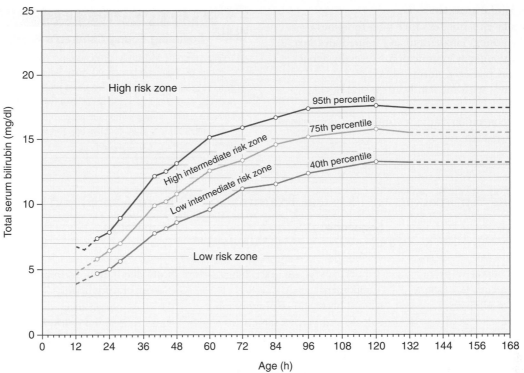

FIGURE **1-3** Nomogram for designation of risk in 2840 well newborns at 36 or more weeks of gestational age with birth weight of 2000 g (4.4 pounds) or more, or 35 or more weeks of gestational age and birth weight of 2500 g (5.5 pounds) or more, based on the hour-specific serum bilirubin values. (This nomogram should not be used to represent the natural history of neonatal hyperbilirubinemia.) (From Bhutani VK, Johnson L, Sivieri EM: Predictive ability of a predischarge hour-specific serum bilirubin for subsequent significant hyperbilirubinemia in healthy term and near-term newborns, *Pediatrics* 103(1):6-14, 1999.)

If the child refuses to cooperate, use the following techniques:
- Assess reason for uncooperative behavior; consider that a child who is unduly afraid of a male examiner may have had a previous traumatic experience, including sexual abuse.
- Try to involve child and parent in process, or, if appropriate, ask parent to leave.
- Avoid prolonged explanations about examining procedure.
- Use a firm, direct approach regarding expected behavior.
- Perform examination as quickly as possible.
- Have attendant gently restrain child.
- Minimize any disruptions or stimulation:
  - Limit number of people in room.
  - Use isolated room.
  - Use quiet, calm, confident voice.

Begin the examination in a nonthreatening manner for young children or children who are fearful (Atraumatic Care box).
- Use activities that can be presented as games, such as tests for cranial nerves (see p. 73) or parts of developmental testing (see p. 121).
- Use approaches such as "Simon says" to encourage child to make a face, squeeze a hand, stand on one foot, and so on.

- Use the paper-doll technique:
  - Lay the child supine on an examining table or floor that is covered with a large sheet of paper.
  - Trace outline around the child's body.
  - Use the body outline to demonstrate what will be examined, such as drawing a heart and listening with the stethoscope before performing the activity on the child.

If several children in the family will be examined, begin with the most cooperative child.

Involve child in the examination process.
- Provide choices, such as sitting either on the table or on the parent's lap.
- Allow child to handle or hold equipment.
- Encourage child to use equipment on a doll, family member, or examiner.
- Explain each step of the procedure in simple language.

Examine child in a comfortable and secure position.
- Sitting in parent's lap
- Sitting upright if in respiratory distress

Proceed to examine the body in an organized sequence (usually head to toe) with the following exceptions:
- Alter sequence to accommodate needs of different-age children (see p. 30).

- Examine painful areas last.
- In emergency situation, examine vital functions (airway, breathing, circulation) and injured area first.

Reassure child throughout examination, especially about bodily concerns that arise during puberty.

Discuss the findings with the family at the end of the examination.

Praise child for cooperation during examination; give reward such as an inexpensive toy or paper sticker.

### ATRAUMATIC CARE

**Reducing Young Children's Fears**

Young children, especially preschoolers, fear intrusive procedures because of their poorly defined body boundaries. Therefore avoid invasive procedures, such as measuring rectal temperature, whenever possible. Also, avoid using the word "take" when measuring vital signs, because young children interpret words literally and may think that their temperature or other function will be taken away. Instead, say, "I want to know how warm you are."

## Age-Specific Approaches to Physical Examination During Childhood

| Position | Sequence | Preparation |
|---|---|---|
| **Infant** | | |
| Before sits alone: supine or prone, preferably in parent's lap; before 4-6 months: can place on examining table<br>After sits alone: sit in parent's lap whenever possible<br>If on table, place with parent in full view | If quiet, auscultate heart, lungs, abdomen.<br>Record heart and respiratory rates.<br>Palpate and percuss same areas.<br>Proceed in usual head-to-toe direction.<br>Perform traumatic procedures last (eyes, ears, mouth [while infant is crying]).<br>Elicit reflexes as body part examined.<br>Elicit Moro reflex last. | Completely undress infant if room temperature permits.<br>Leave diaper on male.<br>Gain cooperation with distraction, bright objects, rattles, talking.<br>Have older infants hold a small block in each hand; until voluntary release develops toward end of the first year, infants will be unable to grasp other objects (e.g., stethoscope, otoscope).<br>Smile at infant; use soft, gentle voice.<br>Pacify with bottle of sugar water or feeding.<br>Enlist parent's aid in restraining to examine ears, mouth.<br>Avoid abrupt, jerky movements. |
| **Toddler** | | |
| Sitting or standing on or by parent<br>Prone or supine in parent's lap | Inspect body area through play: count fingers, tickle toes.<br>Use minimal physical contact initially.<br>Introduce equipment slowly.<br>Auscultate, percuss, palpate whenever quiet.<br>Perform traumatic procedures last (same as for infant). | Have parent remove child's outer clothing.<br>Remove underwear as body part is examined.<br>Allow child to inspect equipment; demonstrating use of equipment is usually ineffective.<br>If uncooperative, perform procedures quickly.<br>Use restraint when appropriate; request parent's assistance.<br>Talk about examination if cooperative; use short phrases.<br>Praise for cooperative behavior. |
| **Preschool Child** | | |
| Prefers standing or sitting<br>Usually cooperative prone or supine<br>Prefers parent's closeness | If cooperative, proceed in head-to-toe direction.<br>If uncooperative, proceed as with toddler. | Request self-undressing.<br>Allow to wear underpants.<br>Offer equipment for inspection; briefly demonstrate use.<br>Make up story about procedure: "I'm seeing how strong your muscles are" (blood pressure).<br>Use paper-doll technique.<br>Give choices when possible.<br>Expect cooperation; use positive statements: "Open your mouth." |

## Age-Specific Approaches to Physical Examination During Childhood—cont'd

| Position | Sequence | Preparation |
|---|---|---|
| **School-Age Child** | | |
| Prefers sitting | Proceed in head-to-toe direction. | Request self-undressing. |
| Cooperative in most positions | May examine genitalia last in older | Allow to wear underpants. |
| Younger child prefers parent's | child. | Give gown to wear. |
| presence. | Respect need for privacy. | Explain purpose of equipment and significance |
| Older child may prefer privacy. | | of procedure, such as otoscope to see |
| | | eardrum, which is necessary for hearing. |
| | | Teach about body functioning and care. |
| **Adolescent** | | |
| Same as for school-age child | Same as for older school-age child | Allow to undress in private. |
| Offer option of parent's presence. | | Give gown. |
| | | Expose only area to be examined. |
| | | Respect need for privacy. |
| | | Explain findings during examination: "Your |
| | | muscles are firm and strong." |
| | | Matter-of-factly comment about sexual |
| | | development: "Your breasts are developing |
| | | as they should be." |
| | | Emphasize normalcy of development. |
| | | Examine genitalia as any other body part; may |
| | | leave for end. |

# Outline of a Physical Assessment

**A. Growth measurements**
  1. Length and height
  2. Crown-to-rump length or sitting height
  3. Weight
  4. Head circumference

**B. Physiologic measurements**
  1. Temperature
  2. Pulse
  3. Respiration
  4. Blood pressure
  5. Pain assessment
  6. Pulse oximetry as needed

**C. General appearance**

**D. Skin**

**E. Accessory structures**

**F. Lymph nodes**

**G. Head**

**H. Neck**

**I. Eyes**

**J. Ears**

**K. Nose**

**L. Mouth and throat**

**M. Chest**

**N. Lungs**

**O. Heart**

**P. Abdomen**

**Q. Genitalia**
  1. Male
  2. Female

**R. Anus**

**S. Back and extremities**

**T. Neurologic assessment**
  1. Mental status
  2. Motor functioning
  3. Sensory functioning
  4. Reflexes (deep tendons)
  5. Cranial nerves

## Summary of Physical Assessment of the Child

| Assessment | Procedure |
|---|---|

### Growth Measurements

See Figure 1-4, A and B.

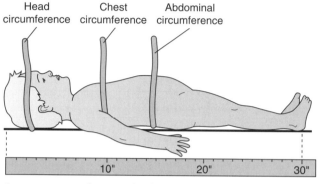

Head circumference  Chest circumference  Abdominal circumference

10"  20"  30"

**A**  Crown-to-heel recumbent length

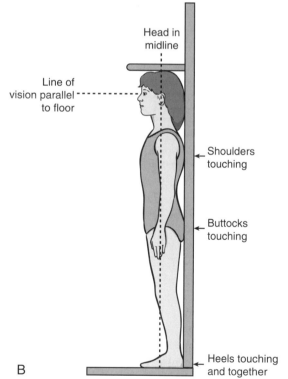

Head in midline

Line of vision parallel to floor

Shoulders touching

Buttocks touching

Heels touching and together

**B**

FIGURE **1-4**  A, Measurement of head, chest, and abdominal circumference and crown-to-heel (recumbent) length. B, Measurement of height (stature). (A, From Price DL: *Pediatric nursing: An introductory text,* ed 10, St Louis, 2007, Saunders. B, From Wilson S: *Health assessment for nursing practice,* ed 4, St Louis, 2009, Mosby.)

Plot length, weight, and head circumference on standard percentile charts.

Charts for 0-36 months and 2-20 years both include children ages 24-36 months; record only recumbent length on 0- to 36-month chart and only stature on 2- to 20-year chart.

The prepubescent charts are appropriate only for plotting values for prepubescent boys and girls, regardless of chronologic age, and not for any child showing signs of pubescence, such as breast budding, testicular enlargement, or growth of axillary or pubic hair.

## Usual Findings

Measurements of length, weight, and head circumference between the 25th and 75th percentiles are likely to represent normal growth (Safety Alert).

Measurements between the 10th and 25th and between the 75th and 90th percentiles may or may not be normal, depending on previous and subsequent measurements and on genetic and environmental factors.

Growth curve remains generally within the same percentile, except during rapid growth periods.

> **! SAFETY ALERT**
>
> The 50th percentile represents the median growth (or midpoint of all the growth measurements for each age). The 5th percentile represents the lowest 5%, and the 95th percentile represents the highest 5% of growth measurements for each age.

## Comments

Questionable results may include the following:

1. Children whose height and weight percentiles are widely disparate, for example, height in the 10th percentile and weight in the 90th percentile, especially with above-average skinfold thickness
2. Children who fail to show the expected gain in height and weight, especially during the rapid growth periods of infancy and adolescence
3. Children who show a sudden increase, except during puberty, or decrease in a previously steady growth pattern

Compare findings with growth patterns of other family members: consider genetic influence on growth determination

Compare children's growth trends (height and weight) with midparental height (MPH). Most children with normal birth weights and heights and normal childhood growth will achieve an adult height within ±2 inches of MPH. Special charts are available for parent-specific adjustments for evaluation of the child's height.

To calculate MPH, use the following formulas:

For girls:
Father's height − 13 cm or 5 inches + Mother's height/2

For boys:
Father's height + 13 cm or 5 inches + Mother's height/2

*Continued*

## Summary of Physical Assessment of the Child—cont'd

| Assessment | Procedure |
|---|---|
| *Length and Height* | Recumbent length in children below 24-36 months: Place supine with head in midline. Grasp knees and push gently toward table to *fully* extend legs. Measure from vertex (top) of head to heels of feet (toes pointing upward). Standing height (stature) in children over 24-36 months: Remove socks and shoes. Have child stand as tall as possible, back straight, head in midline, and eyes looking straight ahead (see Figure 1-4, B.) Check for flexion of knees, slumping shoulders, and raising of heels. Measure from top of head to standing surface. Measure to the nearest cm or $\frac{1}{8}$ inch. |
| *Weight* | Weigh infants and young children nude on platform-type scale; protect infant by placing hand above body to prevent falling off scale. Weigh older children in underwear (and gown if privacy is a concern; no shoes) on standing-type upright scale. Check that scale is balanced before weighing. Cover scale with clean sheet of paper for each child. Measure to the nearest 10 g or $\frac{1}{2}$ ounce for infants and 100 g or $\frac{1}{4}$ pound for children. |
| *Head Circumference* | Measure with paper or steel tape at greatest circumference, from top of the eyebrows and pinna of the ear to occipital prominence of skull. |
| *Chest Circumference* | Measure around chest at nipple line. Ideally, take measurements during inhalation and expiration; record the average of the two values. |
| *Pulse* | Take apical pulse in children younger than 2-3 years. Point of maximum intensity located lateral to nipple at fourth to fifth interspace at or near midclavicular line. Take radial pulse in children older than 2-3 years. Count pulse for 1 full minute, especially if any irregularity is present. For repeated measurement, count pulse for 15 or 30 seconds and multiply by 4 or 2, respectively. |

| Usual Findings | Comments |
|---|---|
| Plot on growth chart.<br>Compare value with percentile for weight.<br>Rule of thumb guide*:<br>At 1 year: 1.5 × birth length<br>2-12 years: Age (years) × 2.5 + 30 = length (inches) | For accurate measurements, use infant-measuring device for recumbent length and stadiometer for standing height.<br>Normally height is less if measured in the afternoon than in the morning. To minimize this variation, apply modest upward pressure under the jaw or the mastoid processes. |

### Expected Growth Rates at Various Ages*

| Age | Expected Growth Rate (cm/year) |
|---|---|
| 1-6 months | 18-22 |
| 6-12 months | 14-18 |
| Second year | 11 |
| Third year | 8 |
| Fourth year | 7 |
| Fifth to tenth years | 5-6 |

*From *Human growth and disorders: An update,* South San Francisco, 1989, Genentech.

| | |
|---|---|
| Plot on growth chart.<br>Compare value with percentile for length.<br>Rule of thumb guides*:<br>At 1 year: 3 × birth weight<br>1-9 years: Age (years) × 5 + 17 = weight (pounds)<br>9-12 years: Age (years) × 9 − 20 = weight (pounds) | Compare weight with appearance, for example, excessive fat; well-developed musculature; flabby, loose skin; bony prominences (for skinfold measurement, see below).<br>Assess nutritional status; compare with weight. |
| Plot on growth chart.<br>Compare percentile with those of height and weight.<br>Compare with chest circumference:<br>At birth, head circumference exceeds chest circumference by 2-3 cm (1 inch).<br>At 1-2 years, head circumference equals chest circumference.<br>During childhood, chest circumference exceeds head circumference by about 5-7 cm (2-3 inches).<br>Compare with head circumference (see earlier in table). | Usually taken in children under 36 months of age<br>Taken in any child whose head size appears abnormal<br><br><br><br><br><br>May be measured during examination of chest |
| (For average pulse rates at rest, see inside front cover.) | Pulse rate normally may increase with inspiration and decrease with expiration (sinus arrhythmia) (See also Box 1-5.)<br>May grade pulses:<br>  **Grade 0**—Not palpable<br>  **Grade +1**—Difficult to palpate; thready, weak, easily obliterated with pressure<br>  **Grade +2**—Difficult to palpate; may be obliterated with pressure<br>  **Grade +3**—Easy to palpate; not easily obliterated with pressure (normal)<br>  **Grade +4**—Strong, bounding; not obliterated with pressure |

*Based on NCHS growth charts for boys, 50th percentile. For explanation of percentiles, see Safety Alert, p. 33.

*Continued*

## Summary of Physical Assessment of the Child—cont'd

| Assessment | Procedure |
|---|---|
| **Respiration** | Observe rate of breathing for 1 full minute. In infants and young children, observe abdominal movement. In older children, observe thoracic movement. |
| **Blood Pressure** | *Selection of Cuff* |

No matter what type of noninvasive technique is used, the most important factor in accurately measuring blood pressure is the use of an appropriately sized cuff (cuff size refers only to the inner inflatable bladder, not the cloth covering) (Table 1-1). A technique to establish an appropriate cuff size is to choose a cuff having a bladder width that is approximately 40% of the arm circumference midway between the olecranon and the acromion. This will usually be a cuff bladder that covers 80% to 100% of the circumference of the arm (Figure 1-5). Researchers have found that selection of a cuff with a bladder width equal to 40% of the upper arm circumference most accurately reflects directly measured radial arterial pressure.

Cuffs that are either too narrow or too wide affect the accuracy of blood pressure measurements. If the cuff size is too small, the reading on the device is falsely high. If the cuff size is too large, the reading is falsely low.

When another site is used, blood pressure measurements using noninvasive techniques may differ. Generally, systolic blood pressure in the lower extremities (thigh or calf) is higher than that in the upper extremities, and systolic blood pressure in the calf is higher than that in the thigh (see Figure 1-5).

| TABLE 1-1 | Recommended Dimensions for Blood Pressure Cuff Bladders | | |
|---|---|---|---|
| Age Range | Width (cm) | Length (cm) | Maximum Arm Circumference (cm)* |
| Newborn | 4 | 8 | 10 |
| Infant | 6 | 12 | 15 |
| Child | 9 | 18 | 22 |
| Small adult | 10 | 24 | 26 |
| Adult | 13 | 30 | 34 |
| Large adult | 16 | 38 | 44 |
| Thigh | 20 | 42 | 52 |

From National High Blood Pressure Education Program Working Group on High Blood Pressure in Children and Adolescents: The fourth report on the diagnosis, evaluation, and treatment of high blood pressure in children and adolescents, *Pediatrics* 114(2 Suppl 4th Report):555-576, 2004.
*Calculated so that the largest arm would still allow the bladder to encircle arm by at least 80%.

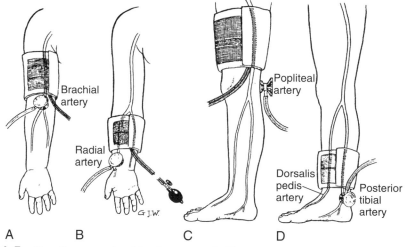

FIGURE **1-5**  Sites for measuring blood pressure. A, Upper arm. B, Lower arm or forearm. C, Thigh. D, Calf or ankle.

## Usual Findings

(For average respiratory rates at rest, see inside front cover.)

> **⚠ SAFETY ALERT**
> Published norms for blood pressure, such as those on the inside front cover, are valid only if the same method of measurement (auscultation and cuff size determination) is used in clinical practice.

> **⚠ SAFETY ALERT**
> When taking blood pressure, use an appropriately sized cuff. When the correct size is not available, use an oversized cuff rather than an undersized one, or use another site that more appropriately fits the cuff size. Do not choose a cuff based on the name of the cuff (e.g., an "infant" cuff may be too small for some infants).

## Comments

Repeat measurements above 95th percentile later during initial visit when child is least anxious; if a high reading persists, repeat measurements at least three times during subsequent visits to detect hypertension.

*Significant hypertension*—Blood pressure persistently between 95th and 99th percentile for age, gender, and height

*Severe hypertension*—Blood pressure persistently at or above 99th percentile for age, gender, and height

Refer children with consistently high blood pressure readings or significant differences in pressure between upper and lower extremities for further evaluation (e.g., in newborns, a calf pressure less than 6-9 mm Hg compared with upper arm pressure).*

Blood pressure readings using oscillometry are generally higher than those using auscultation but correlate better with direct radial artery blood pressure than auscultation readings.†

---

*Park M, Lee D: Normative arm and calf blood pressure values in the newborn, *Pediatrics* 83(2):240-243, 1989.
†Park M, Menard S: Accuracy of blood pressure measurement by the Dinamap monitor in infants and children, *Pediatrics* 79(6):907-914, 1987.

*Continued*

## Summary of Physical Assessment of the Child—cont'd

| Assessment | Procedure |
|---|---|
| **General Appearance** | |
| | Observe the following: |
| |     Facies |
| |     Posture |
| |     Body movement |
| |     Hygiene |
| |     Nutrition |
| |     Behavior |
| |     Development |
| |     State of awareness |
| *Skin* | |
| | Observe skin in natural daylight or neutral artificial light. |
| | *Color*—Most reliably assessed in sclera, conjunctiva, nail beds, tongue, buccal mucosa, palms, and soles |
| | *Texture*—Note moisture, smoothness, roughness, integrity of skin, and temperature. |
| | *Temperature*—Compare each part of body for even temperature. |
| | *Turgor*—Grasp skin on abdomen between thumb and index finger, pull taut, and release quickly. Indent skin with finger. |

| Usual Findings | Comments |
|---|---|
| Evaluated in terms of a comprehensive assessment; often gives clues to underlying problems such as poor hygiene and nutrition from parental neglect or poverty | Record actual observations that lead to a conclusion, such as signs of poor hygiene; give examples of present development milestones.<br>Follow up on clues that may indicate problems, for example, investigate feeding practices of family if child appears undernourished. |
| | Reveals significant clues to problems such as poor hygiene, child abuse, inadequate nutrition, and serious physical disorders. |
| Genetically determined:<br>  Light-skinned—From milky white to rosy colored<br>  Dark-skinned—Various shades of brown, red, yellow, olive, and bluish tones | Observe for abnormalities such as pallor, cyanosis, erythema, ecchymosis, petechiae, and jaundice (Table 1-2).<br>Factors affecting color include natural skin tone, melanin production, edema, hygiene, hemoglobin levels of blood, amount of lighting, color of room, atmospheric temperature, and use of cosmetics. |
| Smooth, slightly dry to touch, with even temperature | Note obvious changes, such as clammy skin, oily skin, obvious lesions, and excessive dryness (Boxes 1-2 and 1-3). |
| Usually same all over body, although exposed parts, such as hands, may be cooler<br>Resumes shape immediately with no tenting, wrinkling, or prolonged depression | Note obvious differences, such as warm upper extremities and cold lower extremities.<br>Good skin turgor indicates adequate hydration and possibly nutrition.<br>Note "tenting" or poor elasticity of the pulled skin (sign of dehydration and/or malnutrition) or obvious pitting of skin on indentation or signs of swelling (signs of edema). |

| TABLE 1-2 | Differences in Color Changes of Racial Groups | |
|---|---|---|
| **Color Change** | **Appearance in Light Skin** | **Appearance in Dark Skin** |
| Cyanosis | Bluish tinge, especially in palpebral conjunctiva (lower eyelid), nail beds, earlobes, lips, oral membranes, soles, and palms | Ashen gray lips and tongue |
| Pallor | Loss of rosy glow in skin, especially face | Ashen gray appearance in black skin<br>More yellowish brown color in brown skin |
| Erythema | Redness easily seen anywhere on body | Much more difficult to assess; palpate for warmth or edema |
| Ecchymoses | Purplish to yellow-green areas; may be seen anywhere on skin | Very difficult to see unless in mouth or conjunctiva |
| Petechiae | Purplish pinpoints most easily seen on buttocks, abdomen, and inner surfaces of the arms or legs | Usually invisible except in oral mucosa, conjunctiva of eyelids, and conjunctiva covering eyeball |
| Jaundice | Yellow staining seen in sclera of eyes, skin, fingernails, soles, palms, and oral mucosa | Most reliably assessed in sclera, hard palate, palms, and soles |

*Continued*

BOX **1-2** | Primary Skin Lesions

**Macule**—flat; nonpalpable; circumscribed; less than 1 cm in diameter; brown, red, purple, white, or tan in color
*Examples:* Freckles; flat moles; rubella; rubeola

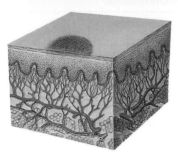

**Plaque**—elevated; flat topped; firm; rough; superficial papule greater than 1 cm in diameter; may be coalesced papules
*Examples:* Psoriasis; seborrheic and actinic keratoses

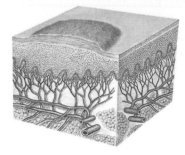

**Patch**—flat; nonpalpable; irregular in shape; macule that is greater than 1 cm in diameter
*Examples:* Vitiligo; port-wine marks

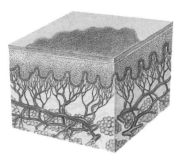

**Wheal**—elevated, irregularly shaped area of cutaneous edema; solid, transient, changing, variable diameter; pale pink with lighter center
*Examples:* Urticaria; insect bites

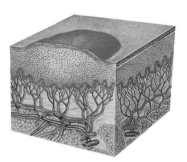

**Papule**—elevated; palpable; firm; circumscribed; less than 1 cm in diameter; brown, red, pink, tan, or bluish red in color
*Examples:* Warts; drug-related eruptions; pigmented nevi

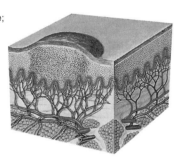

**Nodule**—elevated; firm; circumscribed; palpable; deeper in dermis than papule; 1 to 2 cm in diameter
*Examples:* Erythema nodosum; lipomas

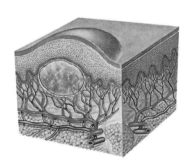

**Vesicle**—elevated; circumscribed; superficial; filled with serous fluid; less than 1 cm in diameter
*Examples:* Blister; varicella

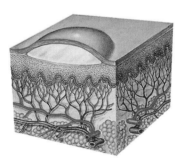

**Pustule**—elevated; superficial; similar to vesicle but filled with purulent fluid
*Examples:* Impetigo; acne; variola

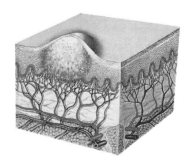

**Bulla**—vesicle greater than 1 cm in diameter
*Examples:* Blister; pemphigus vulgaris

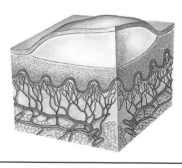

**Cyst**—elevated; circumscribed; palpable; encapsulated; filled with liquid or semisolid material
*Example:* Sebaceous cyst

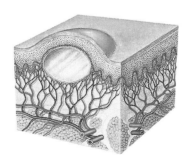

Illustrations from Seidel HM and others: *Mosby's guide to physical examination*, ed 7, St Louis, 2011, Mosby.

## BOX 1-3 | Secondary Skin Lesions

**Scale**—heaped-up keratinized cells; flaky exfoliation; irregular; thick or thin; dry or oily; varied size; silver, white, or tan in color
*Examples:* Psoriasis; exfoliative dermatitis

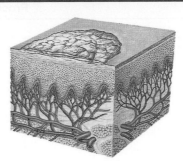

**Crust**—dried serum, blood, or purulent exudate; slightly elevated; size varies; brown, red, black, tan, or straw in color
*Examples:* Scab on abrasion; eczema

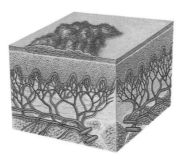

**Lichenification**—rough, thickened epidermis; accentuated skin markings caused by rubbing or irritation; often involves flexor aspect of extremity
*Example:* Chronic dermatitis

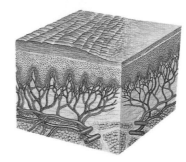

**Scar**—thin to thick fibrous tissue replacing injured dermis; irregular; pink, red, or white in color; may be atrophic or hypertrophic
*Example:* Healed wound or surgical incision

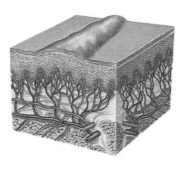

**Keloid**— irregularly shaped, elevated, progressively enlarging scar; grows beyond boundaries of wound; caused by excessive collagen formation during healing
*Example:* Keloid from ear piercing or burn scar

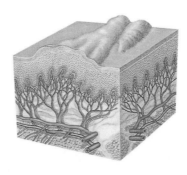

**Excoriation**—loss of epidermis; linear or hollowed-out crusted area; dermis exposed
*Examples:* Abrasion; scratch

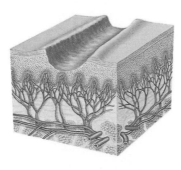

**Fissure**—linear crack or break from epidermis to dermis; small; deep; red
*Examples:* Athlete's foot; cheilosis

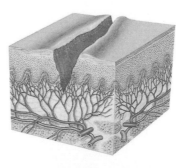

**Erosion**—loss of all or part of epidermis; depressed; moist; glistening; follows rupture of vesicle or bulla; larger than fissure
*Examples:* Varicella; variola following rupture

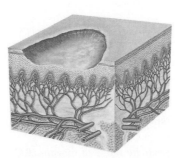

**Ulcer**—loss of epidermis and dermis; concave; varies in size; exudative; red or reddish blue
*Examples:* Decubiti; stasis ulcers

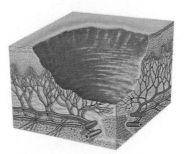

Illustrations from Seidel HM and others: *Mosby's guide to physical examination,* ed 7, St Louis, 2011, Mosby.

## Summary of Physical Assessment of the Child—cont'd

| Assessment | Procedure |
| --- | --- |
| **Accessory Structures** | |
| | *Hair*—Inspect color, texture, quality, distribution, elasticity, and hygiene. |
| | *Nails*—Inspect color, shape, texture, quality, distribution, elasticity, and hygiene. |
| | *Dermatoglyphics*—Observe flexion creases of palm. |
| **Lymph Nodes** | |
| See Figure 1-6. | Palpate using distal portion of fingers. |
| | Press gently but firmly in a circular motion. |
| | Note size, mobility, temperature, tenderness, and any change in enlarged nodes. |
| | *Submaxillary*—Tilt head slightly downward. |
| | *Cervical*—Tilt head slightly upward. |
| | *Axillary*—Have arms relaxed at side but slightly abducted. |
| | *Inguinal*—Place child supine. |
| **Head** | |
| | Note shape and symmetry. |
| | Note head control (especially in infants) and head posture. |
| | Evaluate range of motion (ROM). |
| | Palpate skull for fontanels, nodes, or obvious swellings. |

| Usual Findings | Comments |
|---|---|
| Lustrous, silky, strong, elastic hair | Signs of poor nutrition include stringy, friable, dull, dry, depigmented hair. |
| Genetic factors influence appearance; for example, an African-American child's hair is usually coarser, duller, and curlier. | Note areas of baldness, unusual hairiness, and any evidence of infestation. |
| | During puberty, secondary hair growth indicates normal pubertal changes. |
| Pink, convex, smooth, and flexible; not brittle | Note color changes, such as blueness or yellow tint. |
| In dark-skinned child, color is darker. | Observe for uncut or short, ragged nails (nail biting). |
| | Report any signs of clubbing (base of the nail becomes swollen and feels springy or floating when palpated), a sign of serious respiratory or cardiac dysfunction. |
| Three flexion creases | If pattern differs, draw a sketch to describe it. |
| | Observe for transpalmar crease (one horizontal crease), a characteristic of children with Down syndrome. |

| | |
|---|---|
| Generally not palpable, although small, nontender, movable nodes are normal. | Note tender, enlarged, warm nodes, which usually indicate infection or inflammation proximal to their location. |

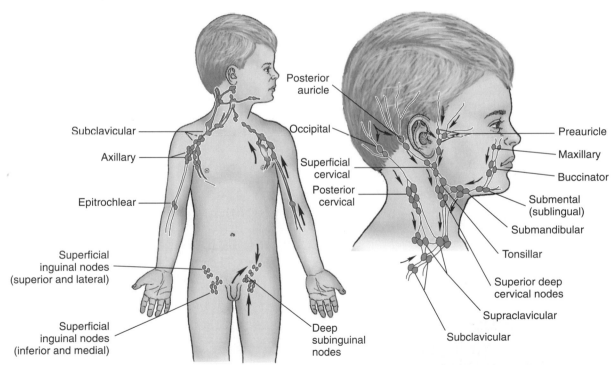

FIGURE **1-6**   Locations of superficial lymph nodes. Arrows indicate directional flow of lymph.

| | |
|---|---|
| Even molding of head, occipital prominence | Report any deviations from expected findings. |
| | Clues to problems include the following: |
| Symmetric facial features | *Uneven molding*—Premature closure of sutures |
| Head control well established by 6 months of age | *Asymmetry*—Paralysis |
| Head in midline | *Head lag*—Retarded motor or mental development |
| Moves head up, down, and from side to side | *Head tilt*—Poor vision |
| Smooth, fused except for fontanels (see p. 20) | *Limited ROM*—Torticollis (wryneck) |
|    Posterior fontanel closes by 2 months | *Resistance to movement and pain*—Meningeal irritation |
|    Anterior fontanel closes by 12-18 months | |

*Continued*

## Summary of Physical Assessment of the Child—cont'd

| Assessment | Procedure |
|---|---|
| **Head—cont'd** | |
| | Transilluminate skull in darkened room; firmly place rubber-collared flashlight against skull at various points. |
| | Examine scalp for hygiene, lesions, infestation, signs of trauma, loss of hair, and discoloration. |
| | Percuss frontal sinuses in children older than 7 years. |
| **Neck** | |
| | Inspect size. |
| | *Trachea*—Palpate for deviation; place thumb and index finger on each side, and slide fingers back and forth. |
| | *Thyroid*—Palpate, noting size, shape, symmetry, tenderness, nodules; place pads of index and middle fingers below cricoid cartilage; feel for isthmus (tissue connecting lobes) rising during swallowing; feel each lobe laterally and posteriorly. |
| | *Carotid arteries*—Palpate on both sides. |
| **Eyes** | |

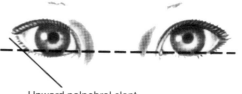

Upward palpebral slant

FIGURE **1-7**   Upward palpebral slant.

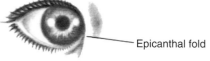

Epicanthal fold

FIGURE **1-8**   Epicanthal fold.

Inspect placement and alignment.
If abnormality is suspected, measure inner canthal distance.
*Palpebral slant*—Draw imaginary line through two points of medial (inner) canthi (Figure 1-7).

*Epicanthal fold*—Observe for excess fold from roof of nose to inner termination of eyebrow (Figure 1-8).
*Lids*—Observe placement, movement, and color (Figure 1-9).

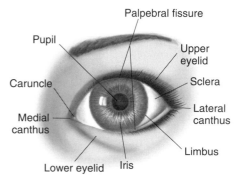

Palpebral fissure
Pupil
Upper eyelid
Caruncle
Sclera
Medial canthus
Lateral canthus
Limbus
Lower eyelid    Iris

FIGURE **1-9**   External structures of the eye.

Palpebral conjunctiva
Pull lower lid down while child looks up.
Evert upper lid by holding lashes and pulling down and forward.
Observe color.
Bulbar conjunctiva—Observe color.

Lacrimal punctum—Observe color.

*Eyelashes and eyebrows*—Observe distribution and direction of growth.
*Sclera*—Observe color (see Figure 1-9).
*Cornea*—Check for opacities by shining light toward eye.

| Usual Findings | Comments |
|---|---|
| Absence of halo around rubber collar | *Halo of light through skull*—Loss of cortex (hydrocephaly) |
| Clean, pink (more deeply pigmented in dark-skinned children) | *Ecchymotic areas on scalp*—Trauma (possibly abuse) |
| | *Loss of hair*—Trauma (hair pulling), lack of stimulation (lying in same position) |
| | *Painful sinuses*—Infection |
| During infancy, normally short with skinfolds | Note any webbing. |
| During early childhood, lengthens | Note any deviation, masses, or nodules when palpating neck structures. |
| In midline; rises with swallowing | |
| In midline; rises with swallowing; lobes equal but often are not palpable | Thyroid is often difficult to palpate. |
| | Inquire if child ever received radiation therapy to neck or upper chest area. |
| Equal bilaterally | Note unequal pulses and protruding neck veins. |
| Placement is symmetric. | Note asymmetry, abnormal spacing (hypertelorism). |
| Inner canthal distance averages 3 cm (1.2 inches). | |
| Usually palpebral fissures lie horizontally on imaginary line; in Asians, there may be an upward slant. | Presence of upward slant and epicanthal folds in children who are not Asian is significant finding in Down syndrome. |
| Often present in Asian children | May give false impression of strabismus |
| When eye is open, falls between upper iris and pupil | Observe for deviations: |
| When eye is closed, sclera, cornea, and palpebral conjunctiva are completely covered. |    Ptosis (upper lid covers part of pupil or lower iris) |
| |    Setting sun sign (upper lid above iris) |
| Symmetric blink |    Inability to completely close eye |
| Color is same as surrounding skin. |    Entropion (turning in) |
| |    Asymmetric, excessive, or infrequent blinking |
| |    Signs of inflammation along lid margin or on lid |
| Pink and glossy | Note any signs of inflammation. |
| Vertical yellow striations along edge near hair follicle | Excessive pallor may indicate anemia. |
| Transparent and white color of underlying sclera | A reddened conjunctiva may indicate eye strain, fatigue, infection, or irritation such as from excessive rubbing or exposure to environmental irritants. |
| Same color as lid | Excessive discharge, tearing, pain, redness, or swelling indicates dacryocystitis. |
| Eyelashes curl away from eye. | Note inward growth of lashes and unusual hairiness of brows. |
| Eyebrows are above eye; do not meet in midline. | |
| White | Note any yellow staining, which may indicate jaundice. |
| Tiny black marks normal in deeply pigmented children | Note any opacities or ulcerations. |
| Transparent | |

*Continued*

## Summary of Physical Assessment of the Child—cont'd

| Assessment | Procedure |
|---|---|
| Eyes—cont'd | |

*Pupils* (see Figure 1-9)

Compare size, shape, and movement.

Test reaction to light; shine light source toward and away from eye.

Test accommodation; have child focus on object from distance, and bring object close to face.

*Iris*—Observe shape, color, size, and clarity (see Figure 1-9).

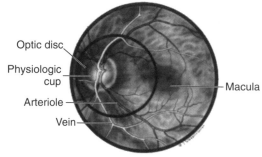

Optic disc
Physiologic cup
Arteriole
Vein
Macula

FIGURE **1-10**  Structures of the fundus. Interior circle represents approximate size of area seen with ophthalmoscope.

*Lens*—Inspect.

*Fundus* (Figure 1-10)

Examine with ophthalmoscope set at 0; approach child from a 15-degree angle; change to plus or minus diopters to produce clear focus.

Measure structures in relationship to disc's diameter (DD).

To facilitate locating macula, have child momentarily look *directly* at light.

Assess vision (for visual acuity, see pp. 127-130).

Use following tests for binocular vision:

*Corneal light reflex test* (also called *red reflex gemini* or *Hirschberg test*)—Shine light directly into the eyes from a distance of about 40.5 cm (16 inches).

*Cover test*—Have child fixate on near (33 cm [13 inches]) or distant (50 cm [20 inches]) object; cover one eye, and observe movement of the uncovered eye.

*Alternate cover test*—Same as cover test, except rapidly cover one eye then the other eye several times; observe movement of covered eye when it is uncovered.

*Peripheral vision*—Have child look straight ahead; move an object, such as your finger, from beyond child's field of vision into view; ask child to signal as soon as the object is seen; estimate the angle from straight line of vision to first detection of peripheral vision.

*Color vision*—Use Ishihara or Hardy-Rand-Rittler test.

| Usual Findings | Comments |
| --- | --- |
| Round, clear, and equal<br>Pupils constrict when light approaches, dilate when light fades.<br>Pupils constrict as object is brought near face. | *PERRLA* is common notation for pupils equal, round, react to light, and accommodation.<br>Note any asymmetry in size and movement. |
| Round, equal, clear<br>Color varies from shades of brown, green, or blue. | Note asymmetry in size, lack of clarity, coloboma (cleft at limbus [junction of iris and sclera]), absence of color (a pinkish glow is seen in albinism), or black- and-white speckling (Brushfield spots are commonly found in Down syndrome). |
| Should not be seen<br>*Red reflex*—Brilliant, uniform reflection of red; appears darker color in deeply pigmented children, lighter in infants<br>*Optic disc*—Creamy pink but lighter than surrounding fundus; round or vertically oval<br>*Physiologic cup*—Small, pale depression in center of disc<br>*Blood vessels*—Emanate from disc; veins are darker and about one fourth larger than arteries; narrow band of light, the arteriolar light reflex, is reflected from center of arteries, not veins; branches cross each other; may see obvious pulsations<br>*Macula*—1 DD in size, darker in color than disc or surrounding fundus, located 2 DD temporal to the disc<br>*Fovea centralis*—Minute, glistening spot of reflected light in center of macula | Note any opacities.<br>Visualization of red reflex virtually rules out most serious defects of cornea, lens, and aqueous and vitreous chambers.<br>Observe for abnormalities:<br>  Partial red or white reflex<br>  Blurring of disc margins<br>  Bulging of disc<br>  Loss of depression<br>  Dilated blood vessels<br>  Tortuous vessels<br>  Hemorrhages<br>  Absence of pulsations<br>  Notching or indenting at crossing of vessels |
| Binocularity is well established by 3-4 months of age. | Refer any child with nonbinocular vision because of malalignment (strabismus) for further evaluation. |
| Light falls symmetrically within each pupil. | Abnormal if light falls asymmetrically in each pupil |
| Uncovered eye does not move. | Abnormal if uncovered eye moves when other eye is covered |
| Neither eye moves when covered or uncovered. | Abnormal if covered eye moves as soon as occluder is removed |
| In each quadrant, sees object at 50 degrees upward, 70 degrees downward, 60 degrees nasalward, and 90 degrees temporally | Inability to see object until it is brought closer to straight line of vision indicates need for further evaluation |
| Able to see a letter or figure within the colored dots | Each test consists of cards on which a color field composed of spots of a certain "confusion" color is printed; against the field is a number (Ishihara) or symbol (Hardy-Rand-Rittler) similarly printed in dots but of a color likely to be confused with the field color by the person with a color vision deficit.<br>Counsel the affected child and parents about the practical inconveniences caused by the disorder, the mode of genetic transmission, and its irreversibility. |

*Continued*

## Summary of Physical Assessment of the Child—cont'd

| Assessment | Procedure |
|---|---|

**Ears**

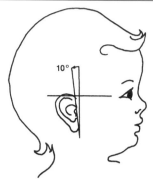

FIGURE **1-11** Placement and alignment of pinna.

*Pinnae*—Inspect placement and alignment (Figure 1-11).

1. Measure height of pinna by drawing an imaginary line from outer orbit of eye to occiput of skull.
2. Measure angle of pinna by drawing a perpendicular line from the imaginary horizontal line and aligning pinna next to this mark.

Observe the usual landmarks of the pinna.

Note presence of any abnormal openings, tags of skin, or sinuses.

Inspect hygiene (odor, discharge, color).

---

### ATRAUMATIC CARE

#### Reducing Distress from Otoscopy in Young Children

Make examining the ear a game by explaining that you are looking for a "big elephant" in the ear. This kind of fairy tale is an absorbing distraction and usually elicits cooperation. After the ear has been examined, clarify that "looking for elephants" was only pretending and thank the child for letting you look in his or her ear. Another great distraction technique is asking the child to put a finger on the opposite ear to keep the light from getting out.

### ! SAFETY ALERT

Sometimes it takes an extra hand to examine a child's ear—one hand to hold the otoscope, a second hand to use the bulb (or a curette), and a third hand to straighten the canal. To gain a third hand, enlist a cooperative child's help. Have the child raise the arm opposite the affected ear up and over the head toward the opposite side. Then ask the child to grasp the upper edge of the earlobe at about the 10 or 1 o'clock position and pull the lobe gently up and back.

Examine external canal and middle ear structures with otoscope (Atraumatic Care box and Safety Alert):

*Child younger than 3 years*

Position prone with ear to be examined toward ceiling; lean over child, using upper portion of body to restrain arms and trunk and examining hand to restrain the head.

*Alternate position:* Seat child sideways in parent's lap; have parent hug child securely around trunk and arms and top of head.

Introduce speculum between 3 o'clock and 9 o'clock position in a *downward* and *forward* slant.

Pull pinna *down* and *back* to the 6 o'clock to 9 o'clock range (Figure 1-12, A).

*Child over 3 years*

Examine while seated with head tilted slightly away from examiner (if child needs restraining, use one of the previously mentioned positions).

Pull pinna *up* and *back* toward a 10 o'clock position (see Figure 1-12, B).

Insert speculum $\frac{1}{4}$ to $\frac{1}{2}$ inch; use widest speculum that diameter of canal easily accommodates.

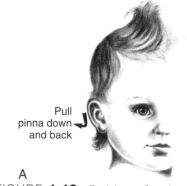

Pull pinna down and back

Pull pinna up and back

A          B

FIGURE **1-12** Positions of eardrum. A, Infant. B, Child over 3 years of age.

| Usual Findings | Comments |
|---|---|
| Slightly crosses or meets this line | Low-set ears are commonly associated with renal anomalies or mental retardation. |
| Lies within a 10-degree angle of the vertical line | |
| Extends slightly forward from the skull | Flattened ears may indicate infrequent change of positioning from a side-lying placement; masses or swelling may make the pinna protrude. |
| Prominences and depressions symmetric | Abnormal landmarks are often signs of possible middle ear anomalies. |
| Adherent lobule (normal variation) | If abnormal opening is present, note any discharge. |
| Soft, yellow cerumen | If ear needs cleaning, discuss hygiene with parent or child. |
| | If ear is free of wax, ascertain the method of cleaning; advise against the use of cotton-tipped applicators or sharp or pointed objects in the canal. |
| *External canal*—Pink (more deeply colored in dark-skinned child); outermost portion lined with minute hairs, some soft yellow cerumen | Note signs of irritation; infection; foreign bodies; and desiccated, packed wax (may interfere with hearing). |
| | If discharge is present, change speculum to examine other ear. |
| Tympanic membrane (Figure 1-13) | Note the following: |
| Translucent, light pearly pink or gray color | Red, tense, bulging drum |
| Slight redness seen normally in infants and children as a result of crying | Dull, transparent gray color |
| | Black areas |
| *Light reflex*—Cone-shaped reflection, normally points away from face at 5 o'clock or 7 o'clock position | Absence of light reflex or bony prominences |
| Bony landmarks present | Retraction of drum with abnormal prominence of landmarks |

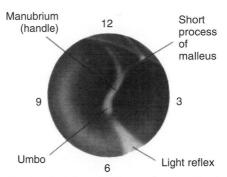

FIGURE **1-13**  Landmarks of tympanic membrane with clock superimposed.

*Continued*

## Summary of Physical Assessment of the Child—cont'd

| Assessment | Procedure |
|---|---|

### Ears—cont'd

Assess hearing (see also pp. 130-132).

*Rinne test*—Place vibrating stem and tuning fork against mastoid bone until child no longer hears sound; move prongs close to auditory meatus.

*Weber test*—Hold tuning fork in midline of head or forehead.

### Nose

See Figure 1-14.

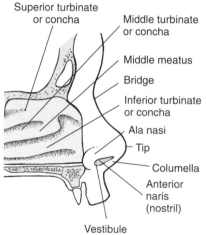

Superior turbinate or concha
Middle turbinate or concha
Middle meatus
Bridge
Inferior turbinate or concha
Ala nasi
Tip
Columella
Anterior naris (nostril)
Vestibule

FIGURE **1-14**  External landmarks and internal structures of the nose.

Inspect size, placement, and alignment; draw imaginary vertical line from center point between eyes to notch of upper lip.

*Anterior vestibule*—Tilt head backward; push tip of nose up, and illuminate cavity with flashlight; to detect perforated septum, shine light into one naris and observe for admittance of light through perforation.

### Mouth and Throat

*Lips*—Note color, texture, and any obvious lesions.

Internal structures (Figure 1-15)

Ask cooperative child to open mouth wide and say "Ahh"; usually not necessary to use tongue blade (Atraumatic Care box).

With young child, place supine with both arms extended along side of head; have parent maintain arm position to immobilize head; may be necessary to use a tongue blade, but avoid eliciting gag reflex by depressing only toward the side of the tongue; use flashlight for good illumination.

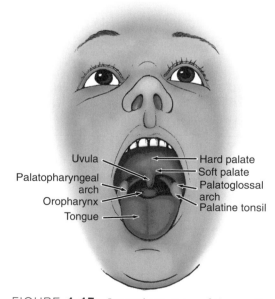

Uvula
Palatopharyngeal arch
Oropharynx
Tongue
Hard palate
Soft palate
Palatoglossal arch
Palatine tonsil

FIGURE **1-15**  Internal structures of the mouth.

**ATRAUMATIC CARE**

**Encouraging Opening the Mouth for Examination**

Perform the examination in front of a mirror.

Let child first examine someone else's mouth, such as the parent, the nurse, or a puppet; then examine child's mouth.

Instruct child to tilt the head back slightly, breathe deeply through the mouth, and hold the breath; this action lowers the tongue to the floor of the mouth without using a tongue blade.

| Usual Findings | Comments |
|---|---|
| Hears sound when prongs are brought close to ear | Rinne and Weber tests distinguish between bone and air conduction; both tests require cooperation and are better suited to children of school age or older. |
| Hears sound equally in both ears | Note abnormal results: <br> *Rinne positive*—Sound is not audible through ear. <br> *Weber positive*—Sound is heard better in affected ear. |
| Both nostrils equal in size <br> Bridge of nose flattened in African-American or Asian children <br> Mucosal lining—Redder than oral membranes; moist, but no discharge | Note any deviation to one side, inequality in size of nostrils, or flaring of alae nasi (sign of respiratory distress). <br><br> Note the following: <br> Abnormally pale, grayish pink, swollen, and boggy membranes <br> Red, swollen membranes <br> Any discharge |
| Turbinate and meatus—Same color as mucosal lining <br><br> Septum—In midline | Foreign object in nose <br> Deviated septum <br> Perforated septum |
| More deeply pigmented than surrounding skin; smooth, moist | Note cyanosis, pallor, lesions, or cracks, especially at corners. |
| *Mucous membranes*—Bright pink, glistening, smooth, uniform, and moist | Note lesions, bleeding, sensitivity, or odor. |
| *Gingiva*—Firm, coral pink, and stippled; margins are "knife-edged" | Note redness, puffiness (especially at margin), or tendency to bleed. |
| *Teeth*—Number appropriate for age, white, good occlusion of upper and lower jaws <br> General rule for estimating number of teeth in children: <br> Under 2 years: Age (in months) minus 6 (e.g., 12 months minus 6 = 6 teeth) | Note loss of teeth, delayed eruption, malocclusion, or obvious discoloration. <br> Compare dental findings with parental report of dental hygiene. <br> ⊜ Assess need for further dental counseling: <br> Eating habits, such as bottle-feeding or prolonged breast-feeding during day for use as "pacifier" or at bedtime, excessive sugar <br> Toothbrushing <br> Sources of fluoride, need for supplementation <br> Periodic, regular examinations by dentist |
| Tongue—Rough texture, freely movable, tip extends to lips, no lesions or masses under tongue | Note smoothness, fissuring, coating on the tongue, excessive redness, swelling, or inability to move the tongue forward to lips; can interfere with speech. |
| Palate—Intact, slightly arched | Note presence of any clefts. |
| Uvula—Protrudes from back of soft palate, moves upward during gag reflex | Note if a bifid (divided in midline) uvula is present. |

*Continued*

Patient and Family Education, Spanish Translations—Caring for Your Child's Teeth

## Summary of Physical Assessment of the Child—cont'd

| Assessment | Procedure |
| --- | --- |

**Mouth and Throat—cont'd**

**Chest**

See Figure 1-16.

Inspect size, shape, symmetry, and movement.

Describe findings according to geographic and imaginary landmarks (Figure 1-17).

Locate intercostal space (ICS), the space directly below rib, by palpating chest inferiorly from second rib.

Other landmarks:

   Nipples usually at fourth ICS

   Tip of eleventh rib felt laterally

   Tip of twelfth rib felt posteriorly

   Tip of scapula at eighth rib or ICS

Inspect breast development.

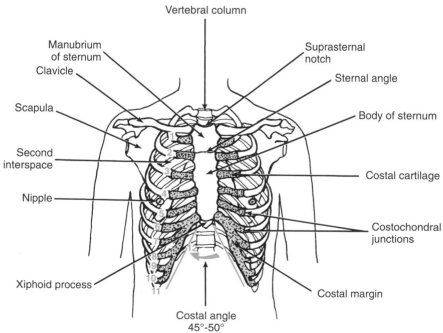

FIGURE **1-16**   Structures of the rib cage.

| Usual Findings | Comments |
| --- | --- |
| Palatine tonsils—Same color as surrounding mucosa, glandular rather than smooth, may be large in prepubertal children | Note exudate and enlargement that could become obstructive. |
| Posterior pharynx—Same color as surrounding mucosa, smooth, moist | Assess for signs of infection (erythema, edema, white lesions, or exudate). |
| In infants, shape is almost circular; with growth, lateral diameter increases in proportion to anteroposterior diameter. | Measurement of chest and palpation of axillary nodes may be done here. |
| Both sides of chest symmetric | Note deviations: |
| Points of attachment between ribs and costal cartilage smooth |   Barrel-shaped chest |
| |   Asymmetry |
| Movement—During inspiration, chest expands, costal angle increases, and diaphragm descends; during expiration, reverse occurs. |   Wide or narrow costal angle<br>  Bony prominences<br>  ***Pectus carinatum (pigeon breast)***—Sternum protrudes outward. |
| Nipples—Darker pigmentation, located slightly lateral to mid-clavicular line between fourth and fifth ribs |   ***Pectus excavatum (funnel chest)***—Lower portion of sternum is depressed.<br>  Retractions (Figure 1-18)<br>  Asymmetric or decreased movement |
| Breast development depends on age; no masses. | Compare breast development with expected stage for age (see p. 118).<br>Discuss importance of monthly breast self-examination with female adolescents. |

## Summary of Physical Assessment of the Child—cont'd

| Assessment | Procedure |
|---|---|

### Chest—cont'd

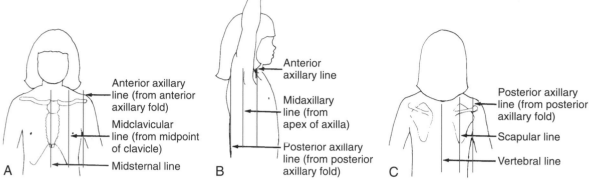

FIGURE **1-17** Imaginary landmarks of the chest. A, Anterior. B, Right lateral. C, Posterior.

### Lungs

See Figure 1-19.

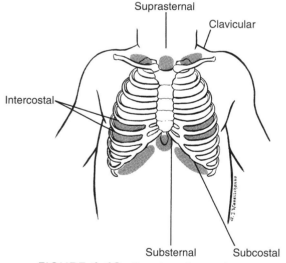

FIGURE **1-18** Location of retractions.

Evaluate respiratory movements for rate, rhythm, depth, quality, and character. (See Atraumatic Care box below)

With child sitting, place each hand flat against back or chest with thumbs in midline along lower costal margins.
*Vocal fremitus*—Palpate as above, and have child say "99," "eee."

Percuss each side of chest in sequence from apex to base (Figure 1-20):
   For anterior aspects of lungs, child sitting or supine
   For posterior aspects of lungs, child sitting

Auscultate breath and voice sounds for intensity, pitch, quality, and relative duration of inspiration and expiration.

---

**👫 ATRAUMATIC CARE**

**Encouraging Deep Breaths**

Ask child to "blow out" the light on an otoscope or pocket flashlight; discreetly turn off the light on the last try so that the child feels successful.

Place a cotton ball in child's palm; ask child to blow the ball into the air and have parent catch it.

Place a small tissue on the top of a pencil and ask child to blow the tissue off.

Have child blow a pinwheel, a party horn, or bubbles.

| Usual Findings | Comments |
|---|---|

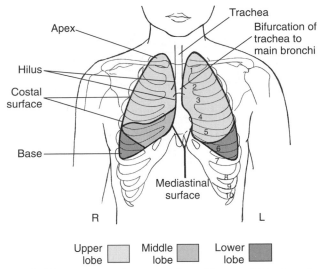

FIGURE **1-19** Location of anterior lobes of lungs within thoracic cavity.

| Usual Findings | Comments |
|---|---|
| Rate expected for age (see inside front cover); regular, effortless, and quiet | Note abnormal rate; irregular rhythm; shallow depth; difficult breathing; or noisy, grunting respirations (Box 1-4). |
| Moves symmetrically with each breath; posterior base descends 5-6 cm (2-2.3 inches) during deep inspiration | |
| Vibrations are symmetric and most intense in thoracic area and least intense at base. | Note asymmetric vibrations or sudden absence or decrease in intensity. Note abnormal vibrations, such as pleural friction rub or crepitation. Note deviation from expected sounds. |
| Lobes are resonant except for (see Figure 1-20): Dullness at fifth interspace right midclavicular line (liver) Dullness from second to fifth interspace over left sternal border to midclavicular line (heart) Tympany below left fifth interspace (stomach) | |
| *Vesicular breath sounds*—Heard over entire surface of lungs except upper intrascapular area and beneath manubrium; inspiration louder, longer, and of higher pitch than expiration | Note deviations from expected breath sounds, particularly if diminished; note absence of sounds. Note adventitious sounds. |

---

### BOX **1-4** | Various Patterns of Respiration

**Tachypnea**—Increased rate
**Bradypnea**—Decreased rate
**Dyspnea**—Distress during breathing
**Apnea**—Cessation of breathing
**Hyperpnea**—Increased depth
**Hypoventilation**—Decreased depth (shallow) and irregular rhythm
**Hyperventilation**—Increased rate and depth
**Kussmaul breathing**—Hyperventilation, gasping, and labored respiration, usually seen in respiratory acidosis (e.g., diabetic coma)

**Cheyne-Stokes respiration**—Gradually increasing rate and depth with periods of apnea
**Biot breathing**—Periods of hyperpnea alternating (similar to Cheyne-Stokes except that the depth remains constant)
**Seesaw (paradoxic) respirations**—Chest falls on inspiration and rises on expiration
**Agonal breathing**—Last gasping breaths before death

*Continued*

## Summary of Physical Assessment of the Child—cont'd

| Assessment | Procedure |
| --- | --- |

### Lungs—cont'd

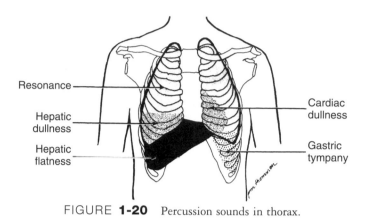

FIGURE **1-20**   Percussion sounds in thorax.

### Heart

See Figure 1-21.

*General Instructions*

Begin with inspection, followed by palpation, then auscultation.

Percussion is not done because it is of limited value in defining the borders or the size of the heart.

Palpate to determine the location of the apical impulse, the most lateral cardiac impulse that may correspond to the apex.

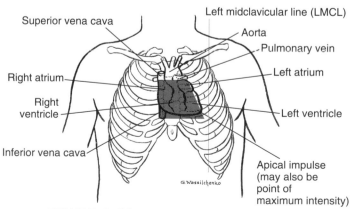

FIGURE **1-21**   Position of heart within thorax.

| Usual Findings | Comments |
|---|---|
| Bronchovesicular breath sounds—Heard in upper intrascapular area and manubrium; inspiration and expiration almost equal in duration, pitch, and intensity | *Crackles*—Discrete, noncontinuous crackling sound, heard primarily during inspiration from passage of air through fluid or moisture; if crackles clear with deep breathing, they are not pathologic |
| Bronchial breath sounds—Heard only over trachea near suprasternal notch; expiration longer, louder, and of higher pitch than inspiration | *Wheezes*—Continuous musical sounds; caused by air passing through narrowed passages, regardless of cause (e.g., exudate, inflammation, foreign body, spasm, tumor) |
| | *Audible inspiratory wheeze (stridor)*—Sonorous, musical wheeze heard without a stethoscope; indicates a high obstruction (e.g., epiglottitis) |
| | *Audible expiratory wheeze*—Whistling, sighing wheeze heard without a stethoscope; indicates a low obstruction |
| | *Pleural friction rub*—Crackling, grating sound during inspiration and expiration; occurs from inflamed pleural surfaces; not affected by coughing |
| Voice sounds—Heard, but syllables are indistinct | Consolidation of lung tissue produces three types of abnormal voice sounds: |
| | *Whispered pectoriloquy*—The child whispers words, and the nurse hears the syllables. |
| | *Bronchophony*—The child speaks words that are not distinguishable, but the vocal resonance is increased in intensity and clarity. |
| | *Egophony*—The child says "ee," which is heard as the nasal sound "ay" through the stethoscope. |
| Symmetric chest wall apical impulse sometimes apparent (in thin children) | Note obvious bulging. Infant's heart is larger in proportion to chest size and lies more centrally. |
| Just lateral to the left MCL and fourth ICS in children >7 years of age | Although the apical impulse gives a general idea of the size of the heart (with enlargement, the apex is lower and more lateral), its normal location is quite variable, making it a rather unreliable indicator of heart size; **point of maximum intensity (PMI)**, area of most intense pulsation, usually is located at same site as apical impulse but it can occur elsewhere. For this reason, the two terms should not be used synonymously. |
| At the left MCL and fifth ICS in children >7 years of age | |
| | During palpation, may feel abnormal vibrations called **thrills** that are similar to cat's purring; they are produced by blood flowing through narrowed or abnormal opening, such as stenotic valve or septal defect. |
| Capillary refilling in 1-2 seconds | Refilling taking longer than 2 seconds is abnormal and indicates impaired skin perfusion; cool temperature prolongs capillary refill time. |

*Continued*

## Summary of Physical Assessment of the Child—cont'd

| Assessment | Procedure |
|---|---|

**Heart—cont'd**

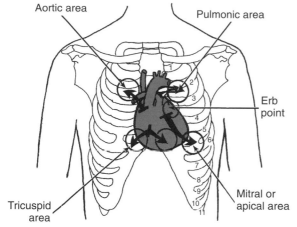

FIGURE **1-22** Directions of heart sounds from anatomic valve sites.

Palpate skin for capillary filling time:
  Lightly press skin on central site, such as forehead, and peripheral site, such as top of hand or foot, to produce slight blanching.
  Assess time it takes for blanched area to return to original color.
Auscultate for heart sounds:
  Listen with child in sitting and reclining positions.
  Use both diaphragm and bell chest pieces.
  Evaluate sounds for quality, intensity, rate, and rhythm (Box 1-5).
Follow sequence (Figure 1-22):
*Aortic area*—Second right intercostal space close to sternum
*Pulmonic area*—Second left intercostal space close to sternum
*Erb point*—Second and third left intercostal spaces close to sternum
*Tricuspid area*—Fifth right and left intercostal spaces close to sternum
*Mitral or apical area*—Fifth intercostal space, left midclavicular line (third to fourth intercostal space and lateral to left midclavicular line [MCL] in infants)

---

### BOX 1-5 | Various Patterns of Heart Rate or Pulse

**Tachycardia**—Increased rate
**Bradycardia**—Decreased rate
**Pulsus alternans**—Strong beat followed by weak beat
**Pulsus bigeminus**—Coupled rhythm in which beat is felt in pairs because of premature beat
**Pulsus paradoxus**—Intensity or force of pulse decreases with inspiration

**Sinus arrhythmia**—Rate increases with inspiration, decreases with expiration
**Water-hammer or Corrigan's pulse**—Especially forceful beat caused by a very wide pulse pressure (systolic blood pressure minus diastolic blood pressure)
**Dicrotic pulse**—Double radial pulse for every apical beat
**Thready pulse**—Rapid, weak pulse that seems to appear and disappear

---

**Abdomen**

*General Instructions*
Inspection is followed by auscultation, percussion, and palpation, which may distort the normal abdominal sounds.
Palpation may be uncomfortable for the child; deep palpation causes a feeling of pressure, and superficial palpation causes a tickling sensation.
To minimize any discomfort and encourage cooperation, use the following:
Position child supine with legs flexed at hips and knees.
Distract child with statements such as "I am going to guess what you ate by feeling your tummy."
Have child "help" with palpation by placing own hand over examiner's palpating hand.
Have child place own hand on abdomen with fingers spread wide apart and palpate between the fingers.

| Usual Findings | Comments |
|---|---|
| $S_1$-$S_2$—Clear, distinct, rate equal to radial pulse; rhythm regular and even | To distinguish $S_1$ from $S_2$, palpate for carotid pulse, which is synchronous with $S_1$. |
| Aortic area—$S_2$ louder than $S_1$ | A normal arrhythmia is **sinus arrhythmia**, in which heart rate increases with inspiration and decreases with expiration. |
| Pulmonic area—Splitting of $S_2$ heard best (normally widens on inspiration) | Identify abnormal sounds; note presence of adventitious sounds such as pericardial friction rubs (similar to pleural friction rubs but not affected by change in respiration). |
| Erb point—Frequent site of innocent murmurs | Record murmurs in relation to the following: |
| Tricuspid area—$S_1$ louder sound preceding $S_2$ | Area best heard |
| Mitral or apical area—$S_1$ heard loudest; splitting of $S_1$ may be audible | Timing within $S_1$-$S_2$ cycle |
| Quality—Clear and distinct | Change with position |
| Intensity—Strong, but not pounding | Loudness and quality |
| Rate—Same as radial pulse | |
| Rhythm—Regular and even | |

Usual findings of innocent murmurs:

Timing within *S1-S2 cycle*—Systolic, that is, they occur with or after S1

Quality—Usually of a low-pitched, musical, or groaning quality

Loudness—Grade III or less in intensity and do not increase over time

Area best heard—Usually loudest in the pulmonic area with no transmission to other areas of the heart

Change with position—Audible in the supine position but absent in the sitting position

Other physical signs—Not associated with any physical signs of cardiac disease

Grading of the intensity of heart murmurs:

I—Very faint, frequently not heard if child sits up

II—Usually readily heard, slightly louder than grade I, audible in all positions

III—Loud but not accompanied by a thrill

IV—Loud, accompanied by a thrill

V—Loud enough to be heard with the stethoscope barely on the chest, accompanied by a thrill

VI—Loud enough to be heard with the stethoscope not touching the chest, often heard with the human ear close to the chest, accompanied by a thrill

*Continued*

## Summary of Physical Assessment of the Child—cont'd

| Assessment | Procedure |
| --- | --- |
| Abdomen—cont'd | |

Inspect contour, size, and tone

Note condition of skin.
Note movement.

Inspect umbilicus for herniation, fistulas, hygiene, and discharge.

Observe for hernias (Figure 1-23):
*Inguinal*—Slide little finger into external inguinal ring at base of scrotum; ask child to cough.
*Femoral*—Place finger over femoral canal (located by placing index finger over femoral pulse and middle finger against skin toward midline).
Auscultate for bowel sounds and aortic pulsations.

Percuss the abdomen.

Palpate abdominal organs (Figure 1-24):
Place one hand flat against back, and use palpating hand to "feel" organs between both hands.
Proceed from lower quadrants *upward* to avoid missing edge of enlarged organ.

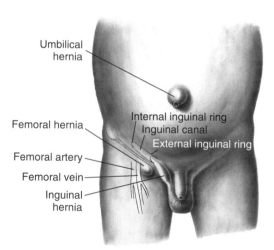

Umbilical hernia
Internal inguinal ring
Inguinal canal
External inguinal ring
Femoral hernia
Femoral artery
Femoral vein
Inguinal hernia

FIGURE **1-23**  Locations of hernias.

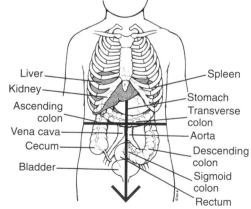

Liver
Kidney
Ascending colon
Vena cava
Cecum
Bladder
Spleen
Stomach
Transverse colon
Aorta
Descending colon
Sigmoid colon
Rectum

FIGURE **1-24**  Locations of structures in abdomen.

1 - ASSESSMENT

| Usual Findings | Comments |
|---|---|
| *Infants and young children*—Cylindric and prominent in erect position, flat when supine | Contour, size, and tone are good indicators of nutritional status and muscular development.Note deviations: |
| *Adolescents*—Characteristic adult curves, fairly flat when erect |   Prominent, flabby |
| Circumference decreases in relation to chest size with age. |   Distention |
| Firm tone; muscular in adolescent males |   Concave |
| |   Tense, boardlike |
| |   Loose, wrinkled |
| |   Midline protrusion |
| |   Silvery, whitish striae |
| |   Distended veins |
| Smooth, uniformly taut | |
| In children under 7 or 8 years, rises with inspiration and synchronous with chest movement | Paradoxic respirations (chest rises while abdomen falls) |
| In older children, less respiratory movement | Visible peristaltic waves |
| In thin children, visible pulsations from descending aorta sometimes seen in epigastric region | |
| Flat to slight protrusion; no herniation or discharge | If herniation is present, palpate for abdominal contents. |
| | Discuss with parents any home remedies used to reduce the herniation, especially umbilical hernias (e.g., belly binders, taping umbilicus flat). |
| None | |
| *Bowel sounds*—Short, metallic, tinkling sounds like gurgles, clicks, or growls heard every 10-30 seconds | Bowel sounds may be stimulated by stroking abdominal wall with a fingertip. |
| *Aortic pulsations*—Heard in epigastrium, slightly left of midline | Note hyperperistalsis or absence of bowel sounds. |
| Tympany over stomach on left side and most of abdomen, except for dullness or flatness just below right costal margin (liver) | Note percussion sounds other than those expected. |
| *Liver*—1-2 cm below right costal margin in infants and young children | Usually not palpable in older children |
| | Considered enlarged if 3 cm below costal margin |
| | Normally descends with inspiration; should not be considered a sign of enlargement |
| | Usually not palpable in older children |
| *Spleen*—Sometimes 1-2 cm below left costal margin in infants and young children | Considered enlarged if more than 2 cm below left costal margin; also descends with inspiration |
| | Other structures that sometimes are palpable include kidneys, bladder, cecum, and sigmoid colon; know their location to avoid mistaking them for abnormal masses; most common palpable mass is feces. |
| | In sexually active females, consider a palpable mass in the lower abdomen a pregnant uterus. |

*Continued*

## Summary of Physical Assessment of the Child—cont'd

| Assessment | Procedure |
|---|---|

### Abdomen—cont'd

Use imaginary lines at umbilicus to divide the abdomen into quadrants (see Figure 1-24):
  Right upper quadrant (RUQ)
  Right lower quadrant (RLQ)
  Left upper quadrant (LUQ)
  Left lower quadrant (LLQ)
Palpate femoral pulses simultaneously—Place tips of two or three fingers about midway between iliac crest and pubic symphysis.
Elicit abdominal reflex—Scratch skin from side to midline in each quadrant.

### Genitalia

#### *Male*

See Figure 1-25.

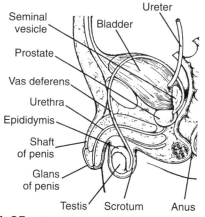

FIGURE **1-25**   Major structures of genitalia in circumcised prepubertal male.

Labels: Seminal vesicle, Ureter, Bladder, Prostate, Vas deferens, Urethra, Epididymis, Shaft of penis, Glans of penis, Testis, Scrotum, Anus

#### *General Instructions*

Proceed in same manner as examination of other areas; explain procedure and its significance before doing it, such as palpating for testes.
Respect privacy at all times.
Use opportunity to discuss concerns about sexual development with older child and adolescent.
Use opportunity to discuss sexual safety with young children: that this is their private area, and if someone touches them in a way that is uncomfortable they should always tell their parent or some other trusted person.
If in contact with body substances, wear gloves.
*Penis*—Inspect size.

*Glans and shaft*—Inspect for signs of swelling, skin lesions, and inflammation.
*Prepuce*—Inspect in uncircumcised male.

*Urethral meatus*—Inspect location, and note any discharge.

*Scrotum*—Inspect size, location, skin, and hair distribution.

*Testes*—Palpate each scrotal sac using thumb and index finger.

| Usual Findings | Comments |
|---|---|
| Equal and strong bilaterally | Note absence of femoral pulse. Normally may be absent in children under 1 year of age |
| Umbilicus moves toward quadrant that was stroked. | Examination may be anxiety producing for older children and adolescents; may be left for end of physical examination. |
| Generally, size is insignificant in prepubescent male. Compare growth with expected sexual development during puberty (see p. 117). None | Note large penis, possible sign of precocious puberty. In obese child, penis may be obscured by fat pad over pubic symphysis. |
| Easily retracted to expose glans and urethral meatus | In infants, prepuce is tight for up to 3 years and should not be retracted. |
| Centered at tip of glans No discharge | Discuss importance of hygiene. Note location on ventral or dorsal surface of penis, possible sign of ambiguous genitalia, hypospadias, or epispadias. Whenever possible, note strength and direction of urinary stream. |
| May appear large in infants Hangs freely from perineum behind penis One sac hangs lower than other. Loose, wrinkled skin, usually redder and coarser in adolescents Compare hair distribution with that expected for pubertal stage; typical mature male pattern forms a diamond shape from umbilicus to anus (see p. 117). Small ovoid bodies about 1.5-2 cm long Double in size during puberty | Note scrota that are small, close to perineum, with any degree of midline separation. Well-formed rugae indicate descent of testes. Prevent cremasteric reflex that retracts testes by: Warming hands Having child sit in tailor fashion or squat Blocking pathway of ascent by placing thumb and index finger over upper part of scrotal sac along inguinal canal Note failure to palpate testes after taking these precautions. Discuss testicular self-examination with adolescent male. |

*Continued*

## Summary of Physical Assessment of the Child—cont'd

| Assessment | Procedure |
|---|---|
| **Abdomen—cont'd** | |

*Female*

See Figure 1-26.

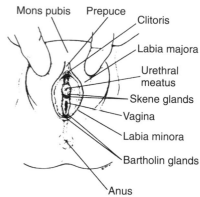

FIGURE **1-26**  External structures of genitalia in prepubertal female. Labia are spread to reveal deep structures.

*External genitalia*—Inspect structures; place young child in semireclining position in parent's lap with knees bent and soles of feet in apposition.

*Labia*—Palpate for any masses.

*Urethral meatus*—Inspect for location; identified as V-shaped slit by wiping downward from clitoris to perineum.

*Skene glands*—Palpate or inspect

*Vaginal orifice*—Internal examination usually not performed; inspect for obvious opening.

*Bartholin glands*—Palpate or inspect

---

**Anus**

*Anal area*—Inspect for general firmness, condition of skin.

*Anal reflex*—Elicit by gently pricking or scratching perianal area.

---

**Back and Extremities**

Inspect curvature and symmetry of spine (Figure 1-27).

Test for scoliosis:
    Have child stand erect; observe from behind, and note asymmetry of shoulders and hips.
    Have child bend forward at the waist until back is parallel to floor; observe from side, and note asymmetry or prominence of rib cage.
Note mobility of spine.

Inspect each extremity joint for symmetry, size, temperature, color, tenderness, and mobility.
Test for developmental dysplasia of the hip.

| Usual Findings | Comments |
|---|---|
| Mons pubis—Fat pad over symphysis pubis; covered with hair in adolescence; usual hair distribution is triangular (see p. 119) | |
| Clitoris—Located at anterior end of labia minora; covered by small flap of skin (prepuce) | Note evidence of enlargement (may be small phallus). |
| Labia majora—Two thick folds of skin from mons to posterior commissure; inner surface pink and moist | Note any palpable masses (may be testes), evidence of fusion, enlargement, or signs of female circumcision. |
| Labia minora—Two folds of skin interior to labia majora, usually invisible until puberty; prominent in newborn | |
| Located posterior to clitoris and anterior to vagina | Note opening from clitoris or inside vagina. |
| Surround meatus; no lesions | Common sites of cysts and venereal warts (condylomata acuminata) |
| Located posterior to urethral meatus; may be covered by crescent-shaped or circular membrane (**hymen**); discharge usually clear or whitish | Note excessive, foul-smelling, or colored discharge. |
| Surround vaginal opening; no lesions, secrete clear mucoid fluid | |
| Buttocks—Firm; gluteal folds symmetric | Note evidence of diaper rash; inquire about hygiene and type of diaper (cloth or ultraabsorbent paper; the latter can decrease diaper dermatitis). |
| Quick contraction of external anal sphincter; no protrusion of rectum | Note:  Fissures  Polyps  Rectal prolapse  Hemorrhoids  Warts |
| Rounded or **C**-shaped in the newborn | Note any abnormal curvatures and presence of masses or lesions. |
| Cervical secondary curve forms at about 3 months of age. | Other signs of scoliosis:  Slight limp |
| Lumbar secondary curve forms at about 12-18 months, resulting in typical double-**S** curve | Crooked hem or waistline  Complaint of backache |
| Lordosis normal in young children but decreases with age | |
| Shoulders, scapula, and iliac crests symmetric | |
| Flexible, full range of motion, no pain or stiffness | Note stiffness and pain on movement of neck or back; requires immediate evaluation. |
| Symmetric length | Note any deviations. |
| Equal size | Note warmth, swelling, tenderness, and immobility of joints. |
| Correct number of digits | |
| Nails pink | |
| Temperature equal, although feet may be cooler than hands | |
| Full range of motion | |

*Continued*

## Summary of Physical Assessment of the Child—cont'd

| Assessment | Procedure |
| --- | --- |

### Back and Extremities—cont'd

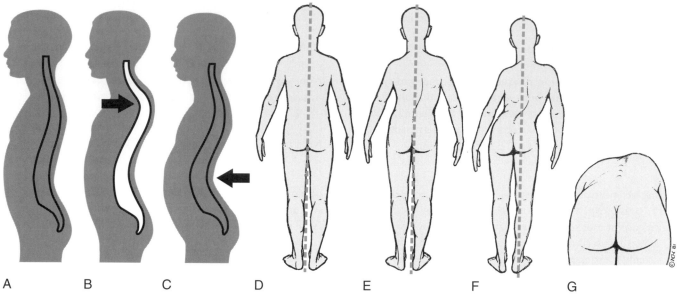

FIGURE **1-27** Defects of spinal column. A, Normal spine. B, Kyphosis. C, Lordosis. D, Normal spine in balance. E, Mild scoliosis in balance. F, Severe scoliosis not in balance. G, Rib hump and flank asymmetry seen in flexion caused by rotary component. (Redrawn from Hilt NE, Schmitt EW: *Pediatric orthopedic nursing,* St Louis, 1975, Mosby.)

Assess shape of bones:

> Measure distance between the knees when child stands with malleoli in apposition.
>
> Measure distance between the malleoli when child stands with knees together.
>
> Inspect position of feet; test if foot deformity at birth is result of fetal position or development by scratching outer, then inner, side of sole; if self-correctable, foot assumes right angle to leg.

Inspect gait:

> Have child walk in straight line.
>
> Estimate angle of gait by drawing imaginary line through center of foot and line of progression.

*Plantar reflex*—Elicit by stroking lateral sole from heel upward to little toe across to hallux.

Inspect development and tone of muscles.

Test strength:

*Arms*—Have child raise arms while applying counterpressure with your hands.

*Legs*—Have child sit with legs dangling; proceed as with arms.

*Hands*—Have child squeeze your fingers as tightly as possible.

*Feet*—Have child plantar flex (push soles toward floor) while applying counterpressure to soles.

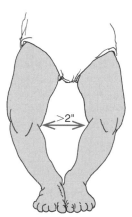

>2"

FIGURE **1-28**  Genu varum (bowleg).

**Usual Findings**

**Comments**

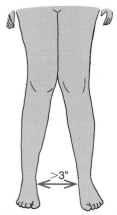

FIGURE **1-29**   Genu valgum (knock knee).

---

| BOX **1-6** | Types of Foot and Ankle Deformities |

**Pes planus (flatfoot)**—Normal finding in infancy; may be result of muscular weakness in older child

**Pes valgus**—Eversion (turning outward) of entire foot, but sole rests on ground

**Pes varus**—Inversion (turning inward) of entire foot, but sole rests on ground

**Metatarsus valgus**—Eversion of forefoot while heel remains straight; also called toeing out or duck walk

**Talipes valgus**—Eversion of foot so that only inner side of foot rests on ground

**Talipes varus**—Inversion of foot so that only outer sole of foot rests on ground

**Talipes equinus**—Extension or plantar flexion of foot so that only ball and toes rest on ground; commonly combined with talipes varus (most common of clubfoot deformities)

**Talipes calcaneus**—Dorsal flexion of foot so that only heel rests on ground

---

Less than 5 cm (2 inches) in children over 2 years of age

Less than 7.5 cm (3 inches) in children over 7 years of age

Held at right angle to leg; pointed straight ahead or turned slightly outward when standing

Fat pads on sole give appearance of flat feet; arch develops after child is walking.

"Toddling" or broad-based gait normal in young children; gradually assumes graceful gait with feet close together.

Feet turn outward less than 30 degrees and inward less than 10 degrees.

Flexion of toes in children older than 1 year

Symmetric
Increase in tone during muscle contraction
Equal bilaterally

Greater distance indicates **genu varum (bowleg)** (Figure 1-28).

Greater distance indicates **genu valgum (knock knee)** (Figure 1-29).

Note foot and ankle deformities (Box 1-6).

Note abnormal gait:
   Waddling
   Scissor
   Toeing-in
   Broad-based in older children
Babinski reflex seen in younger children (see p. 25)

Note atrophy, hypertrophy, spasticity, flaccidity, rigidity, or weakness.

*Continued*

## Summary of Physical Assessment of the Child—cont'd

| Assessment | Procedure |
|---|---|
| **Neurologic Assessment** | |
| *Mental Status* | Observe behavior, mood, affect, general orientation to surroundings, and level of consciousness (see pp. 86-88). |
| *Motor Functioning* | Test muscle strength, tone, and development (see p. 121).<br><br>Test cerebellar functioning:<br>*Finger-to-nose test*—With child's arm extended, have child touch nose with the index finger.<br>*Heel-to-shin test*—With child standing, have child run the heel of one foot down the shin of the other leg.<br>*Romberg test*—Have child stand erect with feet together and eyes closed.<br>Have child touch tip of each finger to thumb in rapid succession.<br>Have child pat leg with first one side, then the other side of hand in rapid sequence.<br>Have child tap your hand with ball of foot as quickly as possible. |
| *Sensory Functioning* | Test vision and hearing (see pp. 127-132).<br>*Sensory intactness*—Touch skin lightly with a pin, and have child point to stimulated area while keeping eyes closed.<br><br>Sensory discrimination:<br>Touch skin with pin and cotton; have child describe the sensation as sharp or dull.<br>Touch skin with cold and warm object (e.g., metal and rubber heads of reflex hammer); have child differentiate between temperatures.<br>Using two pins, touch skin simultaneously with both or only one pin; have child discriminate when one or two pins are used. |
| *Reflexes (Deep Tendon)* | *Biceps*—Hold child's arm by placing the partially flexed elbow in your hand with the thumb over the antecubital space; strike your thumbnail with the hammer.<br>*Triceps*—Bend the arm at the elbow, and rest the palm in your hand; strike the triceps tendon.<br>*Alternate procedure*—If child is supine, rest arm over chest and strike the triceps tendon. |

| Usual Findings | Comments |
| --- | --- |
|  | Subjective impressions are based on observation throughout the examination. |
|  | Objective findings can be attained through developmental testing, such as Denver II. |
| Performs each test successfully with eyes opened and closed | May be difficult to test in children younger than preschool age |
| During heel-to-shin and Romberg tests, stand close to child to prevent falls. | Note any awkwardness or lack of coordination in performance. |
| **Romberg test**—Does not lean to side or fall | Falling or leaning to one side is abnormal and is called the **Romberg sign**. |
| Localizes pinprick | Use sterile pin or other sharp object (e.g., toothpick), being careful not to puncture skin. |
|  | Compare sensation in symmetric areas at both distal and proximal points. |
| Able to distinguish types of sensation and temperature | Note difficulty in performing test, especially in older child. |
| Minimal distance for discrimination on finger is about 2-3 mm. |  |
| *Biceps*—Partial flexion of forearm | Use distraction techniques to prevent child from inhibiting reflex activity: |
|  | For upper extremity reflexes, ask child to clench teeth or to squeeze thigh with the hand on the side not being tested. Rest upper arm in palm of hand. |
| *Triceps*—Partial extension of forearm | For lower extremity reflexes, have child lock fingers and pull one hand against the other or grip hands together. Usual grading of reflexes: |
|  | **Grade 0**—Absent |
|  | **Grade 1**— Diminished |
|  | **Grade 2**—Normal, average |
|  | **Grade 3**—Brisker than normal |
|  | **Grade 4**—Hyperactive (clonus) |
|  | Note asymmetric, absent, diminished, or hyperactive reflexes. |

*Continued*

## Summary of Physical Assessment of the Child—cont'd

| Assessment | Procedure |
|---|---|
| **Neurologic Assessment—cont'd** | |
| | *Brachioradialis*—Rest forearm on the lap or abdomen, with the arm flexed at the elbow and palm down; strike the radius about 1 inch (depending on child's size) above the wrist. |
| | *Knee jerk or patellar reflex*—Sit child on the edge of the examining table or on parent's lap with the lower legs flexed at the knee and dangling freely; tap the patellar tendon just below the knee cap. |
| | *Achilles*—Use the same position as for the knee jerk; support the foot lightly in your hand, and strike the Achilles tendon. |
| | *Ankle clonus*—See p. 25. |
| | *Kernig sign*—Flex child's leg at hip and knee while supine; note pain or resistance. |
| | *Brudzinski sign*—With child supine, flex the head; note pain and involuntary flexion of hip and knees. |
| *Cranial Nerves* | (See Assessment of Cranial Nerves, p. 73.) |

| Usual Findings | Comments |
| --- | --- |

*Brachioradialis*—Flexion of the forearm and supination (turning upward) of the palm

*Patellar*—Partial extension of lower leg

*Achilles*—Plantar flexion of foot (foot pointing downward)

*Ankle clonus*—Absence of beats
*Kernig*—Absence of pain or resistance

*Brudzinski*—Absence of pain or associated movements

These special reflexes are elicited when meningeal irritation is suspected.

Signs of pain, resistance, or associated movements require immediate referral.

Testing of cranial nerves may be done as part of the neurologic examination or integrated into assessment of each system, such as cranial nerves II, III, IV, and VI with the eye.

Cranial nerves can usually be tested in children of preschool age and older.

Note inability to perform any of the items correctly.

## Temperature Measurement Locations for Infants and Children

### Oral

Place tip under tongue in right or left posterior sublingual pocket, not in front of tongue. Have child keep mouth closed, without biting on thermometer.

Pacifier thermometers measure intraoral or supralingual temperature and are available but lack support in the literature.

Several factors affect mouth temperature: eating and mastication, hot and cold beverages, open-mouth breathing, ambient temperature.

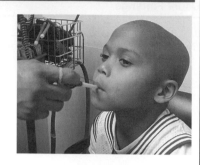

### Axillary

Place tip under arm in center of axilla and keep close to skin, not clothing. Child's arm must be held firmly against side.

May be affected by poor peripheral perfusion (results in lower value), clothing or swaddling, use of radiant warmer, or amount of brown fat in cold-stressed neonate (results in higher value).

Advantage: avoids intrusive procedure and eliminates risk of rectal perforation.

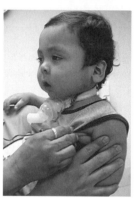

### Aural or Ear Based

An infrared probe, small enough to be deeply inserted into the canal to allow the sensor to obtain the measurement. The size of the probe (most are 8 mm) may influence accuracy of the result. In young children this may be a problem because of the small diameter of the canal. Proper placement of the ear is controversial with regard to whether the pinna should be pulled as during otoscopy.

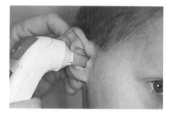

### Rectal

Place well-lubricated tip at maximum 2.5 cm (1 inch) into rectum for children and 1.5 cm for infants; securely hold thermometer close to anus.

Child may be placed in side-lying, supine, or prone position (i.e., supine with knees flexed toward abdomen); cover penis, as procedure may stimulate urination. A small child may be placed prone across parent's lap.

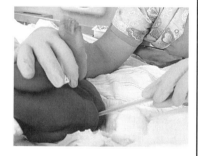

### Temporal Artery

An infrared sensor probe scans across the forehead, capturing the heat from the arterial blood flow. The only artery close enough to the skin's surface to provide access for accurate temperature measurement is the temporal artery.

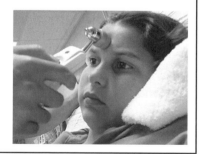

Adapted from Martin SA, Kline AM: Can there be a standard for temperature measurement in the pediatric intensive care unit? *AACN Clin Issues* 15(2): 254-266, 2004; Falzon A, Grech V, Caruana B, and others: How reliable is axillary temperature measurement? *Acta Pediatr* 92(3):309-313, 2003.

1 - ASSESSMENT

## Assessment of Cranial Nerves

| Cranial Nerve | Distribution or Function | Test |
|---|---|---|
| I—Olfactory (S)* | Olfactory mucosa of nasal cavity | With child's eyes closed, have child identify odors such as coffee, alcohol, or other smells from a swab; test each nostril separately. |
| II—Optic (S) | Rods and cones of retina, optic nerve | Check for perception of light, visual acuity, peripheral vision, color vision, and normal optic disc. |
| III—Oculomotor (M) | Extraocular muscles (EOM) of eye:<br>*Superior rectus (SR)*—Moves eyeball up and in<br>*Inferior rectus (IR)*—Moves eyeball down and in<br>*Medial rectus (MR)*—Moves eyeball nasally<br>*Inferior oblique (IO)*—Moves eyeball up and out | Have child follow an object (toy) or light in the six cardinal positions of gaze (Figure 1-30). |
| | Pupil constriction and accommodation | Perform PERRLA (see p. 47). |
| | Eyelid closing | Check for proper placement of lid (see p. 44). |
| IV—Trochlear (M) | *Superior oblique (SO) muscle*—Moves eye down and out | Have child look down and in (see Figure 1-30). |
| V—Trigeminal (M, S) | Muscles of mastication | Have child bite down hard and open jaw; test symmetry and strength. |
| | Sensory: Face, scalp, nasal and buccal mucosa | With child's eyes closed, see if child can detect light touch in the mandibular and maxillary regions.<br>Test corneal and blink reflex by touching cornea lightly (approach child from the side so that child does not blink before cornea is touched). |
| VI—Abducens (M) | *Lateral rectus (LR) muscle*—Moves eye temporally | Have child look toward temporal side (see Figure 1-30). |
| VII—Facial (M, S) | Muscles for facial expression | Have child smile, make funny face, or show teeth to see symmetry of expression. |
| | Anterior two thirds of tongue (sensory) | Have child identify a sweet or salty solution; place each taste on anterior section and sides of protruding tongue; if child retracts tongue, solution will dissolve toward posterior part of tongue. |
| | Nasal cavity and lacrimal gland, sublingual and submandibular salivary glands | Not tested |
| VIII—Auditory, Acoustic, or Vestibulocochlear (S) | Internal ear<br>Hearing, balance | Test hearing; note any loss of equilibrium or presence of vertigo (dizziness). |

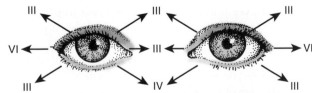

FIGURE **1-30**   Checking extraocular movements in the six cardinal positions indicates the functioning of cranial nerves III, IV, and VI. (From Ignatavicius DD, Workman ML: *Medical-surgical nursing: Patient-centered collaborative care*, ed 6, St Louis, 2009, Saunders.)

*S, Sensory; M, motor.

*Continued*

## Assessment of Cranial Nerves—cont'd

| Cranial Nerve | Distribution or Function | Test |
|---|---|---|
| IX—Glossopharyngeal (M, S) | Pharynx, tongue | Stimulate posterior pharynx with a tongue blade; the child should gag. |
| | Posterior one third of tongue (sensory) | Test sense of sour or bitter taste on posterior segment of tongue. |
| X—Vagus (M, S) | Muscles of larynx, pharynx, some organs of gastrointestinal system, sensory fibers of root of tongue, heart, lung, and some organs of gastrointestinal system | Note hoarseness of the voice, gag reflex, and ability to swallow. |
| | | Check that uvula is in midline; when stimulated with a tongue blade, should deviate upward and to the stimulated side. |
| XI—Accessory (M) | Sternocleidomastoid and trapezius muscles of shoulder | Have child shrug shoulders while applying mild pressure; with the hands placed on shoulders, have child turn head against opposing pressure on either side; note symmetry and strength. |
| XII—Hypoglossal (M) | Muscles of tongue | Have child move tongue in all directions; have child protrude tongue as far as possible; note any midline deviation. |
| | | Test strength by placing tongue blade on one side of tongue and having child move it away. |

# Nursing Assessment of Specific Health Problems

## ⊖The Child with Acute Respiratory Infection

*Acute respiratory infection*—An inflammatory process caused by viral, bacterial, or atypical (mycoplasma) infection or aspiration of foreign substances, which involves any or all parts of the respiratory tract

*Lower respiratory tract*—Consists of the bronchi and bronchioles (which constitute the reactive portion of the airway because of their smooth muscle content and ability to constrict) and the alveoli

*Croup syndromes*—Consist of the epiglottis, larynx, and trachea (the structurally stable, nonreactive portion of the airway)

*Upper respiratory tract (upper airway)*—Consists of the nose and pharynx

### Assessment

Assist with diagnostic procedures and tests (e.g., radiography, throat culture, thoracentesis, venipuncture for blood analysis).

Observe for general clinical manifestations of acute respiratory tract infection (Box 1-7).

Identify factors affecting type of illness and response to acute respiratory infection (e.g., age and size of child, ability to resist infection, contact with infected children, coexisting disorders affecting respiratory tract).

Assess respiratory status.

Monitor respirations for rate, depth, pattern, presence of retractions, and flaring nares.

Auscultate lungs.
- Evaluate breath sounds (type and location).
- Detect presence of crackles or wheezes.
- Detect areas of consolidation.
- Evaluate effectiveness of chest physiotherapy.

Observe for presence or absence of retractions, nasal flaring.

Observe color of skin and mucous membranes for pallor and cyanosis.

Observe for presence of hoarseness, stridor, and cough.

Monitor heart rate and regularity.

Observe behavior.
- Restlessness
- Irritability
- Apprehension

Observe for signs of the following:
- Chest pain
- Abdominal pain
- Dyspnea

Observe for clinical manifestations of respiratory infection (specific).

### Upper Respiratory Tract Infections

*Nasopharyngitis*—Viral infection, acute rhinitis or coryza, equivalent of the common cold in adults

Edema and vasodilation of mucosa

**BOX  1-7** | Signs and Symptoms Associated with Respiratory Infections in Infants and Small Children

### Fever
May be absent in newborn infants
Greatest at ages 6 months to 3 years
- Temperature may reach 39.5° to 40.5° C (103° to 105° F), even with mild infections
Often appears as first sign of infection
Child may be listless and irritable, or somewhat euphoric and more active than normal temporarily; some children talk with unaccustomed rapidity
Tendency to develop high temperatures with infection in certain families
- May precipitate febrile seizures
- Febrile seizures uncommon after 3 or 4 years of age

### Meningismus
Meningeal signs without infection of the meninges
Occurs with abrupt onset of fever
Accompanied by:
- Headache
- Pain and stiffness in the back and neck
- Presence of Kernig and Brudzinski signs
Subsides as temperature drops

### Anorexia
Common with most childhood illnesses
Frequently the initial evidence of illness
Almost invariably accompanies acute infections in small children
Persists to a greater or lesser degree throughout febrile stage of illness; often extends into convalescence

### Vomiting
Small children vomit readily with illness
A clue to the onset of infection
May precede other signs by several hours
Usually short-lived but may persist during the illness

### Diarrhea
Usually mild, transient diarrhea but may become severe
Often accompanies viral respiratory infections
Is frequent cause of dehydration

### Abdominal Pain
Common complaint
Sometimes indistinguishable from pain of appendicitis
Mesenteric lymphadenitis may be a cause
Muscle spasms from vomiting may be a factor, especially in nervous, tense children

### Nasal Blockage
Small nasal passages of infants easily blocked by mucosal swelling and exudation
Can interfere with respiration and feeding in infants
May contribute to the development of otitis media and sinusitis

### Nasal Discharge
Frequent occurrence
May be thin and watery (rhinorrhea) or thick and purulent, depending on the type and/or stage of infection
Associated with itching
May irritate upper lip and skin surrounding the nose

### Cough
Common feature
May be evident only during the acute phase
May persist several months after a disease

### Respiratory Sounds
Sounds associated with respiratory disease
- Cough
- Hoarseness
- Grunting
- Stridor
- Wheezing
Auscultation
- Wheezing
- Crackles
- Absence of sound

### Sore Throat
Frequent complaint of older children
Younger children (unable to describe symptoms) may not complain, even when throat highly inflamed
- Often child will refuse to take oral fluids or solids

---

## Assessment
Younger child
- Fever
- Irritability, restlessness
- Sneezing
- Vomiting and/or diarrhea, sometimes
- Decreased appetite
- Decreased activity
Older child
- Low-grade fever
- Dryness and irritation of nose and throat

- Sneezing, chilly sensations
- Muscular aches
- Irritating nasal discharge
- Cough, sometimes

*Pharyngitis*—Throat (including the tonsils) is principal anatomic site of pharyngitis (sore throat).

## Assessment
Younger child
- Fever
- General malaise

- Anorexia
- Moderate sore throat
- Headache
- Mild to moderate hyperemia
- Abdominal pain

Older child

- Fever (may reach 40° C [104° F])
- Headache
- Anorexia
- Dysphagia
- Vomiting
- Mild to fiery red, edematous pharynx
- Hyperemia of tonsils and pharynx; may extend to soft palate and uvula
- Often abundant follicular exudate that spreads and coalesces to form pseudomembrane on tonsils
- Cervical glands enlarged and tender

*Influenza (flu)*—Caused by three antigenically distinct orthomyxoviruses: types A and B, which cause epidemic disease, and type C, which is epidemiologically unimportant.

May be subclinical, mild, moderate, or severe

Overt illness

## Assessment

- Dry throat and nasal mucosa
- Dry cough
- Tendency toward hoarseness
- Sudden onset of fever and chills
- Flushed face
- Photophobia
- Myalgia
- Hyperesthesia
- Prostration (sometimes)
- Subglottal croup common (especially in infants)

### Croup Syndromes

*Croup* is a general term applied to a symptom complex characterized by hoarseness, a resonant cough described as barking (croupy), varying degrees of inspiratory stridor, and varying degrees of respiratory distress resulting from swelling or obstruction in the region of the larynx.

*Acute laryngitis*—Infection is usually viral; primary clinical manifestation is hoarseness; common illness of older children and adolescents.

May be accompanied by other upper respiratory symptoms: coryza, sore throat, nasal congestion

May be accompanied by systemic manifestations: fever, headache, myalgia, malaise

Symptoms vary with the infecting virus.

*Acute laryngotracheobronchitis (LTB)*—Viral infection; most common of the croup syndromes; usually occurs in children age 3 months to 8 years

Onset is slowly progressive.

## Assessment

- (Upper respiratory infection [URI]; several days of coryza)
- URI
- Inspiratory stridor
- Barking (seal-like) cough
- Hoarseness
- Dyspnea
- Suprasternal retractions
- Restlessness
- Irritability
- Low-grade fever
- Nontoxic appearance
- May progress to hypoxia and respiratory failure

*Acute spasmodic laryngitis (spasmodic croup)*—Viral infection with allergic and psychogenic factors in some cases; distinguished from laryngitis and LTB by characteristic paroxysmal attacks of laryngeal obstruction that occur chiefly at night; usually occurs in children age 3 months to 3 years

Onset is sudden, at night.

## Assessment

- URI
- Croupy cough
- Stridor
- Hoarseness
- Dyspnea
- Restlessness
- Child appears anxious, frightened.
- Symptoms waken child.
- Symptoms disappear during day.
- Tends to recur

*Acute epiglottitis (supraglottitis)*—Bacterial (usually *Haemophilus influenzae*) infection; serious obstructive inflammatory process that requires immediate attention; occurs principally in children between 2 and 5 years of age but can occur from infancy to adulthood; LTB and epiglottitis do not occur together. Onset is abrupt, rapidly progressive.

## Assessment

- Sore throat
- Drooling
- Absence of spontaneous cough
- Agitation
- Throat is red, inflamed with distinctive large, cherry-red, edematous epiglottitis (Safety Alert)
- High fever
- Toxic appearance
- Rapid pulse and respirations
- Stridor aggravated when supine
- Child will sit upright, leaning forward, with chin thrust out, mouth open, and tongue protruding; tripod position
- Thick, muffled voice
- Croaking, froglike sound on inspiration

- Anxious and frightened expression
- Suprasternal and substernal retractions possibly visible
- Child seldom struggles to breathe (breathing slowly and quietly provides better air exchange)
- Sallow color of mild hypoxia to frank cyanosis

> **! SAFETY ALERT**
>
> Avoid throat examination or culture in suspected epiglottitis because this can precipitate further or complete obstruction. Throat inspection should be attempted only when immediate intubation can be performed if needed.

*Acute tracheitis*—Bacterial (usually *Staphylococcus aureus*) infection of the mucosa of the upper trachea; is a distinct entity with features of both croup and epiglottitis; may cause airway obstruction severe enough to cause respiratory arrest; occurs in children ages 1 month to 6 years. Onset is moderately progressive.

## Assessment

- Follows previous URI
- Begins with signs and symptoms similar to those of LTB
- Croupy cough
- Stridor unaffected by position
- Copious purulent secretions—may be severe enough to cause respiratory arrest
- Toxic appearance
- High fever
- No response to LTB therapy

### Lower Respiratory Tract Infections

*Asthmatic bronchitis*—Exaggerated response of bronchi to infection; most commonly caused by viruses but may be by any variety of URI pathogens; bronchospasm, exudation, and edema of bronchi are similar to asthma in older children; occurs in late infancy and early childhood.

## Assessment

- Previous URI
- Wheezing
- Productive cough
- (See also assessment of bronchial asthma, p. 79.)

*Viral-induced bronchitis*—Inflammation of large airways (trachea and bronchi); usually occurs in association with viral URI, but other agents (e.g., bacteria, fungi, allergic disorders, airborne irritants) can trigger symptoms; seldom occurs as an isolated entity in childhood; affects children in first 4 years of life.

## Assessment

- Persistent dry, hacking cough (worse at night), becoming productive in 2 to 3 days
- Tachypnea
- Low-grade fever

*Respiratory syncytial virus (RSV)/bronchiolitis*—Acute viral infection with maximum effect at the bronchiolar level;

usually affects children age 2 to 12 months; rare after age 2 years

## Assessment

- Begins as simple URI with serous nasal discharge
- May be accompanied by mild fever
- Gradually causes increasing respiratory distress
- Dyspnea
- Paroxysmal, nonproductive cough
- Tachypnea with flaring nares and retractions
- Emphysema
- Possible wheezing

### Pneumonias

Pneumonia, inflammation of the pulmonary parenchyma, is common throughout childhood but occurs more frequently in infancy and early childhood. Clinically, pneumonia may occur either as a primary disease or as a complication of another illness. Morphologically, the following types of pneumonias are recognized:

*Lobar pneumonia*—All or a large segment of one or more pulmonary lobes is involved. When both lungs are affected, it is known as bilateral or double pneumonia.

*Bronchopneumonia*—Begins in the terminal bronchioles, which become clogged with mucopurulent exudate to form consolidated patches in nearby lobules; also called lobular pneumonia

*Interstitial pneumonia*—The inflammatory process is more or less confined within the alveolar walls (interstitium) and the peribronchial and interlobular tissues.

Pneumonitis is a localized acute inflammation of the lung without the toxemia associated with lobar pneumonia.

The pneumonias are more often classified according to the etiologic agent: viral, atypical (mycoplasma pneumonia), or bacterial pneumonia, or pneumonia caused by aspiration of foreign substances. Pneumonia may be caused less often by histomycosis, coccidioidomycosis, and other fungi.

*Viral pneumonia*—Occurs more frequently than bacterial pneumonia; seen in children of all age-groups; often associated with viral URIs, and RSV accounts for the largest percentage.

Onset may be acute or insidious.

Symptoms variable

*Mild*—Low-grade fever, slight cough, malaise

*Severe*—High fever, severe cough, prostration

Cough usually unproductive early in disease

A few wheezes or crackles heard on auscultation

*Atypical pneumonia*—Etiologic agent is mycoplasma; occurs principally in fall and winter months; more prevalent in crowded living conditions.

## Assessment

Onset may be sudden or insidious.

General systemic symptoms

- Fever
- Chills (older children)
- Headache
- Malaise
- Anorexia
- Myalgia

Followed by:

- Rhinitis
- Sore throat
- Dry, hacking cough
  - Nonproductive early, then seromucoid sputum, to mucopurulent or blood-streaked
  - Fine crepitant crackles over various lung areas

*Bacterial pneumonia*—Includes pneumococcal, staphylococcal, streptococcal, and chlamydial pneumonias; clinical manifestations differ from other types of pneumonia; individual microorganisms produce a distinct clinical picture.

Onset abrupt

- Usually preceded by viral infection
- Toxic, acutely ill appearance
- Fever, usually high
- Malaise
- Rapid, shallow respirations
- Cough
- Chest pain often exaggerated by deep breathing
- Pain may be referred to abdomen
- Chills
- Meningismus

### Pulmonary Tuberculosis

Caused by *Mycobacterium tuberculosis;* other factors that influence development of tuberculosis (TB) include the following: heredity (resistance to the infection may be genetically transmitted); gender (morbidity and mortality higher in adolescent girls); age (lower resistance in infants, higher incidence during adolescence); stress (emotional or physical); nutritional state; and intercurrent infection (especially human immunodeficiency virus [HIV], measles, pertussis).

Extremely variable

May be asymptomatic or produce a broad range of symptoms

- Fever
- Malaise
- Anorexia
- Weight loss
- Cough may or may not be present (progresses slowly over weeks to months).
- Aching pain and tightness in the chest
- Hemoptysis (rare)

With progression

- Respiratory rate increase
- Poor expansion of lung on the affected side
- Diminished breath sounds and crackles
- Dullness to percussion
- Persistence of fever

- Generalized symptoms manifested (especially infants)
- Child develops pallor, anemia, weakness, and weight loss

### Aspiration of Foreign Substances

Inflammation of lung tissue can occur as the result of irritation from foreign material (e.g., vomitus, small objects, oral secretions, inhalation of smoke) and aspiration of food. Young children are especially prone to aspiration of foreign substances, and weak and debilitated children are subject to aspiration of food, vomitus, or secretions.

*Foreign body (FB) aspiration*—Clinical manifestations and changes produced depend on the degree and location of obstruction and type of FB.

- Choking
- Gagging
- Sternal retractions
- Wheezing
- Cough
- Inability to speak or breathe (larynx)
- Decreased airway entry, dyspnea (bronchi)

Signs of acute distress requiring immediate and quick action

- Cannot speak
- Becomes cyanotic
- Collapses

*Aspiration pneumonia*—May result from aspiration of fluids, food, vomitus, nasopharyngeal secretions, amniotic fluid and debris (during birth process), hydrocarbons, lipids, and talcum powder. Aspiration of fluid or food substances is a particular hazard in children who have difficulty with swallowing; are unable to swallow because of paralysis, weaknesses, debility, congenital anomalies, or absent cough reflex; or are force-fed, especially while crying or breathing rapidly. Irritated mucous membranes become a site for secondary bacterial infection.

*Inhalation injury*—Results from inhalation of smoke (noxious substances are primarily products of incomplete combustion) or other noxious gases. Local injury (smoke)

## Assessment

- Suspected with a history of flames in a closed space whether burns are present or not
- Sooty material around nose, in sputum
- Singed nasal hairs
- Mucosal burns of nose, lips, mouth, or throat
- Hoarse voice
- Cough
- Inspiratory and expiratory stridor
- Signs of respiratory distress (tachypnea, tachycardia, diminished or abnormal breath sounds)

Systemic injury

- Gases that are nontoxic to the airways (e.g., carbon monoxide [CO], hydrogen cyanide) can cause injury and death by interfering with or inhibiting cellular respiration.

Mild CO poisoning
- Headache
- Visual disturbances
- Irritability
- Nausea

Severe CO poisoning
- Confusion
- Hallucinations
- Ataxia
- Coma
- Pallor
- Cyanosis
- Possibly bright, cherry-red lips and skin

## ⊝ The Child with Asthma

*Asthma*—A reversible obstructive process characterized by an increased responsiveness and inflammation of the airways, especially the lower airway. It is a complex, chronic disorder involving biochemical, immunologic, infectious, endocrine, and psychologic factors.

Status asthmaticus is an acute, severe, and prolonged asthma attack in which respiratory distress continues despite vigorous therapeutic measures, especially the administration of sympathomimetics.

### Assessment

Obtain a family history, especially regarding presence of atopy in family members.

Obtain a health history, including any evidence of atopy (e.g., eczema, rhinitis); evidence of possible precipitating factor(s); previous episodes of shortness of breath, wheezing, and coughing; and any complaints of prodromal itching at the front of neck or upper part of back.

Observe for manifestations of bronchial asthma.

**Cough**
- Hacking, paroxysmal, irritative, and nonproductive
- Becomes rattling and productive of frothy, clear, gelatinous sputum

**Respiratory-related signs**
- Coughing in absence of respiratory infection, especially at night
- Shortness of breath
- Prolonged expiratory phase
- Audible wheeze
- Often appears pale
- May have a malar flush and red ears
- Lips deep, dark, red color
- May progress to cyanosis of nail beds and skin, especially circumoral

- Restlessness
- Apprehension
- Anxious facial expression
- Sweating may be prominent as the attack progresses
- During infancy retractions may occur; clinical symptoms of asthma may be less obvious
- Older children may sit upright with shoulders in a hunched-over position, hands on the bed or chair, and arms braced
- Speaks with panting and short or broken phrases

**Chest**
- Hyperresonance on percussion
- Coarse, loud breath sounds
- Wheezes throughout the lung fields
- Prolonged expiration
- Crackles
- Generalized inspiratory and expiratory wheezing; increasingly high pitched

**With repeated episodes**
- Barrel chest
- Elevated shoulders
- Use of accessory muscles of respiration
- Facial appearance—Flattened malar bones, circles beneath the eyes, narrow nose, prominent upper teeth

Observe for manifestations of severe respiratory distress and impending respiratory failure.
- Profuse sweating
- Child sits upright; refuses to lie down
- Suddenly becomes agitated
- Suddenly becomes quiet when previously agitated

Assist with diagnostic procedures and tests (e.g., blood gases, electrolytes, pH; oximetry; urine specific gravity; radiography; pulmonary function tests).

Assess environment for presence of possible allergenic factors.

## ⊝ The Child with Fluid and Electrolyte Disturbance

Dehydration
  *Isotonic (isoosmotic, isonatremic)*—Electrolyte and water deficits present in approximately balanced proportions
  *Hypertonic (hyperosmotic, hypernatremic)*—Water loss in excess of electrolyte loss
  *Hypotonic (hypoosmotic, hyponatremic)*—Electrolyte deficit exceeds water deficit

Fluid excess
  *Edema*—Excess fluid in the interstitial spaces
  *Water intoxication*—Excessive intake of fluid

### Assessment

Take a careful health history, especially regarding current health problem (e.g., length of illness, events that may have precipitated symptoms).

*Vomitus*—Assess for volume, frequency, and type of vomiting

*Sweating*—Can be only estimated from frequency of clothing and linen changes

Perform a physical assessment.

Observe for manifestations of fluid and electrolyte disturbances

*Vital signs*—Temperature (normal, elevated, or lowered depending on degree of dehydration), pulse, and blood pressure

*Skin*—Assess for color, temperature, feel, turgor, and presence or absence of edema

*Mucous membranes*—Assess for moisture, color, and presence and consistency of secretions; condition of tongue

*Fontanel (infants)*—Sunken, soft, normal

*Behavior*—Irritability, lethargy, comatose condition, characteristics of cry (infant), activity level, restlessness

Perform specific assessments.

*Intake and output*—Accurate measurements of fluid intake and output are vital to the assessment of dehydration. This includes oral and parenteral intake and losses from urine, stools, vomiting, fistulas, nasogastric suction, sweat, and wound drainage.

*Body weight*—Measure regularly and at same time of day, usually each morning, to detect decreased or increased weight.

*Urine*—Assess frequency, volume, and color of urine.

*Sensory alterations*—Assess for presence of thirst.

*Stools*—Assess frequency, volume, and consistency of stools.

Assist with diagnostic procedures and tests (e.g., urinalysis, blood chemistry, complete blood count [CBC], blood gases).

## The Child with Acute Diarrhea (Gastroenteritis)

*Acute diarrhea (gastroenteritis)*—An inflammation of the stomach and intestines caused by various bacterial, viral, and parasitic pathogens

### Assessment

Obtain a careful history of illness including the following:

- Possible ingestion of contaminated food or water
- Possible infection elsewhere (e.g., respiratory or urinary tract infection)

Perform a routine physical assessment.

Observe for manifestations of acute gastroenteritis.

Assess state of dehydration (Tables 1-3 and 1-4)

*Record fecal output*—number, volume, characteristics.

*Observe and record presence of associated signs*—tenesmus, cramping, vomiting.

Assist with diagnostic procedures (e.g., collect specimens as needed; stools for pH, blood, sugar, frequency; urine for pH, specific gravity, frequency; CBC, serum electrolytes, creatinine, blood urea nitrogen [BUN]).

Detect source of infection (e.g., examine other members of household, and refer for treatment where indicated).

| TABLE 1-3 | Clinical Manifestations of Dehydration | | |
|---|---|---|---|
| | Isotonic (Loss of Water and Salt) | Hypotonic (Loss of Salt in Excess of Water) | Hypertonic (Loss of Water in Excess of Salt) |
| **Skin** | | | |
| *Color* | Gray | Gray | Gray |
| *Temperature* | Cold | Cold | Cold or hot |
| *Turgor* | Poor | Very poor | Fair |
| *Feel* | Dry | Clammy | Thickened, doughy |
| **Mucous membranes** | Dry | Slightly moist | Parched |
| **Tearing and salivation** | Absent | Absent | Absent |
| **Eyeball** | Sunken and soft | Sunken | Sunken |
| **Fontanel** | Sunken | Sunken | Sunken |
| **Body temperature** | Subnormal or elevated | Subnormal or elevated | Subnormal or elevated |
| **Pulse** | Rapid | Very rapid | Moderately rapid |
| **Respirations** | Rapid | Rapid | Rapid |
| **Behavior** | Irritable to lethargic | Lethargic to comatose; convulsions | Marked lethargy with extreme hyperirritability on stimulation |

**TABLE 1-4**    Signs Associated with Isotonic Dehydration in Infants

| | DEGREE OF DEHYDRATION | | |
| --- | --- | --- | --- |
| | Mild | Moderate | Severe |
| Fluid volume loss | <50 ml/kg | 50-90 ml/kg | ≥100 mg/kg |
| Skin color | Pale | Gray | Mottled |
| Skin elasticity | Decreased | Poor | Very poor |
| Mucous membranes | Dry | Very dry | Parched |
| Urinary output | Decreased | Oliguria | Marked oliguria and azotemia |
| Blood pressure | Normal | Normal or lowered | Lowered |
| Pulse | Normal or increased | Increased | Rapid and thready |
| Capillary filling time | <2 seconds | 2-3 seconds | >3 seconds |

**TABLE 1-5**    Comparison of Clinical Features of Hepatitis Types A, B, and C

| Characteristics | Type A | Type B | Type C |
| --- | --- | --- | --- |
| Onset | Usually rapid, acute | More insidious | Usually insidious |
| Fever | Common and early | Less frequent | Less frequent |
| Anorexia | Common | Mild to moderate | Mild to moderate |
| Nausea and vomiting | Common | Sometimes present | Mild to moderate |
| Rash | Rare | Common | Sometimes present |
| Arthralgia | Rare | Common | Rare |
| Pruritus | Rare | Sometimes present | Sometimes present |
| Jaundice | Present (many cases anicteric) | Present | Present |

## The Child with Acute Hepatitis

*Hepatitis*—An acute or chronic inflammation of the liver
Hepatitis of viral origin is caused by at least six types of virus.

- Hepatitis A virus (HAV)
- Hepatitis B virus (HBV)
- Hepatitis C virus (HCV, previously designated *parenterally transmitted non-A, non-B hepatitis virus*)
- Hepatitis D virus (HDV, occurs in children already infected with HBV)
- Hepatitis E virus (enterically transmitted non-A, non-B hepatitis virus)
- Hepatitis G virus (HGV, blood-borne)

### Assessment

Perform a routine physical assessment.
Take a careful health history, especially regarding the following:

- Contact with persons known to have hepatitis
- Unsafe sanitation practices (e.g., drinking impure water)
- Eating certain foods (e.g., raw shellfish taken from polluted water)
- Previous blood transfusions
- Ingestion of hepatotoxic drugs (e.g., salicylates, sulfonamides, antineoplastic agents, acetaminophen, anticonvulsants)
- Parenteral administration of illicit drugs, or sexual contact with persons who use these drugs

Observe for manifestations of hepatitis (Table 1-5).
Assist with diagnostic procedures and tests (e.g., blood examination for presence of antibodies, liver function tests).

## ⊖ The Child with Appendicitis

*Appendicitis*—An inflammation of the vermiform appendix (blind sac at the end of the cecum)

### Assessment

Take a careful history of illness.
Observe for clinical manifestations of appendicitis as follows:

- Initially abdominal pain is usually colicky, cramping, and located around umbilicus

- Pain progresses and becomes constant
- Right lower quadrant abdominal pain (McBurney point)
- Fever
- Rigid abdomen
- Decreased or absent bowel sounds
- Nausea and vomiting (commonly follows onset of pain)
- Constipation or diarrhea may be present

Nursing Care Plan—The Child with Appendicitis

- Anorexia
- Tachycardia; rapid, shallow breathing
- Pallor
- Lethargy
- Irritability
- Stooped posture

Observe for signs of peritonitis as follows:

- Fever
- Sudden relief from pain (after perforation)
- Subsequent increase in pain, which is usually diffuse and accompanied by rigid guarding of the abdomen

- Progressive abdominal distention
- Tachycardia
- Rapid, shallow breathing
- Pallor
- Chills
- Irritability
- Restlessness

Assist with diagnostic procedures (e.g., white blood count, abdominal radiography).

## The Child with Cardiovascular Dysfunction

*Cardiac dysfunction*—Dysfunction, congenital or acquired, of the heart or the blood vessels

*Cardiovascular system*—Consists of the heart and blood vessels

### Assessment

Assess general appearance, behavior, and function.

- Inspection
  *Nutritional state*—Failure to thrive, poor weight gain, poor feeding habits, fatigue during feeding, or sweating during feeding is associated with heart disease.
  *Color*—Cyanosis is a common feature of congenital heart disease, and pallor is associated with anemia, which frequently accompanies heart disease.
  *Chest deformities*—An enlarged heart sometimes distorts the chest configuration.
  *Unusual pulsations*—Visible pulsations are sometimes present.
  *Respiratory excursion*—The ease or difficulty of respirating (e.g., tachypnea, dyspnea, presence of expiratory grunt, shortness of breath, persistent cough) or frequent respiratory infections.
  *Clubbing of fingers*—Associated with some types of congenital heart disease.

- *Behavior*—Assuming knee-chest position or squatting is typical of some types of heart disease; exercise intolerance.
- Palpation and percussion
  *Chest*—Helps discern heart size and other characteristics (e.g., thrills) associated with heart disease.
  *Abdomen*—Hepatomegaly and/or splenomegaly may be evident.
  *Peripheral pulses*—Rate, regularity, and amplitude (strength) may reveal discrepancies.
- Auscultation
  *Heart*—Detect presence of heart murmurs.
  *Heart rate and rhythm*—Observe for discrepancies between apical and peripheral pulses.
  *Character of heart sounds*—Reveals deviations in heart sounds and intensity that help localize heart defects
  *Lungs*—May reveal crackles, wheezes
  *Blood pressure*—Deviations present in some cardiac conditions (e.g., discrepancies between upper and lower extremities)

Assist with diagnostic procedures and tests (e.g., electrocardiography, radiography, echocardiography, fluoroscopy, ultrasonography, angiography, blood analysis [blood count, hemoglobin, packed cell volume, blood gases], exercise stress test, cardiac catheterization).

## The Child with Congenital Heart Disease

*Congenital heart disease*—A structural or functional defect of the heart or great vessels present at birth

### Assessment

Perform physical assessment with special emphasis on color, pulse (apical, peripheral), respiration, blood pressure, and examination and auscultation of chest.

Take careful health history, including evidence of poor weight gain, poor feeding, exercise intolerance, unusual posturing, or frequent respiratory tract infections.

Observe child for manifestations of congenital heart disease.

Infants

- *Cyanosis*—Generalized, especially mucous membranes, lips and tongue, conjunctiva; highly vascularized areas
- Cyanosis during exertion such as crying, feeding, straining, or when immersed in water; peripheral or central
- Dyspnea, especially following physical effort such as feeding, crying, straining
- Fatigue
- Poor growth and development (failure to thrive)
- Frequent respiratory tract infections

- Feeding difficulties
- Hypotonia
- Excessive sweating
- Syncopal attacks such as paroxysmal hyperpnea, anoxic spells

Older children
- Impaired growth
- Delicate, frail body build

- Fatigue
- Effort dyspnea
- Orthopnea
- Digital clubbing
- Squatting for relief of dyspnea
- Headache
- Epistaxis
- Leg fatigue

## ⊖ The Child with Congestive Heart Failure

*Congestive heart failure*—The inability of the heart to pump an adequate amount of blood to the systemic circulation at normal filling pressures to meet the metabolic demands of the body

### Assessment
Perform a physical assessment.
Perform a cardiac assessment.
Take a careful health history, especially regarding previous cardiac problems.
Observe for manifestations of congestive heart failure.
Impaired myocardial function
- Tachycardia
- Sweating (inappropriate)
- Decreased urine output
- Fatigue
- Weakness
- Restlessness
- Anorexia
- Pale, cool extremities
- Weak peripheral pulses
- Decreased blood pressure

- Gallop rhythm
- Cardiomegaly

Pulmonary congestion
- Tachypnea
- Dyspnea
- Retractions (infants)
- Flaring nares
- Exercise intolerance
- Orthopnea
- Cough, hoarseness
- Cyanosis
- Wheezing
- Grunting

Systemic venous congestion
- Weight gain
- Hepatomegaly
- Peripheral edema, especially periorbital
- Ascites
- Neck vein distention (children)
- Assist with diagnostic procedures and tests (e.g., radiography, electrocardiography, echocardiography).

## ⊖ The Child in Shock (Circulatory Failure)

*Shock (circulatory failure)*—A clinical syndrome characterized by tissue perfusion that is inadequate to meet the metabolic demands of the body, resulting in cellular dysfunction and eventual organ failure.

### Stages of Shock
*Compensated shock*—Vital organ function is maintained by intrinsic compensatory mechanisms; blood flow is usually normal or increased but generally uneven or maldistributed in the microcirculation.
*Decompensated shock*—Efficiency of the cardiovascular system gradually diminishes until perfusion in the microcirculation becomes marginal despite compensatory adjustments.
*Irreversible, or terminal, shock*—Damage to vital organs such as the heart or brain, of such magnitude that the entire organism will be disrupted regardless of therapeutic intervention; death occurs even if cardiovascular measurements return to normal levels with therapy.

### Types of Shock
#### Cardiogenic Shock
Characteristic
- Decreased cardiac output

Most frequent causes
- Following surgery for congenital heart disease
- **Primary pump failure**—Myocarditis, myocardial trauma, biochemical derangements, congestive heart failure
- **Dysrhythmias**—Paroxysmal atrial tachycardia, atrioventricular block, and ventricular dysrhythmias; secondary to myocarditis or biochemical abnormalities

#### Distributive Shock
Characteristics
- Reduction in peripheral vascular resistance
- Profound inadequacies in tissue perfusion
- Increased venous capacity and pooling

- Acute reduction in return blood flow to the heart
- Diminished cardiac output

Most frequent causes

- **Anaphylaxis (anaphylactic shock)**—Extreme allergy or hypersensitivity to a foreign substance
- **Sepsis (septic shock, bacteremic shock, endotoxic shock)**—Overwhelming sepsis and circulating bacterial toxins
- **Loss of neuronal control (neurogenic shock)**—Interruption of neuronal transmission (spinal cord injury)
- **Myocardial depression and peripheral dilation**—Exposure to anesthesia or ingestion of barbiturates, tranquilizers, narcotics, antihypertensive agents, or ganglionic blocking agents

### Hypovolemic Shock

Characteristics

- Reduction in size of vascular compartment
- Falling blood pressure
- Poor capillary filling
- Low central venous pressure (CVP)

Most frequent causes

- *Blood loss (hemorrhagic shock)*—Trauma, gastrointestinal (GI) bleeding, intracranial hemorrhage
- *Plasma loss*—Increased capillary permeability associated with sepsis and acidosis, hypoproteinemia, burns, peritonitis
- *Extracellular fluid loss*—Vomiting, diarrhea, glycosuric diuresis, sunstroke

## Assessment

Maintain vigilance in situations that predispose the patient to shock (e.g., trauma, burns, overwhelming sepsis, diarrhea, vomiting).

Observe for manifestations of shock.

Early clinical signs (compensated shock)

- Apprehension
- Irritability
- Unexplained tachycardia
- Normal blood pressure
- Narrowing pulse pressure
- Thirst
- Pallor
- Diminished urinary output
- Reduced perfusion of extremities

Advanced shock (decompensated shock)

- Confusion and somnolence
- Tachypnea
- Tachycardia
- Moderate metabolic acidosis
- Oliguria
- Cool, pale extremities
- Decreased skin turgor
- Poor capillary filling

Impending cardiopulmonary arrest (irreversible shock)

- Thready, weak pulse
- Hypotension
- Periodic breathing or apnea
- Anuria
- Stupor or coma

Monitor vital signs, CVP, capillary filling, intake and output, and cardiac function, on admission and continuously or very frequently.

Assist with diagnostic procedures and tests (e.g., blood count, blood gases, pH, liver function tests, coagulation studies, renal function tests, cultures, electrolytes, electrocardiography).

# ⊖ The Child with Anemia

*Anemia*—A condition in which the number of red blood cells (RBCs) and/or the hemoglobin concentration is reduced below normal

## Assessment

Perform a physical assessment.

Take a health history, including a careful dietary history, to identify any deficiencies (e.g., evidence of pica, the eating of nonfood substances such as clay, ice, or paste).

Observe for manifestations of anemia.

General manifestations

- Muscle weakness
- Easy fatigability (frequent resting, shortness of breath, poor sucking in infants)
- Pale skin (waxy pallor seen in severe anemia)
- Pica

Central nervous system manifestations

- Headache
- Dizziness
- Lightheadedness
- Irritability
- Slowed thought processes
- Decreased attention span
- Apathy
- Depression

Shock (blood loss anemia)

- Poor peripheral perfusion
- Skin moist and cool
- Low blood pressure and CVP
- Increased heart rate
- Assist with diagnostic tests (e.g., analysis of blood elements)

## ⊜The Child with Acute Renal Failure

*Acute renal failure (ARF)*—A condition that results when the kidneys suddenly are unable to excrete urine of sufficient volume or adequate concentration to maintain normal body fluid balance

## Assessment
### Initial Assessment
Perform a physical assessment.

Take a careful health history, especially regarding evidence of glomerulonephritis, obstructive uropathy, and exposure to or ingestion of toxic chemicals (including heavy metals, carbon tetrachloride, or other organic solvents; and nephrotoxic drugs).

Observe for manifestations of acute renal failure.
  Specific
  - Oliguria
  - Anuria uncommon (except in obstructive disorders)

Nonspecific (may develop)
  - Nausea
  - Vomiting
  - Drowsiness
  - Edema
  - Hypertension
  - Cardiac arrhythmia

Ongoing Assessment

Careful monitoring of the following:
  - Urinary output (insert Foley catheter)
  - Blood pressure, pulse, and respiration
  - Cardiac function
  - Neurologic function
  - Observe for signs of fluid overload
  - Manifestations of underlying disorder or pathology

Assist with diagnostic tests (e.g., urinalysis, BUN, nonprotein nitrogen, creatinine, serum electrolytes, CBC, blood gases, and specific tests to determine cause of renal failure).

## The Child with Chronic Renal Failure

*Chronic renal failure (CRF)*—Occurs when the diseased kidneys are unable to maintain the chemical composition of body fluids within normal limits under normal conditions until more than 50% of functional renal capacity is destroyed by disease or injury

The final stage is end-stage renal disease (ESRD), which is irreversible.

Various biochemical substances accumulate in the blood as a result of diminished renal function and produce complications such as the following:

Anemia caused by hematologic dysfunction, including shortened life span of RBCs, impaired RBC production related to decreased production of erythropoietin, prolonged bleeding time, and nutritional anemia

Calcium and phosphorus disturbances resulting in altered bone metabolism, which in turn causes bone demineralization, growth arrest or retardation, bone pain, and deformities known as renal osteodystrophy

Growth disturbance, probably caused by such factors as poor nutrition, anorexia, renal osteodystrophy, biochemical abnormalities, corticosteroid treatment, tissue resistance to growth hormone, and mineral and vitamin deficiencies

Hyperkalemia of dangerous levels; occurrence uncommon until the end stage

Metabolic acidosis of a sustained nature because of continual hydrogen ion retention and bicarbonate loss

Retention of waste products, especially BUN and creatinine

Water and sodium retention, which contribute to edema and vascular congestion

## Assessment
### Initial Assessment
Perform a routine physical assessment with special attention to measurements of growth parameters.

Take a health history, especially regarding renal dysfunction, eating behavior, frequency of infections, and energy level.

Observe for evidence of manifestations of chronic renal failure.
  Early signs
  - Loss of normal energy
  - Increased fatigue on exertion
  - Pallor, subtle (may not be noticed)
  - Elevated blood pressure (sometimes)
  - Growth delay

  As the disease progresses
  - Decreased appetite (especially at breakfast)
  - Less interest in normal activities
  - Increased or decreased urinary output with compensatory intake of fluid
  - Pallor more evident
  - Sallow, muddy appearance of skin

  Possible complaints
  - Headache
  - Muscle cramps
  - Nausea

  Other signs and symptoms
  - Weight loss
  - Facial edema
  - Malaise
  - Bone or joint pain
  - Growth retardation
  - Dryness or itching of the skin

- Bruised skin
- Sensory or motor loss (sometimes)
- Amenorrhea (common in adolescent girls)

Uremic syndrome (untreated)
- Gastrointestinal (GI) symptoms
  - Anorexia
  - Nausea and vomiting
- Bleeding tendencies
  - Bruises
  - Bloody, diarrheal stools
  - Stomatitis
  - Bleeding from lips and mouth
- Intractable itching
- Uremic frost (deposits of urea crystals on skin)
- Unpleasant uremic breath odor
- Deep respirations
- Hypertension
- Congestive heart failure

- Pulmonary edema
- Neurologic involvement
  - Progressive confusion
  - Dulled sensorium
  - Coma (ultimately)
  - Tremors
  - Muscular twitching
  - Seizures

### Ongoing Assessment

Take a history for new or increasing symptoms.

Carry out frequent physical assessments with particular attention to blood pressure, signs of edema, and neurologic dysfunction.

Assess psychologic responses to the disease and its therapies.

Assist with diagnostic procedures and tests (e.g., urinalysis, CBC, blood chemistry, and renal biopsy).

## ⊖ The Child with Nephrotic Syndrome

*Nephrotic syndrome*—A clinical state characterized by an increased permeability of the glomerular membrane to protein, which results in massive urinary protein loss

## Assessment

Perform a physical assessment, including assessment of extent of edema.

Take a careful health history, especially relative to recent weight gain or renal dysfunction.

Observe for manifestations of nephrotic syndrome.
- Weight gain
- Edema
- Puffiness of face, especially around the eyes
  - Apparent on arising in the morning
  - Subsides during the day

Abdominal swelling (ascites)

Respiratory difficulty (pleural effusion)

Labial or scrotal swelling

Edema of intestinal mucosa causes the following:
- Diarrhea
- Anorexia
- Poor intestinal absorption

Extreme skin pallor (often)

Irritability

Easily fatigued

Lethargic

Blood pressure normal or slightly decreased

Susceptibility to infection

Urine alterations
- Decreased volume
- Darkly opalescent
- Frothy

Assist with diagnostic procedures and tests (e.g., urinalysis for protein, casts, and RBCs; blood analysis for serum protein [total, albumin/globulin ratio, cholesterol]; hemoglobin; hematocrit; serum sodium; renal biopsy).

## ⊖ The Child with Neurologic Dysfunction

*Cerebral dysfunction*—Concerns disorders affecting cerebral structure and function

## Assessment
### Initial Assessment

Take a careful history.
- Family history, for evidence of genetic disorders with neurologic manifestations
- Health history, especially for clues regarding the cause of dysfunction (e.g., injury, short febrile illness, encounter with an animal or insect, ingestion of neurotoxic substances, inhalation of chemicals, past illness, or known diabetes mellitus or sickle cell disease)

- Sudden or progressive alterations in movement (e.g., ataxia, seizures) or mental ability
- Headache, nausea, vomiting, double vision, bowel or bladder incontinence in a previously continent child
- Unusual behavior, including nature and frequency

Perform physical assessment with special emphasis on the following:
- Neurologic assessment (see p. 68)
- Assessment of cranial nerves (see p. 33)
- Developmental assessment (see p. 121)

Perform physical evaluation of infant.
- Size and shape of the head
- Spontaneous activity and postural reflex activity

- Sensory responses
- **Attitude**—Normal flexed posture, extreme extension, opisthotonos, hypotonia
- Symmetry in movement of extremities
- Excessive tremulousness or frequent twitching movements
- Altered expiratory cycle
  - Prolonged apnea
  - Ataxic breathing
  - Paradoxic chest movement
  - Hyperventilation
- Skin and hair texture
- Distinctive facial features
- Presence of a high-pitched, piercing cry
- Abnormal eye movements
- Inability to suck or swallow
- Lip smacking
- Asymmetric contraction of facial muscles
- Yawning (may indicate cranial nerve involvement)
- Muscular activity and coordination
- Level of development

Observe for speed of movement and the presence and location of any tremors, twitching, tics, or other unusual movements.

Observe gait (e.g., ataxia, spasticity, rigidity).

Note any unusual discharge from body orifices.

Note location, extent, and type of any wound.

Assess level of consciousness.*

    **Full consciousness**—Awake and alert; oriented to time, place, and person; behavior appropriate for age

    **Confusion**—Impaired decision making

    **Disorientation**—Confusion regarding time, place; decreased level of consciousness

    **Lethargy**—Limited spontaneous movement, sluggish speech, drowsiness; falls asleep quickly

    **Obtundation**—Arousable with stimulation

    **Stupor**—Remains in a deep sleep, responsive only to vigorous and repeated stimulation; simple motor or moaning responses to stimuli, responses slow

    **Coma**—No motor or verbal response to noxious or painful stimuli or decerebrate posturing

    **Persistent vegetative state (PVS)**—Permanently lost function of the cerebral cortex; eyes follow objects only by reflex or when attracted to the direction of loud sounds; all four limbs are spastic but can withdraw from painful stimuli; hands show reflexive grasping and groping; the face can grimace; some food may be swallowed; and the child may groan or cry but utters no words.

Observe for evidence of increased intracranial pressure (ICP).

Infants

- Tense, bulging fontanel; lack of normal pulsations
- Separated cranial sutures

- Macewen (cracked-pot) sign
- Irritability
- High-pitched cry
- Increased frontooccipital circumference (FOC)
- Distended scalp veins
- Changes in feeding
- Cries when disturbed
- Setting-sun sign

Children

- Headache
- Nausea
- Forceful vomiting, often without nausea
- Diplopia, blurred vision
- Seizures

Personality and behavior signs

- Irritability, restlessness
- Indifference, drowsiness, or lack of interest
- Decline in school performance
- Diminished physical activity and motor performance
- Increased devoted sleeping
- Memory loss if pressure is markedly increased
- Inability to follow simple commands
- Progression to lethargy and drowsiness

Late signs

- Decreased motor response to command
- Decreased sensory response to painful stimuli
- Alterations in pupil size and reactivity
- Sometimes decerebrate or decorticate posturing
- Cheyne-Stokes respirations
- Papilledema
- Decreased consciousness
- Coma

Assist with diagnostic procedures and tests (e.g., lumbar puncture, subdural tap, ventricular puncture, electroencephalography, radiography, magnetic resonance imaging [MRI], computed tomography [CT], nuclear brain scan, echoencephalography, positron emission transaxial tomography, real-time ultrasonography, digital subtraction angiography; blood biochemistry [pH, blood gases, ammonia, glucose], and any special tests).

### Ongoing Assessment (Extent of Assessment Depends on Condition)

Monitor vital signs, especially noting changes in the following:

- Temperature, pulse, blood pressure
- **Respirations**—Regular or irregular, deep or shallow, pattern of breathing, odor of breath

Eye movements

- **Position of globes**—Divergence, conjugate deviation, skewed
- **Movement of globes**—Extraocular palsy, nystagmus, fixed gaze

---

*Modified from Seidel HM and others, editors: *Mosby's guide to physical examination,* ed 6, St Louis, 2006, Mosby.

- **Pupil size**—Dilated, pinpoint, unequal
- **Pupil reaction**—Sluggish, absent, different
- Doll's head maneuver (only if cervical spine injury has been ruled out)

Motor function

- Voluntary movements of extremities (e.g., purposeful or random)
- Changes in muscular tone
- Changes in position of body and/or head
- Tremor, twitching
- Seizure activity (e.g., generalized or partial)
- Signs of meningeal irritation (e.g., nuchal rigidity or opisthotonos)
- **Spontaneous**—Normal but reduced, involuntary, evoked
- **Evoked**—Purposeful, reflex withdrawal

- **Paresis**—Decorticate, decerebrate; any lateralized difference in function
- **Crying and speech**—Present or absent, conversant or confused, monosyllabic, jargon, type of cry (piercing, difficult to hear)
- Level of consciousness
- Monitor ICP device
- Monitor CVP device
- Monitor fluid intake and output
- Weigh daily or as ordered to detect fluid accumulation or reduction
- **Headache (if information can be elicited)**—Presence or absence, type and location, continuous or intermittent
- In infants:
  - ○ Measure FOC
  - ○ **Assess status of fontanel**—Size and tension

## ⊖ The Child with Seizures

*Epilepsy*—A chronic seizure disorder with recurrent and unprovoked seizures, which requires long-term treatment. Not every seizure is epileptic.

*Seizures*—Brief malfunctions of the brain's electrical system resulting from cortical neuronal discharge. Seizures may manifest as convulsions (involuntary muscular contraction and relaxation); changes in behavior, sensations, or perception; visual and auditory hallucinations; and altered consciousness or unconsciousness.

## Assessment

Obtain a health history, especially regarding prenatal, perinatal, and neonatal events; any instances of infection, apnea, colic, or poor feeding; and any information regarding previous accidents or serious illnesses.

Obtain a history of seizure activity including the following:

- Description of child's behavior during seizure
- Age of onset
- Time when seizure occurred—Time of day, while awake or during sleep, relationship to meals
- Any triggering factors that might have precipitated seizure (e.g., fever, infection); falls that may have caused trauma to the head; anxiety; fatigue; activity (e.g., hyperventilation); environmental events (e.g., exposure to strong stimuli such as bright, flashing lights or loud noises)
- Sensory phenomena child experiences
- Duration, progression, and any postictal feelings or behaviors

Perform a physical and neurologic assessment.

Observe seizure manifestations.

Assist with diagnostic procedures and tests (e.g., electroencephalography, tomography, skull radiography, echoencephalography, brain scan; blood chemistry, serum glucose, BUN, ammonia; and specific tests for metabolic disorders).

### Observe Seizure

Describe the following:

- Only what is actually observed
- Order of events (before, during, and after)

Duration of seizure

- Tonic-clonic: from first signs of event until jerking stops
- Absence: from loss of consciousness until patient regains consciousness
- Complex partial: from first sign of unresponsiveness, motor activity, or automatisms until there is responsiveness to environment

### Onset

Time of onset

**Significant preseizure events**—Bright lights, noise, excitement, emotional outbursts

Behavior

- Change in facial expression, such as fear
- Cry or other sound
- Stereotypic or automatous movements
- Random activity (wandering)

Position of head, body, extremities

- Unilateral or bilateral posturing of one or more extremities
- Body deviation to side

### Movement

Change of position, if any

**Site of commencement**—Hand, thumb, mouth, generalized

**Tonic phase, if present**—Length, parts of body involved

**Clonic phase**—Twitching or jerking movements, parts of body involved, sequence of parts involved, generalized, change in character of movements

Lack of movement or muscle tone of any body part or entire body

### Face

Color change—Pallor, cyanosis, flushing

Perspiration

Mouth—Position, deviation to one side, teeth clenched, tongue bitten, frothing at mouth, flecks of blood or bleeding

Lack of expression

### Eyes

Position—Straight ahead, deviation upward, deviation outward, conjugate or divergent

Pupils (if able to assess)—Change in size, equality, reaction to light, and accommodation

### Respiratory Effort

Presence and length of apnea

Presence of stertor

### Other

Involuntary urination

Involuntary defecation

### Observe Postictally

Duration of postictal period

Method of termination

State of consciousness—Unresponsiveness, drowsiness, confusion

Orientation to time, persons

Sleeping but able to be aroused

Motor ability

- Any change in motor power
- Ability to move all extremities
- Any paresis or weakness
- Ability to whistle (if appropriate to age)

Speech—Changes, peculiarities, type and extent of any difficulties

Sensations

- Complaint of discomfort or pain
- Any sensory impairment of hearing, vision
- Recollection of preseizure sensations, warning of attack
- Awareness that attack was beginning
- Recall of words spoken to child

## The Child with a Head Injury

Head injury—A pathologic process involving the scalp, skull, meninges, or brain as a result of mechanical force

Concussion—A transient and reversible neuronal dysfunction, with instantaneous loss of awareness and responsiveness, that results from trauma to the head

Contusion—Petechial hemorrhages or localized bruising along superficial aspects of the brain at the site of impact (coup injury) or a lesion remote from the site of direct trauma (contrecoup injury)

## Assessment

Assess airway, breathing, and circulation.

Examine head for evidence of injury—bruises, lacerations, swelling, depression, drainage or bleeding from any orifice.

Perform a physical assessment of body for evidence of associated injuries, especially spinal cord injury.

Obtain a history of event and subsequent management.

Observe for manifestations of head injury.

### Minor Injury

May or may not lose consciousness

Transient period of confusion

Somnolence

Listlessness

Irritability

Pallor

Vomiting (one or more episodes)

### Signs of Progression

Altered mental status (e.g., difficulty rousing child)

Mounting agitation

Development of focal lateral neurologic signs

Marked changes in vital signs

### Severe Injury

Signs of increased ICP

- Increased head size (infant)
- Bulging fontanel (infant)

Retinal hemorrhage

Extraocular palsies (especially cranial nerve VI)

Hemiparesis

Quadriplegia

Elevated temperature

Unsteady gait

Papilledema

### Associated Signs

Scalp trauma

Other injuries (e.g., to extremities)

- Observe for additional neurologic data
- Bruises and wounds—Location, extent, type
- Unusual behavior—Note nature and frequency, related circumstances
- Incontinence in toilet-trained child (bowel, bladder); spontaneous or associated with other phenomena (e.g., seizure activity)

Assist with diagnostic procedures and tests. (See assessment of the child with neurologic dysfunction, pp. 86-88.)

### Ongoing Assessment

Perform frequent neurologic (Figure 1-31) assessment including the following:

- ⊖ Level of consciousness

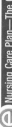

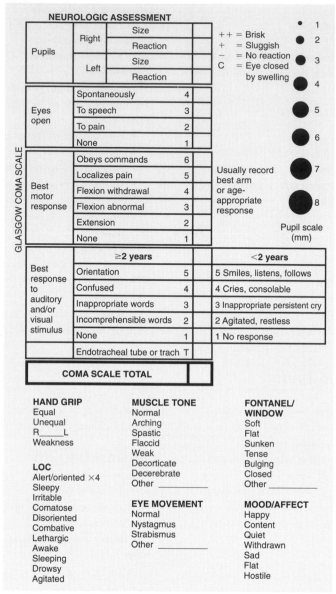

FIGURE **1-31**   Pediatric Glasgow Coma Scale.

- Position and movement
- Presence of headache
- **Young child**—Fussy and restless when handled; rolls head from side to side
- **Older child**—Self-report
- Presence of vertigo
- Child assumes a position and vigorously resists efforts to be moved; forcible movement causes child to vomit and display spontaneous nystagmus.

- Seizures (relatively common in head injury) (see p. 88)
- Presence of drainage from any orifice—Amount and characteristics
- Signs of increased ICP
- Observe for bleeding from nose or ears.
- Test rhinorrhea for glucose (suggests leaking of cerebrospinal fluid [CSF]).

Assist with diagnostic tests (CT scan, MRI, skull x-ray films).

## ⊜ The Child with Acute Bacterial Meningitis

*Acute bacterial meningitis*—A bacterial infection of the meninges and CSF

### Assessment

Obtain a health history, especially regarding a previous infection, injury, or exposure.

Perform a physical assessment.

Observe for the following manifestations of bacterial meningitis.

Children and adolescents
- Usually abrupt onset
- Fever

- Chills
- Headache
- Vomiting
- Alterations in sensorium
- Seizures (often the initial sign)
- Irritability
- Agitation
- May develop:
  o Photophobia
  o Delirium
  o Hallucinations
  o Aggressive behavior
  o Drowsiness
  o Stupor
  o Coma
- Nuchal rigidity
- May progress to opisthotonos
- Positive Kernig and Brudzinski signs (see p. 71)
- Hyperactive but variable reflex responses
- Signs and symptoms peculiar to individual organisms
- Petechial or purpuric rashes (meningococcal infection), especially when associated with a shocklike state
- Joint involvement (meningococcal and *H. influenzae* infection)
- Chronically draining ear (pneumococcal meningitis)

Infants and young children
- Classic picture rarely seen in children between 3 months and 2 years of age
- Fever
- Poor feeding
- Vomiting

- Marked irritability
- Restlessness
- Frequent seizures (often accompanied by a high-pitched cry)
- Bulging fontanel
- Nuchal rigidity may or may not be present.
- Brudzinski and Kernig signs may occur late.
- Subdural empyema (*H. influenzae* infection)

Neonates: specific signs
- Extremely difficult to diagnose
- Manifestations vague and nonspecific
- Well at birth but within a few days begins to look and behave poorly
- Refuses feedings
- Poor sucking ability
- Vomiting or diarrhea
- Poor tone
- Lack of movement
- Poor cry
- Full, tense, and bulging fontanel may appear late in course of illness
- Neck usually supple

Neonates: nonspecific signs
- Hypothermia or fever (depending on the maturity of the infant)
- Jaundice
- Irritability
- Drowsiness
- Seizures
- Respiratory irregularities or apnea
- Cyanosis
- Weight loss

Assist with diagnostic procedures and tests (e.g., lumbar puncture, spinal fluid examination, cultures).

## The Child with Diabetes Mellitus

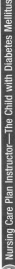

*Diabetes mellitus (DM)*—A chronic disorder involving primarily carbohydrate metabolism and characterized by a partial or complete deficiency of the hormone insulin. DM can be classified into the following three major groups:

Maturity-onset diabetes of youth—Transmitted as an autosomal-dominant disorder that is characterized by impaired insulin secretion with minimal or no defects in insulin action

Type 1 (previously called insulin-dependent diabetes mellitus [IDDM])—Characterized by destruction of the pancreatic beta cells, which produce insulin; this usually leads to absolute insulin deficiency.

Type 2 (previously called non–insulin-dependent diabetes mellitus [NIDDM])—Usually arises because of insulin resistance, in which the body fails to use insulin properly, combined with relative (not absolute) insulin deficiency

### Assessment

Perform a physical assessment.

Obtain a family history, especially regarding other members who have diabetes.

Obtain a health history, especially relative to weight loss, frequency of drinking and voiding, increased appetite, diminished activity level, behavior changes, and other manifestations of type 1 diabetes mellitus as follows:
- The three polys (cardinal signs of diabetes)
  o Polyphagia
  o Polyuria
  o Polydipsia
- Weight loss
- Child may start bed-wetting
- Irritability and "not himself" or "not herself"
- Shortened attention span
- Temper tantrums in young children
- Appears overly tired
- Dry skin

| TABLE 1-6 | Comparison of Manifestations of Hypoglycemia and Hyperglycemia | |
|---|---|---|
| **Variable** | **Hypoglycemia** | **Hyperglycemia** |
| Onset | Rapid (minutes) | Gradual (days) |
| Mood | Labile, irritable, nervous, weepy, combative | Lethargic |
| Mental status | Difficulty concentrating, speaking, focusing, coordinating | Dulled sensorium |
| | | Confused |
| Inward feeling | Shaky feeling, hunger | Thirst |
| | Headache | Weakness |
| | Dizziness | Nausea and vomiting |
| | | Abdominal pain |
| Skin | Pallor | Flushed |
| | Sweating | Signs of dehydration |
| Mucous membranes | Normal | Dry, crusty |
| Respirations | Shallow | Deep, rapid (Kussmaul) |
| Pulse | Tachycardia | Less rapid, weak |
| Breath odor | Normal | Fruity, acetone |
| Neurologic | Tremors | Diminished reflexes |
| | Late: hyperreflexia, dilated pupils, seizure | Paresthesia |
| Ominous signs | Shock, coma | Acidosis, coma |
| **Blood** | | |
| Glucose | Low: below 60 mg/dl | High: 240 mg/dl or more |
| Ketones | Negative or trace | High or large |
| Osmolarity | Normal | High |
| pH | Normal | Low (7.25 or less) |
| Hematocrit | Normal | High |
| $HCO_3$ | Normal | Less than 15 mEq/L |
| **Urine** | | |
| Output | Normal | Polyuria (early) to oliguria (late) |
| Glucose | Negative | High |
| Acetone | Negative or trace | High |

- Blurred vision
- Poor wound healing
- Flushed skin
- Headache
- Frequent infections, including perineal yeast infections and/or thrush
- Hyperglycemia (Table 1-6)
  - Elevated blood glucose levels
  - Glucosuria
- Diabetic ketosis
  - Ketones as well as glucose in urine
  - No noticeable dehydration

- Diabetic ketoacidosis
  - Dehydration
  - Electrolyte imbalance
  - Acidosis
  - Progresses to coma, death

Perform or assist with diagnostic procedures and tests (e.g., fasting blood sugar, serum insulin levels, urine for ketones, blood glucose, serum islet cell antibody level).

# The Child with a Fracture

⊖ *Fracture*—A break in the continuity of a bone caused when the resistance of the bone yields to a stress or force exerted on it

*Comminuted fracture*—Small fragments of bone are broken from fractured shaft and lie in surrounding tissue (rare in children).

**Complete fracture**—Fracture fragments are separated.

**Complicated fracture**—Bone fragments cause damage to other organs or tissues (e.g., lung, bladder).

**Incomplete fracture**—Fracture fragments remain attached.

**Open or compound fracture**—Fracture has an open wound through which the bone has protruded.

**Simple or closed fracture**—Fracture does not produce a break in the skin.

Most frequent fractures in children:

**Bends**—A child's flexible bone can be bent 45 degrees or more before breaking. However, if bent, the bone will straighten slowly, but not completely, to produce some deformity but without the angulation that exists when the bone breaks. Bends occur more commonly in the ulna and fibula, often associated with fractures of the radius and tibia.

**Buckle fracture**—Compression of the porous bone produces a buckle or torus fracture. This appears as a raised or bulging projection at the fracture site. Torus fractures occur in the most porous portion of the bone near the metaphysis (the portion of the bone shaft adjacent to the epiphysis) and are more common in young children.

**Greenstick fracture**—Occurs when a bone is angulated beyond the limits of bending; the compressed side bends and the tension side fails, causing an incomplete fracture similar to the break observed when a green stick is broken.

**Complete fracture**—Divides the bone fragments; they often remain attached by a periosteal hinge, which can aid or hinder reduction.

## Assessment

Obtain a history of event, previous injury, and experience with health personnel.

Observe for manifestations of fracture.

Signs of injury

Generalized swelling

Pain or tenderness

Diminished functional use of affected part (Strongly suspect fracture in small child who refuses to walk or move an upper extremity.)

Bruising

Severe muscular rigidity

Crepitus (grating sensation at fracture site)

Assess for location of fracture. Observe for deformity; instruct child to point to painful area.

Assess for circulation and sensation distal to fracture site.

Assist with diagnostic procedures and tests (e.g., radiography, tomography).

## Assessment of the Extremity in a Cast or Traction

Assess the 5 Ps as follows:

- Pain and point of tenderness
- *Pulselessness*—distal to the fracture site (late and ominous sign)
- Pallor
- *Paresthesia*—sensation distal to the fracture site
- *Paralysis*—movement distal to the fracture site

## The Child Who Is Maltreated

*Child maltreatment*—A broad term that includes intentional physical abuse or neglect, emotional abuse or neglect, and sexual abuse of children, usually by an adult

*Emotional abuse*—The deliberate attempt to destroy or significantly impair a child's self-esteem or competence

*Emotional neglect*—Failure to meet the child's needs for affection, attention, and emotional nurturance

*Physical abuse*—The deliberate infliction of physical injury

*Physical neglect*—The deprivation of necessities, such as food, clothing, shelter, supervision, medical care, and education

*Munchausen syndrome by proxy*—Physical abuse inflicted on a child, usually by the mother, to fabricate or induce an illness that requires medical care for the child

*Sexual abuse*—Contacts or interactions between a child and an adult when the child is being used for the sexual stimulation of that adult or another person

### Assessment

Perform a physical assessment with special attention to manifestations of potential abuse or neglect (Box 1-8).

Obtain a history of event, being alert for discrepancies in descriptions by caregiver and observations.

- Note sequence of events, including times, especially time lapse between occurrence of injury and initiation of treatment.
- Interview child when appropriate, including verbal quotations and information from drawings or other play activities.
- Interview parents, witnesses, and other significant persons, including their verbal quotations.

Observe parent-child interactions (e.g., verbal interactions, eye contact, touching, evidence of parental concern).

Observe or obtain information regarding names, ages, and conditions of other children in the home (if possible).

Perform a developmental test.

Assist with diagnostic procedures and tests (e.g., radiology, collection of specimens for examination).

## BOX 1-8 | Clinical Manifestations of Potential Child Maltreatment

### Physical Neglect
**Suggestive Physical Findings**
Failure to thrive
Signs of malnutrition, such as thin extremities, abdominal distention, lack of subcutaneous fat
Poor personal hygiene
Unclean and/or inappropriate dress
Evidence of poor health care, such as delayed immunization, untreated infections, frequent colds
Frequent injuries from lack of supervision

**Suggestive Behaviors**
Dull and inactive; excessively passive or sleepy
Self-stimulatory behaviors, such as finger-sucking or rocking
Begging or stealing food
Absenteeism from school
Drug or alcohol addiction
Vandalism or shoplifting

### Emotional Abuse and Neglect
**Suggestive Physical Findings**
Failure to thrive
Feeding disorders
Enuresis
Sleep disorders

**Suggestive Behaviors**
Self-stimulatory behaviors such as biting, rocking, sucking
During infancy, lack of social smile and stranger anxiety
Withdrawal
Unusual fearfulness
Antisocial behavior, such as destructiveness, stealing, cruelty
Extremes of behavior, such as overcompliant and passive or aggressive and demanding
Lags in emotional and intellectual development, especially language
Suicide attempts

### Physical Abuse
**Suggestive Physical Findings**
Bruises and welts (may be in various stages of healing)
On face, lips, mouth, back, buttocks, thighs, or areas of torso
Regular patterns descriptive of object used, such as belt buckle, hand, wire hanger, chain, wooden spoon, squeeze or pinch marks
Burns on soles of feet, palms of hands, back, or buttocks
Patterns descriptive of object used, such as round cigar or cigarette burns, sharply demarcated areas from immersion in scalding water, rope burns on wrists or ankles from being bound, burns in the shape of an iron, radiator, or electric stove burner
Absence of "splash" marks and presence of symmetric burns
Fractures and dislocations
Skull, nose, or facial structures
Injury may denote type of abuse, such as spiral fracture or dislocation from twisting of an extremity or whiplash from shaking the child
Multiple new or old fractures in various stages of healing
Lacerations and abrasions on backs of arms, legs, torso, face, or external genitalia

Unusual symptoms, such as abdominal swelling, pain, and vomiting from punching
Descriptive marks such as from human bites or pulling out of hair
Chemical
Unexplained repeated poisoning, especially drug overdose
Unexplained sudden illness, such as hypoglycemia from insulin administration

**Suggestive Behaviors**
Wariness of physical contact with adults
Apparent fear of parents or of going home
Lying very still while surveying environment
Inappropriate reaction to injury, such as failure to cry from pain
Lack of reaction to frightening events
Apprehensiveness when hearing other children cry
Indiscriminate friendliness and displays of affection
Superficial relationships
Acting-out behavior, such as aggression, to seek attention
Withdrawal behavior

### Sexual Abuse
**Suggestive Physical Findings**
Bruises, bleeding, lacerations or irritation of external genitalia, anus, mouth, or throat
Torn, stained, or bloody underclothing
Pain on urination or pain, swelling, and itching of genital area
Penile discharge
Sexually transmitted disease, nonspecific vaginitis, or venereal warts
Difficulty in walking or sitting
Unusual odor in the genital area
Recurrent urinary tract infections
Presence of semen
Pregnancy in young adolescent

**Suggestive Behaviors**
Sudden emergence of sexually related problems, including excessive or public masturbation, age-inappropriate sexual play, promiscuity, or overtly seductive behavior
Withdrawn behavior, excessive daydreaming
Preoccupation with fantasies, especially in play
Poor relationships with peers
Sudden changes, such as anxiety, loss or gain of weight, clinging behavior
In incestuous relationships, excessive anger at mother for not protecting daughter
Regressive behavior, such as bed-wetting or thumb sucking
Sudden onset of phobias or fears, particularly fears of the dark, men, strangers, or particular settings or situations (e.g., undue fear of leaving the house or staying at the daycare center or the baby-sitter's house)
Running away from home
Substance abuse, particularly of alcohol or mood-elevating drugs
Profound and rapid personality changes, especially extreme depression, hostility, and aggression (often accompanied by social withdrawal)
Rapidly declining school performance
Suicidal attempts or ideation

# ⊖The Child with Burns

*Burns*—The destruction of skin caused by thermal, chemical, electric, or radioactive agents

Burn severity criteria

  *Minor burns*—Partial-thickness burns of less than 10% of body surface area (BSA)

  *Moderate burns*—Partial-thickness burns of 10% to 20% of BSA (age-related; see Major, or critical, burns)

  *Major, or critical, burns*

- Burns complicated by respiratory tract injury
- Partial-thickness burns of 20% or more of BSA
- Burns of face, hands, feet, or genitalia, even if they appear to be partial thickness
- All full-thickness burns
- Any child younger than 2 years of age, unless the burn is very small and very superficial (20% or more of BSA considered critical in child younger than 2 years of age)
- Electric burns that penetrate
- Deep chemical burns
- Respiratory tract damage
- Burns complicated by fractures or soft tissue injury

- Burns complicated by concurrent illness, such as obesity, diabetes, epilepsy, or cardiac or renal disease

## Assessment
### Initial Assessments

Assess respiratory status.

Assess for extent of burn injury based on percentage of BSA involved (Figure 1-32).

Assess for depth of burn injury.

  Superficial (first-degree) burns

- Dry, red surface
- Blanches on pressure and refills
- Minimal or no edema
- Painful; sensitive to touch

  Partial-thickness (second-degree) burns

- Blistered, moist
- Serous drainage
- Edema
- Mottled pink or red
- Blanches on pressure and refills
- Very painful; sensitive to touch

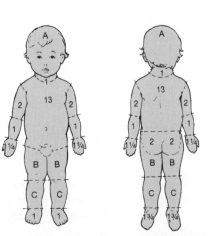

**RELATIVE PERCENTAGES OF AREAS AFFECTED BY GROWTH**

| AREA | BIRTH | AGE 1 YR | AGE 5 YR |
|---|---|---|---|
| A = ½ of head | 9½ | 8½ | 6½ |
| B = ½ of one thigh | 2¾ | 3¼ | 4 |
| C = ½ of one leg | 2½ | 2½ | 2¾ |

A

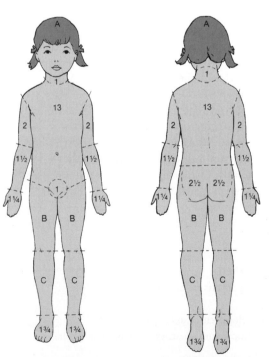

**RELATIVE PERCENTAGES OF AREAS AFFECTED BY GROWTH**

| AREA | AGE 10 YR | AGE 15 YR | ADULT |
|---|---|---|---|
| A = ½ of head | 5½ | 4½ | 3½ |
| B = ½ of one thigh | 4½ | 4½ | 4¾ |
| C = ½ of one leg | 3 | 3¼ | 3½ |

B

FIGURE **1-32** Estimation of distribution of burns in children. A, Children from birth to age 5 years. B, Older children.

Full-thickness (third-degree) burns
- Tough, leathery
- Dull, dry surface
- Marbled, pale white, brown, tan, red, or black
- Does not blanch on pressure
- Edema
- Variable pain, often severe

**Assess for evidence of associated injuries.**
- Check eyes for injury or irritation.
- Check nasopharynx for edema or redness.
- Check for singed hair, including nasal hair.
- Assess for other injuries (e.g., bruises, fractures, internal injuries).

Observe for evidence of respiratory distress.
Assess need for pain medication.
Weigh child on admission; take vital signs.
Assess level of consciousness (see p. 86).
Obtain history of burn injury, especially time of injury, nature of burning agent, duration of contact, whether injury occurred in an enclosed area, and any medication given.

Obtain pertinent history relative to preburn condition—weight, preexisting illnesses, any allergies, and tetanus immunization.
Assist with diagnostic procedures and tests (e.g., blood count, urinalysis, wound cultures, and hematocrit).

### Ongoing Assessments
Monitor vital signs, including blood pressure.
Measure intake and output.
Monitor intravenous (IV) infusion; observe for evidence of overhydration.
Assess circulation of areas peripheral to burns.
Assess for evidence of healing, stability of temporary cover or graft, and infection.
*Observe for evidence of complications*—pneumonia, wound sepsis, Curling (stress) ulcer, central nervous system (CNS) dysfunction (hallucinations, personality changes, delirium, seizures, alterations in sensorium), hypertension.

# ⊖ The Child with Attention Deficit Hyperactivity Disorder

*Attention deficit hyperactivity disorder (ADHD)*—An illness consisting of three primary characteristics: inappropriate degrees of inattention, impulsivity, and hyperactivity. The goals of treatment for ADHD include pharmacologic therapy with CNS stimulants such as methylphenidate (Ritalin, Metadate) and dextroamphetamine (Dexedrine),* home behavior management to reduce impulsive behavior and increase attentiveness, a structured school environment to increase educational success and decrease frustration with learning, and psychologic counseling for the child and family. Coexisting problems sometimes seen in the child with ADHD include speech disorders, anxiety, depression, mood disorders, hearing and vision problems, oppositional defiant disorder, and learning disorders.

## Assessment
Perform a comprehensive age-appropriate physical assessment.
Perform a developmental assessment.
Obtain a developmental history for evidence of the following:
- Aggressive behavior in early childhood
- History of excessive fussiness and irritability as infant and toddler

- History of destructive behavior as small child
- History of disciplinary problems in early childhood

Obtain a family history.
- Some evidence suggests that one parent may have had similar problems as child; therefore a history of parents' childhoods is imperative.
- Note if other children in the family have been diagnosed with ADHD or have behaviors consistent with ADHD.
- Inquire about family daily routines, including mealtimes and time set aside for schoolwork and play time (to rule out the environment as a potential cause for distractions related to learning).

Assist with diagnostic test (e.g., electroencephalogram [EEG], blood lead levels, and thyroid levels to rule out potential organic causes of seizures, lead poisoning, and hyperthyroidism; neurologic evaluation; hearing and vision screening).
Evaluate the effectiveness of therapies prescribed (e.g., structured environment at school and home, pharmacotherapy, and family and child psychotherapy).
Perform and/or assist with psychometric testing.

---

*Note that pharmacotherapy is not limited to these medications.

# ⊖The Child with Poisoning

*Poisoning*—The condition or physical state produced when a substance, in relatively small amounts, is applied to body surfaces, ingested, injected, inhaled, or absorbed and subsequently causes structural damage or disturbance of function

## Assessment

Perform a physical assessment with particular attention to vital signs, breath odor, state of consciousness, skin changes, and neurologic signs.

Obtain a careful and detailed history regarding what, when, and how much of a toxic substance has entered the body.

Look for evidence of poison (e.g., container, plant, vomitus).

Observe for evidence of ingestion, inhalation, or absorption of toxic substances.

Skin manifestations
- Pallor
- Redness
- Evidence of burning
- Pain

Mucous membrane manifestations
- Evidence of irritation
- Red discoloration
- White discoloration
- Swelling

Gastrointestinal manifestations
- Salivation
- Dry mouth
- Nausea and vomiting
- Diarrhea
- Abdominal pain
- Anorexia

Cardiovascular manifestations
- Arrhythmias
- Delayed capillary refill
- Decreased blood pressure
- Increased, weak pulse
- Pallor
- Cool, clammy skin
- Evidence of shock

Respiratory manifestations
- Gagging, choking, coughing
- Increased, shallow respirations
- Bradypnea
- Unexplained cyanosis
- Grunting

Renal manifestations
- Oliguria
- Hematuria

Metabolic and autonomic manifestations
- Sweating
- Hyperthermia
- Hypothermia
- Metabolic acidosis

Neuromuscular manifestations
- Weakness
- Involuntary movements
- Teeth gnashing
- Ataxia
- Dilated pupils
- Constricted pupils
- Seizures

Altered sensorium
- Anxiety, agitation
- Hallucinations
- Loss of consciousness
- Dizziness
- Confusion
- Lethargy, stupor
- Coma

Observe for clinical manifestations characteristic of specific poison.

Assist with diagnostic tests (e.g., blood levels of toxins, radiograph to determine presence of masses of undissolved tablets remaining in GI tract).

Observe for latent symptoms of poisoning.

# The Child with Lead Poisoning

***Lead poisoning***—The chronic ingestion or inhalation of lead-containing substances, resulting in physical and mental dysfunction

## Assessment

Perform a physical assessment.

Obtain a history of possible sources of lead in the child's environment.

Ingested

- Lead-based paint*
  - ○ Interior: walls, windowsills, floors, furniture
  - ○ Exterior: door frames, fences, porches, siding
- Plaster, caulking
- Unglazed pottery
- Colored newsprint
- Painted food wrappers
- Cigarette butts and ashes
- Water from leaded pipes, water fountains
- Foods or liquids from cans soldered with lead
- Household dust
- Soil, especially along heavily trafficked roadways
- Food grown in contaminated soil

- Urban playgrounds
- Folk remedies
- Pewter vessels or dishes
- Food or drinks stored in lead crystal
- Lead bullets
- Lead fishing sinkers
- Lead curtain weights
- Hobby materials (e.g., leaded paint or solder for stained glass windows)

Inhaled

- Sanding and scraping of lead-based painted surfaces*
- Burning of leaded objects
  - ○ Automobile batteries
  - ○ Logs made of colored newspaper
- Automobile exhaust
- Cigarette smoke
- Sniffing leaded gasoline
- Dust
  - ○ Poorly cleaned urban housing
  - ○ Contaminated clothing and skin of household members working in smelting factories or construction

*Most common sources

Obtain a history of pica, or look for evidence of this behavior during assessment.

Obtain a dietary history, especially regarding intake of iron and calcium.

Observe for manifestations of lead poisoning.

General signs
- Anemia
- Acute crampy abdominal pain
- Vomiting
- Constipation
- Anorexia
- Headache
- Fever
- Lethargy
- Impaired growth

CNS signs (early)
- Hyperactivity
- Aggression
- Impulsiveness
- Decreased interest in play
- Lethargy
- Irritability
- Loss of developmental progress
- Hearing impairment
- Learning difficulties
- Short attention span
- Distractibility
- Mild intellectual deficits

CNS signs (late)
- Mental retardation
- Paralysis
- Blindness
- Convulsions
- Coma
- Death

Signs of gasoline sniffing
- Irritability
- Tremor
- Hallucinations
- Confusion
- Lack of impulse control
- Depression
- Impaired perception and coordination
- Sleep disturbances

Assist with diagnostic procedures and tests (e.g., blood-lead concentration, erythrocyte-protoporphyrin level, bone radiography, urinalysis, hemoglobin and CBC, and lead mobilization test).

# ⊖ The Child with a Communicable Disease

*Communicable disease*—An illness caused by a specific infectious agent or its toxic products through a direct or indirect mode of transmission of that agent from a reservoir

## Disease

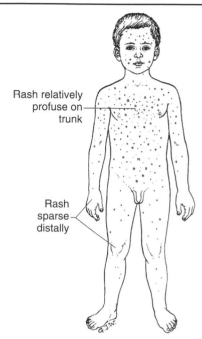

Rash relatively profuse on trunk

Rash sparse distally

*Chickenpox (Varicella) (Figure 1-33)*

**Cause:** Varicella-zoster virus (VZV)

**Source:** Respiratory secretions, to a lesser degree, skin lesions (scabs not infectious)

**Transmission:** Direct contact, droplet (airborne) spread, and contaminated objects

**Incubation period:** 2-3 weeks, usually 13-17 days

**Period of communicability:** 1 day before eruption of lesions (prodromal period) to the time when all lesions have crusted

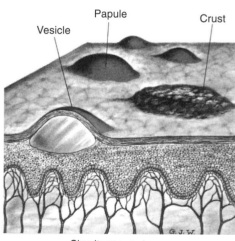

Papule

Vesicle

Crust

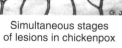

Simultaneous stages of lesions in chickenpox

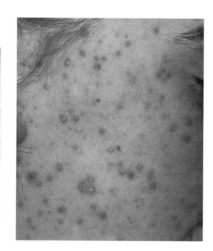

FIGURE **1-33** Chickenpox (varicella). (Clinical view from Habif TP: *Clinical dermatology: A color guide to diagnosis and therapy,* ed 5, St Louis, 2010, Mosby.)

| Clinical Manifestations | Nursing Considerations |
| --- | --- |
| Prodromal stage: Slight fever, malaise, and anorexia for first 24 hours; rash highly pruritic; begins as macule, rapidly progresses to papule and then vesicle (surrounded by erythematous base, breaks easily and forms crusts); all three stages (papule, vesicle, crust) present in varying degrees at one time | Maintain strict isolation in hospital. |
| | Isolate child in home until vesicles have dried, and isolate high-risk children from infected children. |
| | Administer skin care: Give bath and change clothes and linens daily; administer topical application of calamine lotion; keep child's fingernails short and clean; apply mittens if child scratches. |
| Distribution: Centripetal, spreading to face and proximal extremities but sparse on distal limbs and less on areas not exposed to heat (e.g., from clothing or sun) | Administer antihistamines and antiviral agents. |
| | If older child, reason with child regarding danger of scar formation from scratching. |
| Constitutional signs and symptoms: Fever, irritability from pruritus | Avoid use of aspirin; use of acetaminophen controversial. |

*Continued*

## The Child with a Communicable Disease—cont'd

### Disease

### Diphtheria

**Cause:** *Corynebacterium diphtheriae*

**Source:** Respiratory secretions, skin, and other lesions

**Transmission:** Direct contact with infected person, a carrier, or contaminated articles

**Incubation period:** Usually 2-5 days, possibly longer

**Period of communicability:** Variable; until virulent bacilli are no longer present (identified by three negative cultures); usually 2 weeks but as long as 4 weeks

### Erythema Infectiosum (Fifth Disease) (Figure 1-34)

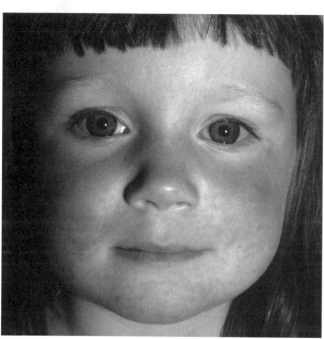

FIGURE **1-34**   Erythema infectiosum. (From Habif TP: *Clinical dermatology: A color guide to diagnosis and therapy,* ed 5, St Louis, 2010, Mosby.)

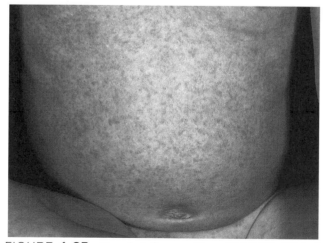

FIGURE **1-35**   Roseola infantum. (From Habif TP: *Clinical dermatology: A color guide to diagnosis and therapy,* ed 5, St Louis, 2010, Mosby.)

### Exanthema subitum (roseola) (Figure 1-35)

**Cause:** Human herpesvirus type 6 (HHV-6)

**Source:** Unknown

**Transmission:** Unknown (occurs between 6 months and 3 years of age)

**Incubation period:** Usually 5-15 days

**Period of communicability:** Unknown

| Clinical Manifestations | Nursing Considerations |
|---|---|
| Vary according to anatomic location of pseudomembrane | Maintain strict isolation in hospital. |
| Nasal: Resembles common cold, serosanguineous mucopurulent nasal discharge without constitutional symptoms; may be frank epistaxis | Participate in sensitivity testing; have epinephrine available. |
| Tonsillar or pharyngeal: Malaise; anorexia; sore throat; low-grade fever; smooth, adherent, white or gray membrane; lymphadenitis | Administer antibiotics; observe for signs of sensitivity to penicillin. |
| | Administer complete care to maintain bed rest. |
| Laryngeal: Fever, hoarseness, cough, with or without previous signs listed; potential airway obstruction, apprehension, dyspnea, cyanosis | Use suctioning as needed to maintain patent airway. Observe respirations for signs of obstruction. Administer humidified oxygen if prescribed. |
| Rash appears in three stages. | |
| I—Erythema on face, chiefly on cheeks, "slapped face" appearance; disappears by 1-4 days | Isolation of child not necessary, except hospitalized child (immunosuppressed or with aplastic crisis) suspected of human papillomavirus (HPV) infection is placed on respiratory isolation. |
| II—About 1 day after rash appears on face, maculopapular red spots appear, symmetrically distributed on upper and lower extremities; rash progresses from proximal to distal surfaces and may last a week or more. | Pregnant women: Need not be excluded from workplace where HPV infection is present; explain low risk of fetal death to those in contact with affected children. |
| III—Rash subsides but reappears if skin is irritated or traumatized (sun, heat, cold, friction). | |
| In child with aplastic crisis, rash is usually absent and prodromal illness includes fever, myalgia, lethargy, nausea, vomiting, and abdominal pain. | |
| Persistent high fever (greater than 38.9° C [102° F]) for 3-4 days in child who appears well | Administer antipyretics as needed. |
| Precipitous drop in fever to normal with appearance of rash (a typical exanthema subitum can occur without rash) | If child is prone to seizures, discuss appropriate precautions, possibility of recurrent febrile seizures. |
| Rash: Discrete rose-pink macules or maculopapules appearing first on trunk, then spreading to neck, face, and extremities; nonpruritic, fades on pressure; appears 2-3 days after onset of fever and lasts 1-2 days | |
| Associated signs and symptoms: Cervical or postauricular lymphadenopathy, injected pharynx, cough, coryza | |

*Continued*

## The Child with a Communicable Disease—cont'd

### Disease

**First day of rash** | **Third day of rash**

Koplik spots on buccal mucosa (see inset)

Confluent maculopapules

Rash discrete

Discrete maculopapules

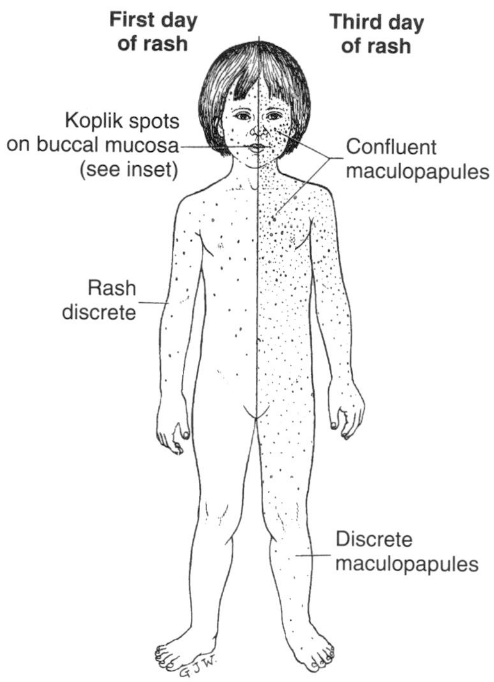

FIGURE **1-36** Measles. (Clinical view from Seidel HM, Ball JW, Dains JE, and others: *Mosby's guide to physical examination*, ed 4, St Louis, 1999, Mosby.)

### Measles (rubeola) (Figure 1-36)

**Cause:** Virus

**Source:** Respiratory secretions, blood, and urine

**Transmission:** Usually by direct contact with droplets from infected person

**Incubation period:** 10-20 days

**Period of communicability:** From 4 days before to 5 days after rash appears, but mainly during prodromal (catarrhal) stage

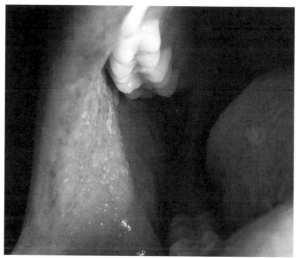

FIGURE **1-37** Koplik's spots. (From Habif TP: *Clinical dermatology: A color guide to diagnosis and therapy*, ed 5, St Louis, 2010, Mosby.)

### Mumps

**Cause:** Paramyxovirus

**Source:** Saliva

**Transmission:** Direct contact or droplet spread from an infected person

**Incubation period:** 14-21 days

**Period of communicability:** Most communicable immediately before and after swelling begins

### Pertussis (whooping cough)

**Cause:** *Bordetella pertussis*

**Source:** Respiratory secretions

**Transmission:** Direct contact or droplet spread from infected person; indirect contact with freshly contaminated articles

**Incubation period:** 5-21 days, usually 10

**Period of communicability:** Greatest during catarrhal stage before onset of paroxysms and may extend to fourth week after onset of paroxysms

| Clinical Manifestations | Nursing Considerations |
|---|---|

Prodromal (catarrhal) stage: Fever and malaise, followed in 24 hours by coryza, cough, conjunctivitis, Koplik spots (small, irregular red spots with a minute, bluish-white center first seen on buccal mucosa opposite molars 2 days before rash; Figure 1-37); symptoms gradually increase in severity until second day after rash appears, when they begin to subside.

Rash: Appears 3-4 days after onset of prodromal stage; begins as erythematous maculopapular eruption on face and gradually spreads downward; more severe in earlier sites (appears confluent) and less intense in later sites (appears discrete); after 3-4 days assumes brownish appearance, and fine desquamation occurs over areas of extensive involvement.

Constitutional signs and symptoms:

Anorexia, malaise, generalized lymphadenopathy

Isolation until fifth day of rash; if hospitalized, institute respiratory precautions.

Maintain bed rest during prodromal stage; provide quiet activity.

Fever: Instruct parents to administer antipyretics; avoid chilling; if child is prone to seizures, institute appropriate precautions. (Fever spikes to 40° C [104° F] between fourth and fifth days.)

Eye care: Dim lights if photophobia present; clean eyelids with warm saline solution to remove secretions or crusts; keep child from rubbing eyes; examine cornea for signs of ulceration.

Coryza/cough: Use cool-mist vaporizer; protect skin around nares with layer of petrolatum; encourage fluids and soft, bland foods.

Skin care: Keep skin clean; use tepid baths as necessary.

---

Prodromal stage: Fever, headache, malaise, and anorexia for 24 hours, followed by jaw or ear pain that is aggravated by chewing

Parotitis: By third day, parotid gland(s) (either unilateral or bilateral) enlarge and reach maximum size in 1-3 days; accompanied by pain and tenderness.

Isolation during period of communicability; institute respiratory precautions during hospitalization.

Maintain bed rest during prodromal phase until swelling subsides.

Give analgesics for pain.

Encourage fluids and soft, bland foods; avoid foods requiring chewing.

Apply hot or cold compresses to neck, whichever is more comforting.

To relieve orchitis, provide warmth and local support with tight-fitting underpants. (Stretch bathing suit works well.)

---

Catarrhal stage: Begins with signs and symptoms of upper respiratory tract infection, such as coryza, sneezing, lacrimation, cough, and low-grade fever; symptoms continue for 1-2 weeks, when dry, hacking cough becomes more severe.

Paroxysmal stage: Cough most often occurs at night and consists of short, rapid coughs followed by sudden inspiration associated with a high-pitched crowing sound or whoop; during paroxysm cheeks become flushed or cyanotic, vomiting frequently follows attack; stage generally lasts 4-6 weeks, followed by convalescent stage.

Isolation during catarrhal stage; if hospitalized, institute respiratory precautions.

Maintain bed rest as long as fever is present.

Provide restful environment and reduce factors that promote paroxysms (e.g., dust, smoke, sudden changes in temperature, chilling, activity, excitement); keep room well ventilated.

Encourage fluids; offer small amounts of fluids frequently; refeed child after vomiting.

Provide high humidity (humidifier or tent); suction as needed.

Observe for signs of airway obstruction (e.g., increased restlessness, apprehension, retractions, cyanosis).

*Continued*

# The Child with a Communicable Disease—cont'd

## Disease

### Poliomyelitis

**Cause:** Enteroviruses, three types: type 1—most frequent cause of paralysis, both epidemic and endemic; type 2—least frequently associated with paralysis; type 3—second most frequently associated with paralysis

**Source:** Feces and oropharyngeal secretions

**Transmission:** Direct contact with person with apparent or inapparent active infection; spread is via fecal-oral and pharyngeal-oropharyngeal routes

**Incubation period:** Usually 7-14 days, with range of 5-35 days

**Period of communicability:** Not exactly known; virus is present in throat and feces shortly after infection and persists for about 1 week in throat and 4-6 weeks in feces

### Rubella (German measles) (Figure 1-38)

**Cause:** Rubella virus

**Source:** Respiratory secretions; virus also present in blood, stool, and urine

**Transmission:** Direct contact and spread via infected person; indirectly via articles freshly contaminated with nasopharyngeal secretions, feces, or urine

**Incubation period:** 14-21 days

**Period of communicability:** 7 days before to about 5 days after appearance of rash

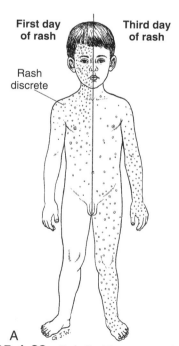
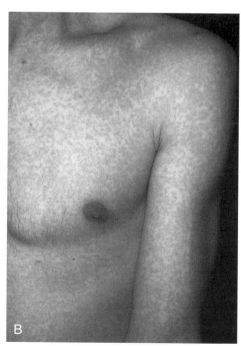

FIGURE **1-38** Rubella (German measles). A, Progression of rash. B, Clinical view. (From Habif TP: *Clinical dermatology: A color guide to diagnosis and therapy*, ed 5, St Louis, 2010, Mosby.)

| Clinical Manifestations | Nursing Considerations |
|---|---|
| May be manifested in three different forms: | Maintain complete bed rest. |
| Abortive or inapparent: Fever, uneasiness, sore throat, headache, anorexia, vomiting, abdominal pain; lasts a few hours to a few days | Administer mild sedatives as necessary to relieve anxiety and promote rest. |
| Nonparalytic: Same manifestations as abortive but more severe, with pain and stiffness in neck, back, and legs | Participate in physiotherapy procedures (use of moist hot packs and range-of-motion exercises). |
| Paralytic: Initial course similar to nonparalytic type, followed by recovery, then signs of CNS paralysis | Position child to maintain body alignment and prevent contractures or decubiti; use footboard. |
| | Encourage child to move; administer analgesics for maximum comfort during physical activity. |
| | Observe for respiratory paralysis (difficulty in talking, ineffective cough, inability to hold breath, shallow and rapid respirations); report such signs and symptoms to practitioner; have tracheostomy tray at bedside. |
| Prodromal stage: Absent in children, present in adults and adolescents; consists of low-grade fever, headache, malaise, anorexia, mild conjunctivitis, coryza, sore throat, cough, and lymphadenopathy; lasts for 1-5 days, subsides 1 day after appearance of rash | Reassure parents of benign nature of illness in affected child. |
| Rash: First appears on face and rapidly spreads downward to neck, arms, trunk, and legs; by end of first day body is covered with a discrete, pinkish-red maculopapular exanthema; disappears in same order as it began and is usually gone by third day | Employ comfort measures as necessary. |
| Constitutional signs and symptoms: Occasionally low-grade fever, headache, malaise, and lymphadenopathy | Isolate child from pregnant women. |

*Continued*

# The Child with a Communicable Disease—cont'd

**Disease**

### *Scarlet fever (Figure 1-39)*

**Cause:** Group A β-hemolytic streptococci

**Source:** Respiratory secretions

**Transmission:** Direct contact with infected person or droplet spread; indirectly by contact with contaminated articles or ingestion of contaminated milk or other food

**Incubation period:** 2-4 days, with range of 1-7 days

**Period of communicability:** During incubation period and clinical illness approximately 10 days; during first 2 weeks of carrier phase, although may persist for months

**First day of rash**

- Flushed cheeks
- White strawberry tongue (see inset)
- Increased density on neck
- Transverse lines (Pastia sign)
- Increased density in groin

**Third day of rash**

- Circumoral pallor
- Red strawberry tongue (see inset)
- Increased density in axilla
- Positive blanching test (Schultz-Charlton)

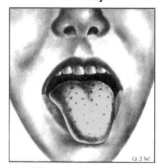

First day

White strawberry tongue

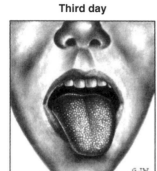

Third day

Red strawberry tongue

FIGURE **1-39**   Scarlet fever.

## Clinical Manifestations

Prodromal stage: High fever, vomiting, headache, chills, malaise, abdominal pain

Enanthema: Tonsils enlarged, edematous, reddened, and covered with patches of exudate; in severe case appearance resembles membrane seen in diphtheria; pharynx is edematous and beefy red; during first 1-2 days tongue is coated and papillae become red and swollen (white strawberry tongue); by fourth or fifth day white coat sloughs off, leaving prominent papillae (red strawberry tongue); palate is covered with erythematous punctate lesions.

Exanthema: Rash appears within 12 hours after prodromal signs; red, pinhead-sized punctate lesions rapidly become generalized but are absent on face, which becomes flushed with striking circumoral pallor; rash is more intense in folds of joints; by end of first week desquamation begins (fine, sandpaper-like on torso; sheetlike sloughing on palms and soles), which may be complete by 3 weeks or longer.

## Nursing Considerations

Institute respiratory precautions until 24 hours after initiation of treatment.

Ensure compliance with oral antibiotic therapy. (Intramuscular benzathine penicillin G [Bicillin] may be given if compliance is questionable.)

Maintain bed rest during febrile phase; provide quiet activity during convalescent period.

Relieve discomfort of sore throat with analgesics, gargles, lozenges, antiseptic throat sprays, and inhalation of cool mist.

Encourage fluids during febrile phase; avoid irritating liquids (citrus juices) or rough foods; when child is able to eat, begin with soft diet.

Advise parents to consult practitioner if fever persists after beginning therapy.

# Family Assessment

Family assessment involves the collection of data about:

*Family structure*—The composition of the family (who lives in the home) and those social, cultural, religious, and economic characteristics that influence the child's and family's overall psychobiologic health

*Family function*—How the family members behave toward one another, the roles family members assume, and the quality of their relationships

In its broadest sense, "family" refers to all those individuals who are significant to the nuclear unit, including relatives, friends, and other social groups, such as the school and church. The more common method of eliciting information on family structure and function is by interviewing family members. However, several family assessment tools can be used to collect and graphically record data about family composition, environment, and relationships. These tools include screening questionnaires and diagrams.

## Indications for Comprehensive Family Assessment

Children receiving comprehensive well-child care

Children experiencing major stressful life events, such as chronic illness, disability, parental divorce, foster care, or death of a family member

Children requiring extensive home care

Children with developmental delays

Children with repeated injuries and those with suspected child abuse

Children with behavioral or physical problems that suggest family dysfunction as the cause

## Cultural Considerations

Who is considered "family"?

Who makes the decisions for the family?

What family members will be involved?

Who helps the family when someone is ill?

What support services are available through the family's cultural community?

## Family Assessment Interview

### General Guidelines for Family Interview

Schedule the interview with the family at a time that is most convenient for all parties; include as many family members as possible; clearly state the purpose of the interview.

Begin the interview by asking each person's name and relationship to others in the family.

Restate the purpose and the objective of the interview.

Keep the initial conversation general to put members at ease and to learn the "big picture" of the family.

Identify major concerns, and reflect these back to the family to be certain that all parties perceive the same message.

Terminate the interview with a summary of what was discussed and a plan for additional sessions if needed.

### Structural Assessment Areas
#### Family Composition

Immediate members of the household (names, ages, relationships)

Significant extended family members

Previous marriages, separations, deaths of spouses, or divorces

### Home and Community Environment

Type of dwelling, number of rooms, occupants

Sleeping arrangements

Number of floors, accessibility of stairs, elevators

Adequacy of utilities

Safety features (fire escape, smoke detector, guardrails on windows, use of car restraint) and firearms

Environmental hazards (e.g., chipped paint, poor sanitation, pollution, heavy street traffic)

Availability and location of health facilities, schools, play areas

Relationship with neighbors

Recent crises or changes in home

Child's reaction and adjustment to recent stresses

### Occupation and Education of Family Members

Types of employment

Work schedules

Work satisfaction

Exposure to environmental or industrial hazards

Sources of income and adequacy

Effect of illness on financial status

Highest degree or grade level attained

### Cultural and Religious Traditions

Religious beliefs and practices

Cultural or ethnic beliefs and practices

Language spoken in home

Assessment questions

- Does the family identify with a particular religious or ethnic group? Are both parents from that group?
- How is religious or ethnic background part of family life?
- What special religious or cultural traditions are practiced in the home (e.g., food choices and preparation)?
- Where were family members born, and how long have they lived in the United States?
- What language does the family speak most frequently?
- Do they speak or understand English?
- What do they believe causes health or illness?
- What religious or ethnic beliefs influence the family's perception of illness and its treatment?
- What methods are used to prevent and treat illness?
- How does the family know when a health problem needs medical attention?
- Who is the person the family contacts when a member is ill?
- Does the family rely on cultural or religious healers or remedies? If so, ask them to describe the type of healer or remedy.
- Who does the family go to for support (clergy, medical healer, relatives)?
- Does the family experience discrimination because of their race, beliefs, or practices? If so, ask them to describe these experiences.

## Functional Assessment Areas
### Family Interactions and Roles

Interactions refer to ways family members relate to one another.

Chief concern is amount of intimacy and closeness among the members, especially spouses.

Roles refer to behaviors of people as they assume a different status or position.

Observations

- Family members' responses to one another (cordial, hostile, cool, loving, patient, short-tempered)
- Obvious roles of leadership versus submission
- Support and attention shown to various members

Assessment questions

- What activities do family members perform together?
- With whom do family members talk to when something is bothering them?
- What are members' household chores?
- Who usually oversees what is happening with the children, such as at school or concerning their health?
- How easy or difficult is it for the family to change or to accept new responsibilities for household tasks?

## Power, Decision Making, and Problem Solving

Power refers to an individual member's control over others in the family; manifested through family decision making and problem solving.

Chief concern is clarity of boundaries of power between parents and children.

One method of assessment involves offering a hypothetical conflict or problem, such as a child failing school, and asking family members how they would handle the situation.

Assessment questions include the following:

- Who usually makes the decisions in the family?
- If one parent makes a decision, can the child appeal to the other parent to change it?
- What input do children have in making decisions or discussing rules?
- Who makes and enforces the rules?
- What happens when a rule is broken?

### Communication

Concerned with clarity and directness of communication patterns

Observations

- Who speaks to whom
- Whether one person speaks for or interrupts another
- Whether members appear disinterested when certain individuals speak
- Whether there is agreement between verbal and nonverbal messages
- Further assessment, such as periodically asking family members if they understood what was just said and to repeat the message

Assessment questions include the following:

- How often do family members wait until others are through talking before "having their say"?
- Do parents or older siblings tend to lecture and preach?
- Do parents tend to talk down to the children?

### Expression of Feelings and Individuality

Concerned with personal space and freedom to grow within limits and structure needed for guidance.

Observing patterns of communication offers clues to how freely feelings are expressed.

Assessment questions include the following:

- Is it acceptable for family members to get angry or sad?
- Who gets angry most of the time? What does this person do?
- If someone is upset, how do other family members try to comfort this person?
- Who comforts specific family members?
- When someone wants to do something, such as try out for a new sport or get a job, what is the family's response (offer assistance, discouragement, or no advice)?

# Nutritional Assessment

A nutritional assessment is an essential part of a complete health appraisal. Its purpose is to evaluate the child's nutritional status—the condition of health as it relates to the state of balance between nutrient intake and nutrient expenditure or need. A thorough nutritional assessment includes information about dietary intake, clinical assessment of nutritional status, anthropometric measures, sociodemographic data, and biochemical status.

Information about dietary intake usually begins with a dietary history (see next section) and may be coupled with a more detailed account of actual food intake. Two methods of recording food intake are a food diary and a food frequency record. A food frequency record provides information about the number of times in a day or week items from MyPyramid for Kids are consumed.

A number of biochemical tests are available for studying nutritional status. Common laboratory procedures related to nutritional status include measurement of hemoglobin, hematocrit, transferrin, albumin, creatinine, and nitrogen. (See Common Laboratory Tests in Unit 6.)

## Dietary History

What are the family's usual mealtimes?
Do family members eat together or at separate times?
Who does the family grocery shopping and meal preparation?
How much money is spent to buy food each week?
How are most foods cooked—baked, broiled, boiled, microwaved, stir-fried, deep-fried, other?
How often does the family or your child eat out?
- What kinds of restaurants do you go to?
- What kinds of food does your child typically eat at restaurants?

Does your child eat breakfast regularly?
Where does your child eat lunch?
What are your child's favorite foods, beverages, and snacks?
- What are the average amounts eaten per day?
- What foods are artificially sweetened?
- What are your child's snacking habits?
- When are sweet foods usually eaten?
- What are your child's toothbrushing habits?

What special cultural practices are followed?
- What ethnic foods are eaten?
- Are there dietary restrictions? What foods and beverages does your child dislike?

How would you describe your child's usual appetite (hearty eater, picky eater)?
What are your child's feeding habits (breast, bottle, cup, spoon, eats by self, needs assistance, any special devices)?
Does your child take vitamins or other supplements; do they contain iron or fluoride? How often are they given?
Are there any known or suspected food allergies; is your child on a special diet?
Has your child lost or gained weight recently?
Are there any feeding problems (excessive fussiness, spitting up, colic, difficulty sucking or swallowing); any dental problems or appliances, such as braces, that affect eating?
What types of exercise does your child do regularly?
Is there a family history of cancer, diabetes, heart disease, high blood pressure, or obesity?

## Cultural Considerations

What are the common foods eaten by the child and family?
Are there dietary patterns that may be contraindicated in the plan of care?

What foods are thought to promote health?
Are there religious food prescriptions and restrictions?

# Sleep Assessment

A sleep history is usually taken during the general health history. However, when sleep problems are identified, a more detailed history of sleep and awake patterns is needed for planning appropriate intervention. The following information includes a summary of a comprehensive sleep history.

# Assessment of Sleep Problems in Children*

## General History of Chief Complaint

Ask parents or child to describe sleep problems; record in their words.

Inquire about onset, duration, character, frequency, and consistency of sleep problems:

Circumstances surrounding onset (e.g., birth of sibling, start of toilet training, death of significant other, move from crib to bed)

Circumstances that aggravate problem (e.g., overtiredness, family conflict, disrupted routine [visitors])

Remedies used to correct problem, and results of interventions

## 24-Hour Sleep History

Time and regularity of meals†
- Family members present
- Activities afterward, especially evening meal

Time of night and day sleep periods
- Hours of sleep and waking
- Hours of being put to bed and taken out of bed
- How bedtime is decided (when child looks tired or at a time decided by parent; do both parents agree on bedtime?)

Prebedtime or prenap rituals (bath, bottle- or breast-feeding, snack, television, active or quiet playing, story)
- Mood before nap or bedtime (wide awake, sleepy, happy, cranky)
- Which parent(s) participates in nap or bedtime rituals?

Nap and bedtime rituals
- Where is child allowed to fall asleep? (own bed or crib, couch, parent's bed, someone's lap, other)
- Is child helped to fall asleep? (rocked; walked; patted; given pacifier or bottle; placed in room with light; television, radio, or tape recorder on; other)
- Are patterns consistent each time, or do they vary?
- Does child wake if sleep aids are changed or taken away (placed in own bed, television turned off, other)?
- Does child verbally insist that parents stay in room?
- Child's behaviors if refuses to go to sleep or stay in room
- If child complains of fears, how convincing are the fears?

Sleep environment
- Number of bedrooms
- Location of bedrooms, especially in relation to parent's (parents') room
- Sensory features (light on, door open or closed, noise level, temperature)

Night wakings
- Time, frequency, and duration
- Child's behavior (calls out; cries; comes out of room; appears frightened, confused, or upset)
- Parental responses (let child cry, go in immediately, take to own bed, feed, pick up, rock, give pacifier, talk, scold, threaten, other)
- Conditions that reestablish sleep
  - Do they always work?
  - How long do the interventions take to work?
  - Which parent intervenes?
  - Do both parents use same or different approach?

Daytime sleepiness
- Occurrence of falling asleep at inappropriate times (circumstances, suddenness and irresistibility of onset, length of sleep, mood on awakening)
- Signs of fatigue (yawning or lying down, as well as overactivity, impulsivity, distractibility, irritability, temper tantrums)

## Past Sleep History

Sleep patterns since infancy, especially ages when started to sleep through the night, stopped daytime naps, began later bedtime

Response to changes in sleep arrangements (crib to bed, different room or house, other)

Sleep behaviors (restlessness, snoring, sleepwalking, nightmares, partial wakings [young child may wake confused, crying, and thrashing but does not respond to parent; falls asleep without intervention if not excessively disturbed])

Parental perception of child's sleep habits (good or poor sleeper, light or deep sleeper, needs little sleep)

Family history of sleep problems (sibling behavior imitated by child; some sleep disorders [e.g., narcolepsy, enuresis] tend to recur in families)

---

*Modified from Ferber R: Assessment procedures for diagnosis of sleep disorders in children. In Noshpitz J, editor: *Sleep disorders for the clinician,* London, 1987, Butterworth, pp 185-193.

†A convenient point to start the 24-hour history is the evening meal.

# Growth Measurements

## General Trends in Physical Growth During Childhood

| Age | Weight* | Height* |
|---|---|---|
| **Infants** | | |
| *Birth to 6 months* | Weekly gain: 140-200 g (5-7 ounces)<br>Birth weight doubles by end of first 6 months† | Monthly gain: 2.5 cm (1 inch) |
| *6-12 months* | Weekly gain: 85-140 g (3-5 ounces)<br>Birth weight triples by end of first year† | Monthly gain: 1.25 cm (0.5 inch)<br>Birth length increases by approximately 50% by end of first year |
| **Toddlers** | Birth weight quadruples by age 2½ years<br>Yearly gain: 2-3 kg (4.4-6.6 pounds) | Height at age 2 years is approximately 50% of eventual adult height<br>Gain during second year: about 12 cm (4.8 inches)<br>Gain during third year: about 6-8 cm (2.4-3.2 inches) |
| **Preschoolers** | Yearly gain: 2-3 kg (4.4-6.6 pounds) | Birth length doubles by age 4 years<br>Yearly gain: 6-8 cm (2.4-3.2 inches) |
| **School-age children** | Yearly gain: 2-3 kg (4.4-6.6 pounds) | Yearly gain after age 6 years: 5 cm (2 inches)<br>Birth length triples by about age 13 years |
| **Pubertal Growth Spurt** | | |
| *Females (10-14 years)* | Weight gain: 7-25 kg (15-55 pounds) | Height gain: 5-25 cm (2-10 inches); approximately 95% of mature height achieved by onset of menarche or skeletal age of 13 years |
| | Mean: 17.5 kg (38.1 pounds) | Mean: 20.5 cm (8.2 inches) |
| *Males (12-16 years)* | Weight gain: 7-30 kg (15-65 pounds) | Height gain: 10-30 cm (4-12 inches); approximately 95% of mature height achieved by skeletal age of 15 years |
| | Mean: 23.7 kg (52.1 pounds) | Mean: 27.5 cm (11 inches) |

*Yearly height and weight gains for each age group represent averaged estimates from a variety of sources.

†A study (Jung E, Czajka-Narins DM: Birth weight doubling and tripling times: An updated look at the effects of birth weight, sex, race, and type of feeding, *Am J Clin Nutr* 42:182-189, 1985) has shown the mean doubling time for birth weight to be 4.7 months and mean tripling time to be 14.7 months.

# Sequence of Tooth Eruption and Shedding

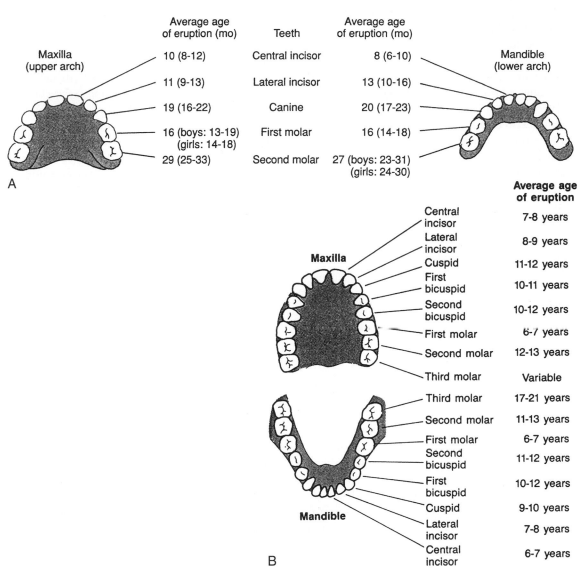

| Maxilla (upper arch) | Average age of eruption (mo) | Teeth | Average age of eruption (mo) | Mandible (lower arch) |
|---|---|---|---|---|
| | 10 (8-12) | Central incisor | 8 (6-10) | |
| | 11 (9-13) | Lateral incisor | 13 (10-16) | |
| | 19 (16-22) | Canine | 20 (17-23) | |
| | 16 (boys: 13-19) (girls: 14-18) | First molar | 16 (14-18) | |
| | 29 (25-33) | Second molar | 27 (boys: 23-31) (girls: 24-30) | |

A

**Maxilla**

| Tooth | Average age of eruption |
|---|---|
| Central incisor | 7-8 years |
| Lateral incisor | 8-9 years |
| Cuspid | 11-12 years |
| First bicuspid | 10-11 years |
| Second bicuspid | 10-12 years |
| First molar | 6-7 years |
| Second molar | 12-13 years |
| Third molar | Variable |

| Tooth | Average age of eruption |
|---|---|
| Third molar | 17-21 years |
| Second molar | 11-13 years |
| First molar | 6-7 years |
| Second bicuspid | 11-12 years |
| First bicuspid | 10-12 years |
| Cuspid | 9-10 years |
| Lateral incisor | 7-8 years |
| Central incisor | 6-7 years |

**Mandible**

B

FIGURE **1-40**   A, Sequence of eruption of primary teeth. Range represents ± standard deviation, or 67% of subjects studied. B, Sequence of eruption of secondary teeth. (Data from Dean JA, McDonald RE, Avery DR: *McDonald and Avery's dentistry for the child and adolescent,* ed 9, St Louis, 2011, Mosby.)

# Growth Charts

The most commonly used growth charts in the United States are from the National Center for Health Statistics (NCHS). The growth charts have been revised to include the body mass index-for-age (BMI-for-age) charts (Figures 1-41 and 1-42), 3rd and 97th smoothed percentiles for all charts, and the 85th percentile for the weight-for-stature and BMI-for-age charts. The data were collected from five national surveys during the period from 1963 to 1994. The revised charts have eliminated the disjunctions between the curves for infants and other children and have been extended for children and adolescents to 20 years (NCHS, 2000).*

The weight for age percentile distributions are now continuous between the infant and the older child charts at 24 to 36 months. The length-for-age to stature-for-age and the weight-for-length to weight-for-stature curves are parallel in the overlapping ages of 24 to 36 months. The revised weight-for-stature charts provide a smoother transition from the weight-for-length charts for preschool-age children.

The most prominent change to the complement of growth charts for older children and adolescents is the addition of the BMI-for-age growth curves. The BMI-for-age charts were developed with national survey data (1963 to 1994), excluding data from the 1988-1994 NHANES III survey for children older than 6 years because an increase in body weight and BMI occurred between NHANES III and previous national surveys. Without this exclusion, the 85th and 95th percentile curves would have been higher, and fewer children and adolescents would have been classified as at risk or overweight. Therefore the BMI-for-age growth curves do not represent the current population of children over 6 years of age.

The gender-specific BMI-for-age charts for ages 2 to 20 years replace the 1977 NCHS weight-for-stature charts that were limited to prepubescent boys under 11½ years of age and statures less than 145 cm and to prepubescent girls under 19 years of age and statures less than 137 cm. BMI-for-age may be used to identify children and adolescents at the upper end of the distribution who are either overweight (≥95th percentile) or at risk for overweight (≥85th and <95th percentiles). The formulas for determining BMI are available at www.cdc.gov and below.

# Versions of the Growth Charts

Three different versions of the charts are available at www.cdc.gov/growthcharts. The first set contains all nine smoothed percentile lines (3rd, 5th, 10th, 25th, 50th, 75th, 90th, 95th, 97th), and the second and third sets contain seven smoothed percentile lines. The second set contains the 5th and 95th percentile lines, and the third set contains the 3rd and 97th percentile lines at the extremes of the distribution. In addition, the charts for weight-for-stature and BMI-for-age contain the 85th percentile. In all the growth charts, age is truncated to the nearest full month; for example, 1 month (1-1.9 months), 11 months (11 to 11.9 months), and 23 months (23-23.9 months).

The three sets of charts are provided to meet the needs of various users. Set 1 shows all the major percentile curves but may have limitations when the curves are close together, especially at the youngest ages. Most users in the United States may wish to use the format shown in set 2 for the majority of routine clinical applications. Pediatric endocrinologists and others dealing with special populations, such as children with failure to thrive, may wish to use the format for set 3.

# Body Mass Index Formula

## English Formula

BMI = [(Weight in pounds ÷ Height in inches) ÷ Height in inches] × 703

Fractions and ounces must be entered as decimal values.*
Example: A 33-pound, 4-ounce child is 37⅝ inches tall.

BMI = [(33.25 pounds ÷ 37.625* inches) ÷ 37.625 inches] × 703 = 16.5

| Fraction | Ounces | Decimal | Fraction | Ounces | Decimal |
|----------|--------|---------|----------|--------|---------|
| ⅛ | 2 | 0.125 | ⅝ | 10 | 0.625 |
| ¼ | 4 | 0.25 | ¾ | 12 | 0.75 |
| ⅜ | 6 | 0.375 | ⅞ | 14 | 0.875 |
| ½ | 8 | 0.5 | | | |

## Metric Formula

BMI = (Weight in kilograms ÷ Height in meters) ÷ Height in meters

or

BMI = [(Weight in kilograms ÷ Height in cm) ÷ Height in cm] × 10,000

Example: A 16.9-kg child is 105.2 cm tall.

BMI = [(16.9 ÷ 105.2 cm) ÷ 105.2 cm] × 10,000 = 15.3

*Kuczmarski RJ and others: CDC growth charts: United States. Advance data from vital and health statistics, no 314, Hyattsville, Md, June 8, 2000, NCHS.

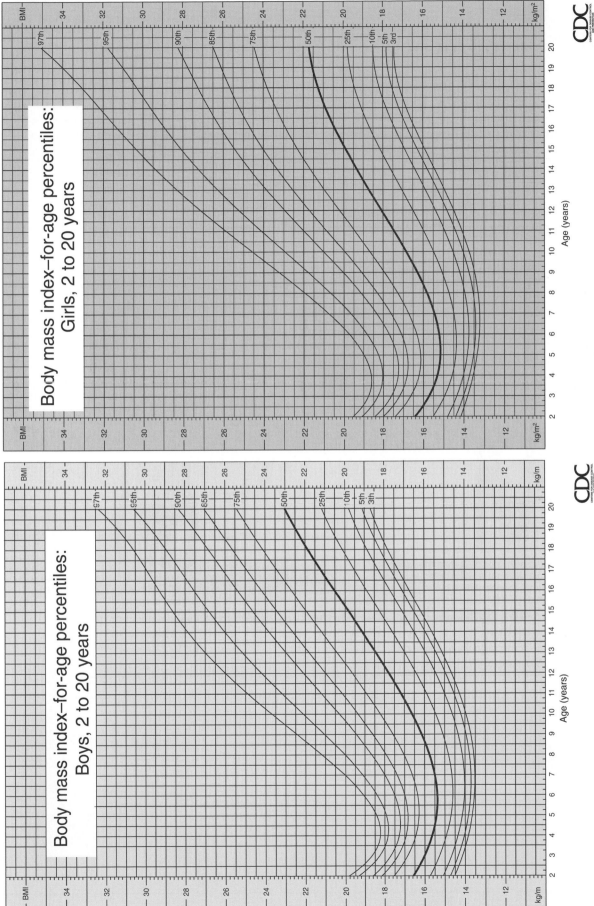

FIGURE **1-42**   Body mass index–for-age percentiles, girls, 2-20 years, CDC growth charts: United States. Developed by the National Center for Health Statistics in collaboration with the National Center for Chronic Disease Prevention and Health Promotion (2000).

FIGURE **1-41**   Body mass index–for-age percentiles, boys, 2-20 years, CDC growth charts: United States. Developed by the National Center for Health Statistics in collaboration with the National Center for Chronic Disease Prevention and Health Promotion (2000).

# Sexual Development

The Tanner stages* were developed by Dr. J.M. Tanner and colleagues. Tanner stages describe the stages of pubertal growth and are numbered from stage 1 (immature) to stage 5 (mature) for both males and females. In females, the Tanner stages describe pubertal development based on breast size and the shape and distribution of pubic hair. In males, the Tanner stages describe pubertal development based on the size and shape of the penis and scrotum and the shape and distribution of pubic hair.

## Sexual Development in Adolescent Males

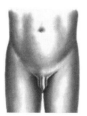

Stage 1
(prepubertal)

No pubic hair; essentially the same as during childhood; no distinction between hair on pubis and over the abdomen

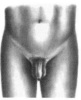

Stage 2 (pubertal)

Initial enlargement of scrotum and testes; reddening and textural changes of scrotal skin; sparse growth of long, straight, downy, and slightly pigmented hair at base of penis

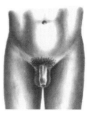

Stage 3

Initial enlargement of penis, mainly in length; testes and scrotum further enlarged; hair darker, coarser, and curly and spread sparsely over entire pubis

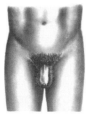

Stage 4

Increased size of penis with growth in diameter and development of glans; glans larger and broader; scrotum darker; pubic hair more abundant with curling but restricted to pubic area

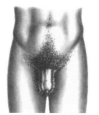

Stage 5

Testes, scrotum, and penis adult in size and shape; hair adult in quantity and type with spread to inner surface of thighs

FIGURE **1-43** Developmental stages of secondary sex characteristics and genital development in boys. Average age span is 12 to 16 years. (Modified from Marshall WA, Tanner JM: Variations in the pattern of pubertal changes in boys, *Arch Dis Child* 45(239):13-23, 1970; Tanner JM: *Growth at adolescence,* Springfield, Ill, 1995, CC Thomas.)

*Tanner JM: *Growth of adolescents,* Oxford, 1962, Blackwell Scientific Publications.

# Sexual Development in Adolescent Females

Stage 1

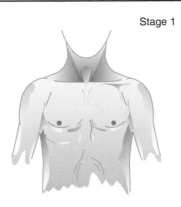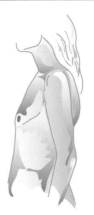

Stage 2
(pubertal)

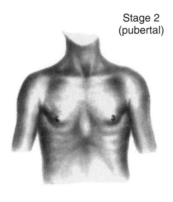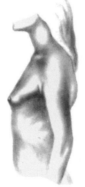

Stage 3

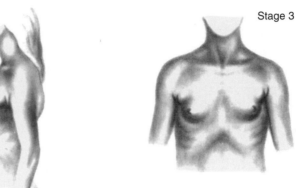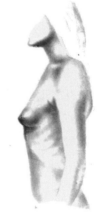

Breast bud stage—small area of
elevation around papilla; enlargement
of areolar diameter

Further enlargement of breast and areola
with no separation of their contours

Stage 4

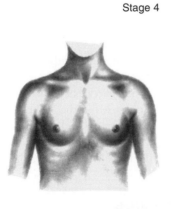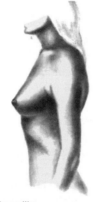

Stage 5

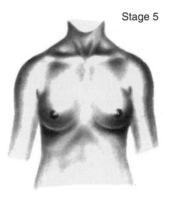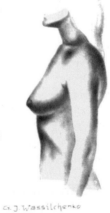

Projection of areola and papilla
to form a secondary mound (may
not occur in all girls)

Mature configuration; projection of papilla
only caused by recession of areola
into general contour

FIGURE **1-44** Development of the breast in girls. Average age span is 11 to 13 years. (Modified from Marshall WA, Tanner JM: Variations in pattern of pubertal changes in girls, *Arch Dis Child* 44(235):291-303, 1969; Tanner JM: *Growth at adolescence*, Springfield, Ill, 1995, CC Thomas.)

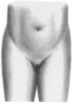

Stage 1
(prepubertal)

No pubic hair; essentially the same as during childhood; no distinction between hair on pubis and over the abdomen

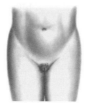

Stage 2

Sparse growth of long, straight, downy, and slightly pigmented hair extending along labia; between stages 2 and 3 begins to appear on pubis

Stage 3

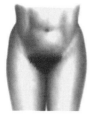

Hair darker, coarser, and curly and spread sparsely over entire pubis in the typical female triangle

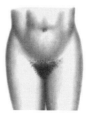

Stage 4

Pubic hair denser, curled, and adult in distribution but less abundant and restricted to the pubic area

Stage 5

Hair adult in quantity, type, and pattern with spread to inner aspect of thighs

FIGURE **1-45**   Growth of pubic hair in girls. Average age span for stages 2 through 5 is 11 to 14 years. (Modified from Marshall WA, Tanner JM: Variations in the pattern of pubertal changes in girls, *Arch Dis Child* 44(235):291-303, 1969; Tanner JM: *Growth at adolescence,* Springfield, Ill, 1955, CC Thomas.)

# Assessment of Development

## Denver II*

The Denver II is a major revision and a restandardization of the Denver Developmental Screening Test (DDST) and the revised Denver Development Screening Test (DDST-R). It differs from the earlier screening tests in items included as well as in the form, the interpretation, and the referral (Figures 1-46 and 1-47). Like the other tests, it assesses gross motor, language, fine motor, adaptive, and personal-social development in children from 1 month to 6 years of age.

### Item Differences

The previous total of 105 items has been increased to 125, including an increase from 21 DDST items to 39 Denver II language items.

Previous items that were difficult to administer and/or interpret have been either modified or eliminated. Many items that were previously tested by parental report now require observation by the examiner.

Each item was evaluated to determine if significant differences existed on the basis of gender, ethnic group, maternal education, and place of residence. Items for which clinically significant differences existed were replaced or, if retained, are discussed in the Technical Manual. When evaluating children delayed on one of these items, the examiner can look up norms for the subpopulations to determine if the delay may be a result of sociocultural differences.

### Test Form Differences

The age scale is similar to the American Academy of Pediatrics suggested periodicity schedule for health maintenance visits. This facilitates use of the Denver II at these times.

In children born prematurely, the age is adjusted only until the child is 2 years old.

---

*To ensure that the Denver II is administered and interpreted in the prescribed manner, it is recommended that those intending to administer it receive the appropriate training, which can be obtained with the forms and instructional manual from Denver Developmental Materials, Inc., PO Box 371075, Denver, CO 80237-5075, 303-355-4729 or 800-419-4729.

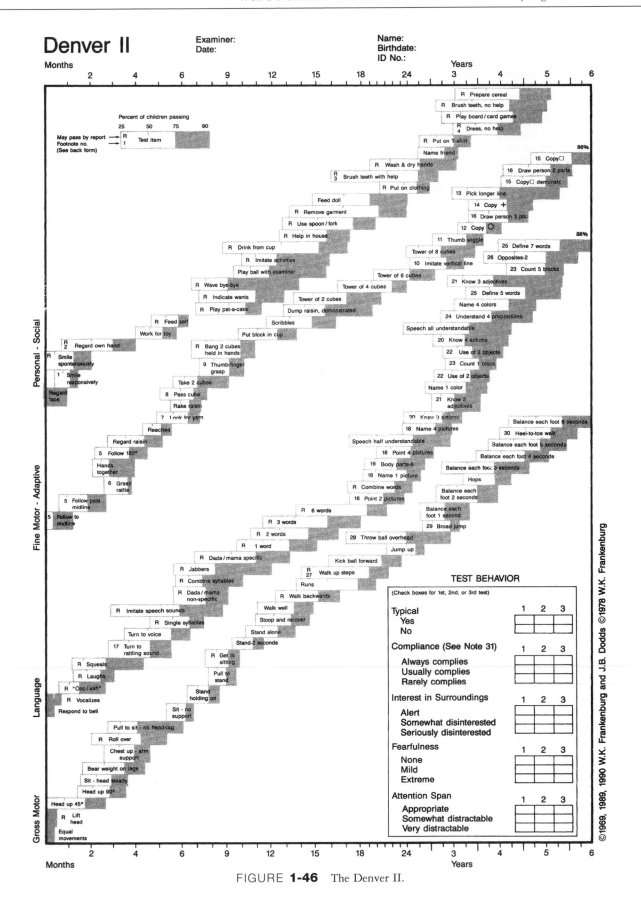

FIGURE **1-46**  The Denver II.

## DIRECTIONS FOR ADMINISTRATION

1. Try to get child to smile by smiling, talking or waving. Do not touch him/her.
2. Child must stare at hand several seconds.
3. Parent may help guide toothbrush and put toothpaste on brush.
4. Child does not have to be able to tie shoes or button/zip in the back.
5. Move yarn slowly in an arc from one side to the other, about 8" above child's face.
6. Pass if child grasps rattle when it is touched to the backs or tips of fingers.
7. Pass if child tries to see where yarn went. Yarn should be dropped quickly from sight from tester's hand without arm movement.
8. Child must transfer cube from hand to hand without help of body, mouth, or table.
9. Pass if child picks up raisin with any part of thumb and finger.
10. Line can vary only 30 degrees or less from tester's line.
11. Make a fist with thumb pointing upward and wiggle only the thumb. Pass if child imitates and does not move any fingers other than the thumb.

 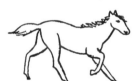 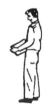 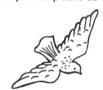

12. Pass any enclosed form. Fail continuous round motions.
13. Which line is longer? (Not bigger.) Turn paper upside down and repeat. (pass 3 of 3 or 5 of 6)
14. Pass any lines crossing near midpoint.
15. Have child copy first. If failed, demonstrate.

When giving items 12, 14, and 15, do not name the forms. Do not demonstrate 12 and 14.

16. When scoring, each pair (2 arms, 2 legs, etc.) counts as one part.
17. Place one cube in cup and shake gently near child's ear, but out of sight. Repeat for other ear.
18. Point to picture and have child name it. (No credit is given for sounds only.)
    If less than 4 pictures are named correctly, have child point to picture as each is named by tester.

    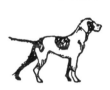

19. Using doll, tell child: Show me the nose, eyes, ears, mouth, hands, feet, tummy, hair. Pass 6 of 8.
20. Using pictures, ask child: Which one flies?... says meow?... talks?... barks?... gallops? Pass 2 of 5, 4 of 5.
21. Ask child: What do you do when you are cold?... tired?... hungry? Pass 2 of 3, 3 of 3.
22. Ask child: What do you do with a cup? What is a chair used for? What is a pencil used for? Action words must be included in answers.
23. Pass if child correctly places <u>and</u> says how many blocks are on paper. (1, 5).
24. Tell child: Put block **on** table; **under** table; **in front of** me, **behind** me. Pass 4 of 4. (Do not help child by pointing, moving head or eyes.)
25. Ask child: What is a ball?... lake?... desk?... house?... banana?... curtain?... fence?... ceiling? Pass if defined in terms of use, shape, what it is made of, or general category (such as banana is fruit, not just yellow). Pass 5 of 8, 7 of 8.
26. Ask child: If a horse is big, a mouse is __? If fire is hot, ice is __? If the sun shines during the day, the moon shines during the __? Pass 2 of 3.
27. Child may use wall or rail only, not person. May not crawl.
28. Child must throw ball overhand 3 feet to within arm's reach of tester.
29. Child must perform standing broad jump over width of test sheet (8 1/2 inches).
30. Tell child to walk forward, ⟨⟨⟩⟩⟩→ heel within 1 inch of toe. Tester may demonstrate. Child must walk 4 consecutive steps.
31. In the second year, half of normal children are non-compliant.

**OBSERVATIONS:**

FIGURE **1-47**    Directions for administration of numbered items on the Denver II. (From Frankenburg WK, and others. *The Denver II training manual*, Denver, Denver Developmental Materials, Inc.)

The items on the test form are arranged in the same format as the DDST-R.

The norms for the distribution bars were updated with the new standardization data but retained the 25th, 50th, 75th, and 90th percentile divisions.

The test form contains a place to rate the child's behavioral characteristics (compliance, interest in surroundings, fearfulness, attention span).

## Interpretation and Referral

Explain to the parents that the Denver II is not an intelligence test but a systematic appraisal of the child's present development. Stress that the child is not expected to perform each item.

To determine relative areas of advancement and areas of delay, sufficient items should be administered to establish the basal and ceiling levels in each sector.

---

**BOX 1-9** | Denver II Scoring

### Interpretation of Denver II Scores
**Advanced**: Passed an item completely to the right of the age line (passed by less than 25% of children at an age older than the child)

**OK**: Passed, failed, or refused an item intersected by the age line between the 25th and 75th percentiles

**Caution**: Failed or refused items intersected by the age line on or between the 75th and 90th percentiles

**Delay**: Failed an item completely to the left of the age line; refusals to the left of the age line may also be considered delays, because the reason for the refusal may be inability to perform the task

### Interpretation of Test
**Normal**: No delays and a maximum of one caution

**Suspect**: One or more delays and/or two or more cautions

**Untestable**: Refusals on one or more items completely to the left of the age line or on more than one item intersected by the age line in the 75th to 90th percentile area

### Recommendations for Referral for Suspect and Untestable Tests
Rescreen in 1 to 2 weeks to rule out temporary factors

If rescreen is suspect or subject is untestable, use clinical judgment based on the following: number of cautions and delays; which items are cautions and delays; rate of past development; clinical examination and history; and availability of referral resources

---

By scoring appropriate items as "pass," "fail," "refusal," or "no opportunity" and relating such scores to the age of the child, each item can be interpreted as described in Box 1-9.

To identify cautions, all items intersected by the age line are administered.

To screen solely for developmental delays, only the items located totally to the left of the child's age line are administered.

Criteria for referral are based on the availability of resources in the community.

## Revised Denver Prescreening Developmental Questionnaire*

The Revised Prescreening Developmental Questionnaire (R-PDQ) is a revision of the original PDQ. Advantages of the R-PDQ include the addition and arrangement of items to be more age-appropriate, simplified parent scoring, and easier comparison with DDST norms for professionals. The R-PDQ is a parent-answered prescreen consisting of 105 questions from the DDST, although only a subset of questions are asked for each age-group. The form may need to be read to less educated caregivers.

Preparation and scoring of the R-PDQ include the following:

1. Calculate the child's age as detailed in the Denver II manual, and choose the appropriate form* for the child: orange (0-9 months), purple (9-24 months), gold (2-4 years), or white (4-6 years). (See sample of 0 to 9 month form, Figure 1-48.)
2. Give the appropriate form to the child's caregiver, and have person note relationship to the child. Have the caregiver answer questions until (1) three "no's" are circled (they do not have to be consecutive), or (2) all the questions on both sides of the form have been answered.
3. Check form to see that all appropriate questions have been answered.
4. Review "yes" and "no" responses. Ensure that the child's caregiver understood each question and scored the items

correctly. Give particular attention to the scoring of questions that require verbal responses by the child and that require the child to draw.

5. Identify delays (items passed by 90% of children at a younger age than the child being screened). Ages at which 90% of children in the DDST sample passed the items are indicated in parentheses in the "For Office Use" column. These ages are shown in months and weeks up to 24 months and in years and months after 24 months. Highlight delays by circling the 90% age in parentheses to the right of the item that the child was not able to perform.
6. Children who have no delays are considered to be developing normally.
7. If a child has one delay, give the caregiver age-appropriate developmental activities to pursue with the child† and schedule the child for rescreening with the R-PDQ 1 month later. If on rescreening 1 month later the child has one or more delays, schedule second-stage screening with the Denver II as soon as possible.
8. If a child has two or more delays on the first-stage screening with the R-PDQ, schedule a second-stage screening with the Denver II as soon as possible. If on second-stage screening with the Denver II the child receives other than normal results, schedule the child for a diagnostic evaluation.

---

*Forms and complete instructions are available from Denver Developmental Materials, Inc., PO Box 371075, Denver, CO 80237-5075, 303-355-4729 or 800-419-4729.

†Suggested Denver Developmental Activities are available from Denver Developmental Materials, Inc.

**0-9 MONTHS (R-PDQ)**

# REVISED DENVER PRESCREENING DEVELOPMENTAL QUESTIONNAIRE

Child's Name _____

Person Completing R-PDQ: _____

Relation to Child: _____

**For Office Use**

Today's Date: _____ yr _____ mo _____ day

Child's Birthdate: _____ yr _____ mo _____ day

Subtract to get Child's Exact Age: _____ yr _____ mo _____ day

R-PDQ Age: (_____ yr _____ mo _____ completed wks)

CONTINUE ANSWERING UNTIL **3 "NOs"** ARE CIRCLED

| | **For Office Use** |
|---|---|

**1. Equal Movements**
When your baby is lying on his/her back, can (s)he move each of his/her arms as easily as the other and each of the legs as easily as the other? Answer **No** if your child makes jerky or uncoordinated movements with one or both of his/her arms or legs.

Yes    No    (0)   FMA

**2. Stomach Lifts Head**
When your baby is on his/her stomach on a flat surface, can (s)he lift his/her head off the surface?

Yes    No    (0-3)   GM

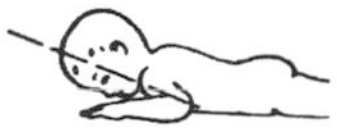

**3. Regards Face**
When your baby is lying on his/her back, can (s)he look at you and watch your face?

Yes    No    (1)   PS

**4. Follows To Midline**
When your child is on his/her back, can (s)he follow your movement by turning his/her head from one side to facing directly forward?

Yes    No    (1-1)   FMA

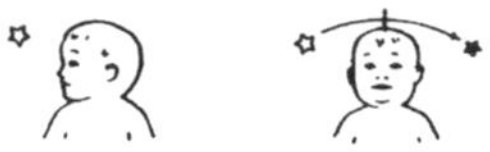

**5. Responds To Bell**
Does your child respond with eye movements, change in breathing or other change in activity to a bell or rattle sounded outside his/her line of vision?

Yes    No    (1-2)   L

**6. Vocalizes Not Crying**
Does your child make sounds other than crying, such as gurgling, cooing, or babbling?

Yes    No    (1-3)   L

**7. Smiles Responsively**
When you smile and talk to your baby, does (s)he smile back at you?

Yes    No    (1-3)   PS

**8. Follows Past Midline**
When your child is on his/her back, does (s)he follow your movement by turning his/her head from one side *almost all the way to the other side?*

Yes    No    (2-2)   FMA

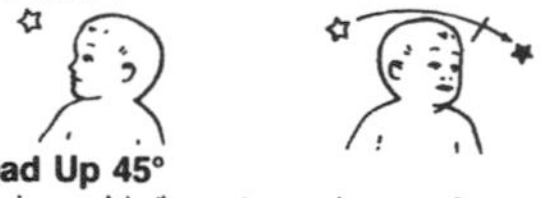

**9. Stomach, Head Up 45°**
When your baby is on his/her stomach on a flat surface, can (s)he lift his/her head 45°?

Yes    No    (2-2)   GM

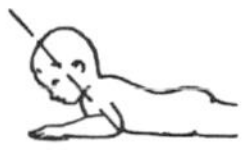

**10. Stomach, Head Up 90°**
When your baby is on his/her stomach on a flat surface, can (s)he lift his/her head 90°?

Yes    No    (3)   GM

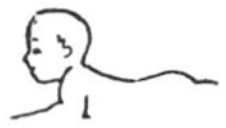

**11. Laughs**
Does your baby laugh out loud without being tickled or touched?

Yes    No    (3-1)   L

**12. Hands Together**
Does your baby play with his/her hands by touching them together?

Yes    No    (3-3)   FMA

**13. Follows 180°**
When your child is on his/her back, does (s)he follow your movement from one side *all the way* to the other side?

Yes    No    (4)   FMA

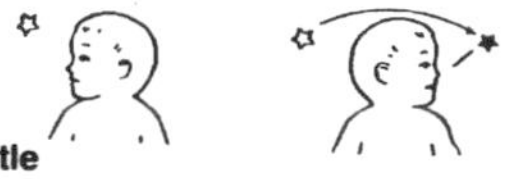

**14. Grasps Rattle**
*It is important that you follow instructions carefully.* Do *not* place the pencil in the palm of your child's hand. When you touch the pencil to the back or tips of your baby's fingers, does your baby grasp the pencil for a few seconds?

Yes    No    (4)   FMA

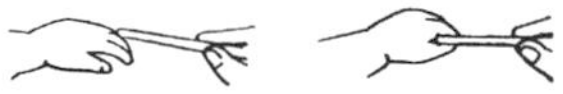

TRY THIS     **NOT** THIS

(Please turn page)

©Wm. K. Frankenburg, M.D., 1975, 1986

FIGURE **1-48** Revised Denver Prescreening Developmental Questionnaire. (The first page is reprinted with permission from William K. Frankenburg, MD, Copyright 1975, 1986, WK Frankenburg, MD.)

# Assessment of Language and Speech

## Major Developmental Characteristics of Language and Speech

| Age (yr) | Normal Language Development | Normal Speech Development | Intelligibility |
|---|---|---|---|
| 1 | Says two or three words with meaning | Omits most final and some initial consonants | Usually no more than 25% intelligible to unfamiliar listener |
| | Imitates sounds of animals | Substitutes consonants *m, w, p, b, k, g, n, t, d,* and *h* for more difficult sounds | Height of unintelligible jargon at age 18 months |
| 2 | Uses two- or three-word phrases | Uses above consonants with vowels, but inconsistently and with much substitution | At age 2 years, 50% intelligible in context |
| | Has vocabulary of about 300 words | Omission of final consonants | |
| | Uses "I," "me," and "you" | Articulation lags behind vocabulary | |
| 3 | Says four- or five-word sentences | Masters *b, t, d, k,* and *g*; sounds *r* and *l* may still be unclear; omits or substitutes *w* | At age 3 years, 75% intelligible |
| | Has vocabulary of about 900 words | | |
| | Uses "who," "what," and "where" in asking questions | Repetitions and hesitations common | |
| | Uses plurals, pronouns, and prepositions | | |
| 4-5 | Has vocabulary of 1500-2100 words | Masters *f* and *v*, may still distort *r, l, s, z, sh, ch, y,* and *th* | Speech is 100% intelligible, although some sounds are still imperfect |
| | Able to use most grammatic forms correctly, such as past tense of verb with "yesterday" | Little or no omission of initial or final consonants | |
| | Uses complete sentences with nouns, verbs, prepositions, adjectives, adverbs, and conjunctions | | |
| 5-6 | Has vocabulary of 3000 words | Masters *r, l,* and *th*; may still distort *s, z, sh, ch,* and *j* (usually mastered by age 7½-8 years) | |
| | Comprehends "if," "because," and "why" | | |

# Assessment of Communication Impairment

Key questions for language disorders
1. How old was your child when he or she spoke his or her first words?
2. How old was your child when he or she began to put words into sentences?
3. Does your child have difficulty in learning new vocabulary words?
4. Does your child omit words from sentences (i.e., do sentences sound telegraphic?) or use short or incomplete sentences?
5. Does your child have trouble with grammar, such as using the verbs is, am, are, was, and were?
6. Can your child follow two or three directions given at once?
7. Do you have to repeat directions or questions?
8. Does your child respond appropriately to questions?
9. Does your child ask questions beginning with who, what, where, and why?
10. Does it seem that your child has made little or no progress in speech and language in the last 6 to 12 months?

Key questions for speech impairment
1. Does your child ever stammer or repeat sounds or words?
2. Does your child seem anxious or frustrated when trying to express an idea?
3. Have you noted certain behaviors, such as blinking, jerking the head, or attempting to rephrase thoughts with different words when your child stammers?
4. What do you do when any of these occurs?
5. Does your child omit sounds from words?
6. Does it seem like your child uses *t, d, k,* or *g* in place of most other consonants when speaking?
7. Does your child omit sounds from words or replace the correct consonant with another one (e.g., "rabbit" with "wabbit")?
8. Do you have any difficulty in understanding your child's speech?
9. Has anyone else ever remarked about having difficulty in understanding your child?
10. Has there been any recent change in the sound of your child's voice?

# Clues for Detecting Communication Impairment

## Language Disability

Assigning meaning to words

- First words not uttered before second birthday
- Vocabulary size reduced for age or fails to show steady increase
- Difficulty in describing characteristics of objects, although may be able to name them
- Infrequent use of modifier words (adjectives, adverbs)
- Excessive use of jargon past age 18 months

Organizing words into sentences

- First sentences not uttered before third birthday
- Short and incomplete sentences
- Tendency to omit words (articles, prepositions)
- Misuse of the "be," "do," and "can" verb forms
- Difficulty understanding and producing questions
- Plateaus at an early developmental level; uses easy speech patterns

Altering word forms

- Omission of endings for plurals and tenses
- Inappropriate use of plurals and tense endings
- Inaccurate use of possessive words

## Speech Impairment

Dysfluency (stuttering)

- Noticeable repetition of sounds, words, or phrases after age 4 years
- Obvious frustration when attempting to communicate
- Demonstration of struggling behavior while talking (head jerks, blinks, retrials, circumlocution)
- Embarrassment about own speech

Articulation deficiency

- Intelligibility of conversational speech absent by age 3 years
- Omission of consonants at beginning of words by age 3 years and at end of words by age 4 years
- Persisting articulation faults after age 7 years
- Omission of a sound where one should occur
- Distortion of a sound
- Substitution of an incorrect sound for a correct one

Voice disorders

- Deviations in pitch (too high or too low, especially for age and gender); monotone
- Deviations in loudness
- Deviations in quality (hypernasality, hyponasality)

# Guidelines for Referral Regarding Communication Impairment

2 years of age

- Failure to speak any meaningful words spontaneously
- Consistent use of gestures rather than vocalizations
- Difficulty in following verbal directions
- Failure to respond consistently to sound

3 years of age

- Speech is largely unintelligible
- Failure to use sentences of three or more words
- Frequent omission of initial consonants
- Use of vowels rather than consonants

5 years of age

- Stutters or has any other type of dysfluency
- Sentence structure noticeably impaired
- Substitutes easily produced sounds for more difficult ones
- Omits word endings (e.g., plurals, tenses of verbs,)

School age

- Poor voice quality (monotonous, loud, or barely audible)
- Vocal pitch inappropriate for age and gender
- Any distortions, omissions, or substitutions of sounds after age 7 years
- Connected speech characterized by use of unusual confusions or reversals

General

- Any child with signs that suggest a hearing impairment
- Any child who is embarrassed or disturbed by own speech
- Parents who are excessively concerned or who pressure the child to speak at a level above that appropriate for age

# Assessment of Vision

## Major Developmental Characteristics of Vision

Birth
- Visual acuity 20/100 to 20/400*
- Pupillary and corneal (blink) reflexes present
- Able to fixate on moving object in range of 45 degrees when held 20 to 25 cm (8 to 10 inches) away
- Cannot integrate head and eye movements well (doll's eye reflex—eyes lag behind if head is rotated to one side)

4 weeks of age
- Can follow in range of 90 degrees
- Can watch parent intently as he or she speaks to infant
- Tear glands begin to function
- Visual acuity is hyperoptic because of less spherical eyeball than in adult

6 to 12 weeks of age
- Has peripheral vision to 180 degrees
- Binocular vision begins at age 6 weeks, is well established by age 4 months
- Convergence on near objects begins by age 6 weeks, is well developed by age 3 months
- Doll's eye reflex disappears

12 to 20 weeks of age
- Recognizes feeding bottle
- Able to fixate on a 1.25-cm (0.5-inch) block
- Looks at hand while sitting or lying on back
- Able to accommodate to near objects

20 to 28 weeks of age
- Adjusts posture to see an object
- Able to rescue a dropped toy
- Develops color preference for yellow and red
- Able to discriminate among simple geometric forms
- Prefers more complex visual stimuli
- Develops hand-eye coordination

28 to 44 weeks of age
- Can fixate on very small objects
- Depth perception begins to develop.
- Lack of binocular vision indicates strabismus.

44 to 52 weeks of age
- Visual acuity 20/40 to 20/60
- Visual loss may develop if strabismus is present.
- Can follow rapidly moving objects

## Clues for Detecting Visual Impairment

### Refractive Errors
#### Myopia
*Nearsightedness*—Ability to see objects clearly at close range but not at a distance
*Pathophysiology*—Results from eyeball that is too long, causing image to fall in front of retina
*Clinical manifestations*
- Rubs eyes excessively
- Tilts head or thrusts head forward
- Has difficulty in reading or performing other close work
- Holds books close to eyes
- Writes or colors with head close to table
- Clumsy; walks into objects
- Blinks more than usual or is irritable when doing close work
- Is unable to see objects clearly
- Does poorly in school, especially in subjects that require demonstration, such as arithmetic
- Dizziness
- Headache
- Nausea following close work

*Treatment*—Corrected with biconcave lenses that focus image on retina

#### Hyperopia
*Farsightedness*—Ability to see objects at a distance but not at close range
*Pathophysiology*—Results from eyeball that is too short, causing image to focus beyond retina
*Clinical manifestations*
- Because of accommodative ability, child can usually see objects at all ranges.
- Most children normally hyperopic until about 7 years of age
*Treatment*—If correction is required, use convex lenses to focus rays on retina.

#### Astigmatism
Unequal curvatures in refractive apparatus
*Pathophysiology*—Results from unequal curvatures in cornea or lens that cause light rays to bend in different directions

---

*Measurement of visual acuity varies according to testing procedures.

*Clinical manifestations*
- Depend on severity of refractive error in each eye
- May have clinical manifestations of myopia

*Treatment*—Corrected with special lenses that compensate for refractive errors

### Anisometropia

Different refractive strengths in each eye

*Pathophysiology*—May develop amblyopia because weaker eye is used less

*Clinical manifestations*
- Depend on severity of refractive error in each eye
- May have clinical manifestations of myopia

*Treatment*—Treated with corrective lenses, preferably contact lenses, to improve vision in each eye so they work as a unit

## Amblyopia

*Lazy eye*—Reduced visual acuity in one eye

*Pathophysiology*
- Condition results when one eye does not receive sufficient stimulation (e.g., from refractive errors, cataract, or strabismus).
- Each retina receives different images, resulting in diplopia (double vision).
- Brain accommodates by suppressing less intense image.
- Visual cortex eventually does not respond to visual stimulation, with loss of vision in that eye.

*Clinical manifestation*—Poor vision in affected eye

*Treatment*—Preventable if treatment of primary visual defect, such as anisometropia or strabismus, begins before 6 years of age

## Strabismus

*"Squint" or cross-eye*—Malalignment of eyes
  *Esotropia*—Inward deviation of eye
  *Exotropia*—Outward deviation of eye

*Pathophysiology*
- May result from muscle imbalance or paralysis, from poor vision, or as congenital defect.
- Because visual axes are not parallel, brain receives two images and amblyopia can result.

*Clinical manifestations*
- Squints eyelids together or frowns
- Has difficulty focusing from one distance to another
- Inaccurate judgment in picking up objects
- Unable to see print or moving objects clearly
- Closes one eye to see
- Tilts head to one side
- If combined with refractive errors, may see any of the manifestations listed for refractive errors
- Diplopia

- Photophobia
- Dizziness
- Headache
- Cross-eye

*Treatment*
- Depends on cause of strabismus
- May involve occlusion therapy (patching stronger eye) or surgery to increase visual stimulation to weaker eye
- Early diagnosis essential to prevent vision loss

## Cataracts

Opacity of crystalline lens

*Pathophysiology*—Prevents light rays from entering eye and being refracted on retina

*Clinical manifestations*
- Gradually less able to see objects clearly
- May lose peripheral vision
- Nystagmus (with complete blindness)
- Gray opacities of lens
- Strabismus
- Absence of red reflex

*Treatment*
- Requires surgery to remove cloudy lens and replace lens (intraocular lens implant, removable contact lens, prescription glasses)
- Must be treated early to prevent blindness from amblyopia

## Glaucoma

Increased intraocular pressure

*Pathophysiology*
- Congenital type results from defective development of some component related to flow of aqueous humor.
- Increased pressure on optic nerve causes eventual atrophy and blindness.

*Clinical manifestations*
- Mostly seen in acquired types; loses peripheral vision
- May bump into objects not directly in front
- Sees halos around objects
- May complain of mild pain or discomfort (severe pain, nausea, vomiting, if sudden rise in pressure)
- Redness
- Excessive tearing (epiphora)
- Photophobia
- Spasmodic winking (blepharospasm)
- Corneal haziness
- Enlargement of eyeball (buphthalmos)

*Treatment*
- Requires surgical treatment (goniotomy) to open outflow tracts
- May require more than one procedure

## Special Tests of Visual Acuity and Estimated Visual Acuity at Different Ages

| Test | Description | Birth | 4 Months | 1 Year | Age of 20/20 Vision (months) |
|---|---|---|---|---|---|
| Optokinetic nystagmus | A striped drum is rotated or a striped tape is moved in front of infant's eyes. Presence of nystagmus indicates vision. Acuity is assessed by using progressively smaller stripes. | 20/400 | 20/200 | 20/60 | 20-30 |
| Forced-choice preferential looking* | Either a homogeneous field or a striped field is presented to infant; an observer monitors the direction of the eyes during presentation of pattern. Acuity is assessed by using progressively smaller striped fields. | 20/400 | 20/200 | 20/50 | 18-24 |
| Visually evoked potentials | Eyes are stimulated with bright light or pattern, and electrical activity to visual cortex is recorded through scalp electrodes. Acuity is assessed by using progressively smaller patterns. | 20/100 to 20/200 | 20/80 | 20/40 | 6-12 |

Data from Hoyt CS, Nickel BL, Billson FA: Ophthalmological examination of the infant: Development aspects, *Surv Ophthalmol* 26(4):177-189, 1982.

*One type of preferential looking test is the *Teller Acuity Card Test,* in which a set of rectangular cards containing different black-and-white patterns or grading is presented to the child as an observer looks through a central peephole in the card. The observer, who is hidden from view, observes the variety of visual cues, such as fixation, eye movements, head movements, or pointing. The finest grading the child is judged to be able to see is taken as the acuity estimate. The test is appropriate for children from birth to 24-36 months of age. (Teller DY and others: Assessment of visual acuity in infants and children: The acuity card procedure, *Dev Med Child Neurol* 28(6):779-789, 1986.)

## Snellen Screening*

### Preparation

1. Hang the Snellen chart (Figure 1-49) on a light-colored wall so that the 20- to 30-foot lines are at eye level when children 6 to 12 years old are tested in the standing position.
2. Secure the chart to the wall with double-stick tape on the back side of all four corners. If the chart must be reversed for use of the letter or E chart, secure it at the top and bottom with tacks. Make sure that the chart does not swing when in place.
3. The illumination intensity on the chart should be 10 to 30 foot-candles, without any glare from windows or light fixtures. The illumination should be checked with a light meter.
4. Mark an exact 20-foot distance from the chart. Mark the floor with a piece of tape or "footprints" positioned so that the heels touch the 20-foot line.

### Procedure

1. Place the child at the 20-foot mark, with the heel edging the line if child is standing or with the back of the chair placed at the marker if the child is seated.

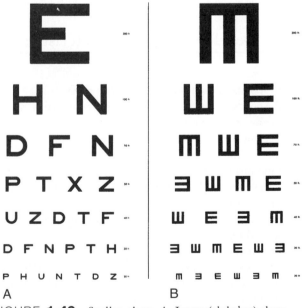

FIGURE **1-49**  Snellen chart. A, Letter (alphabet) chart. B, Symbol E chart.

*Modified from recommendations of *Prevent Blindness America:* Guide to testing distance visual acuity, Schaumburg, Ill, 1995, Prevent Blindness America.

2. If the E chart is used, accustom the child to identifying which direction the legs of the E are pointing. Use a demonstration E card for this purpose.
3. Teach the child to use the occluder to cover one eye. Instruct child to keep both eyes open during the test. Provide a clean cover card for each child, and discard after use.
4. If the child wears glasses, test only with glasses on.
5. Test both eyes together, then right eye, then left eye.
6. Begin with the 40- or 30-foot line, and proceed with test to include the 20-foot line.
7. With a child suspected to have low vision, begin with the 20-foot line and proceed until the child can no longer correctly read three out of four or four out of six symbols on a line.
8. Use covers on the Snellen chart to expose only one symbol or one line at a time. When screening kindergarten-age or older children, expose one line, but a pointer may be used to point to one symbol at a time.

## Recording and Referral

1. Record the last line the child read correctly (three out of four or four out of six symbols).

2. Record visual acuity as a fraction. The numerator represents the distance from the chart, and the denominator represents the last line read correctly. For example, 20/30 means that the child read the 30-foot line at a 20-foot distance.
3. Observe the child's eyes during testing, and record any evidence of squinting, head tilting, thrusting the head forward, excessive blinking, tearing, or redness.
4. Make referrals only after a second screening has been made on children who are potential candidates for referral.
5. The following children should be referred for a complete eye examination:
   a. Three-year-old children with vision in either eye of 20/50 or less (inability to correctly identify one more than half the symbols on the 40-foot line) or a two-line difference in visual acuity between the eyes in the passing range; for example, 20/20 in one eye and 20/40 in the other
   b. All other ages and grades with vision in either eye of 20/40 or less (inability to correctly identify one more than half the symbols on the 30-foot line)
   c. All children who consistently show any of the signs of possible visual disturbances, regardless of visual acuity

# Assessment of Hearing

## Major Developmental Characteristics of Hearing

Birth
- Responds to loud noise with startle reflex
- Responds to sound of human voice more readily than to any other sound
- Becomes quiet with low-pitched sounds, such as lullaby, metronome, or heartbeat

2 to 3 months of age
- Turns head to side when sound is made at level of ear

3 to 4 months of age
- Locates sound by turning head to side and looking in same direction

4 to 6 months of age
- Can localize sounds made below ear, which is followed by localization of sound made above ear; will turn head to side and then look up or down
- Begins to imitate sounds

6 to 8 months of age
- Locates sounds by turning head in a curving arc
- Responds to own name

8 to 10 months of age
- Localizes sounds by turning head diagonally and directly toward sound

10 to 12 months of age
- Knows several words and their meanings, such as "no" and the names of family members
- Learns to control and adjust own response to sound, such as listening for sound to occur again

18 months of age
- Begins to discriminate between harshly dissimilar sounds, such as the sounds of a doorbell and a train

24 months of age
- Refines gross discriminative skills

36 months of age
- Begins to distinguish more subtle differences in speech sounds, such as between "e" and "er"

48 months of age
- Begins to distinguish between similar sounds such as *f* and *th* or between *f* and *s*
- Listening becomes considerably refined
- Able to be tested with an audiometer

# Assessment of Child for Hearing Impairment

Family history
- Genetic disorders associated with hearing impairment
- Family members, especially siblings, with hearing disorders

Prenatal history
- Miscarriages
- Illnesses during pregnancy (rubella, syphilis, diabetes)
- Drugs taken
- Exposure to childhood diseases
- Eclampsia

Delivery
- Duration of labor, type of delivery
- Fetal distress
- Presentation (especially breech)
- Drugs used
- Blood incompatibility

Birth history
- Birth weight <1500 g
- Hyperbilirubinemia at level exceeding indications for exchange transfusion
- Severe asphyxia
- Prematurity
- Congenital perinatal viral infection (cytomegalovirus, rubella, herpes, syphilis, toxoplasmosis)
- Congenital anomalies involving head and neck

Past health history
- Immunizations
- Serious illness (e.g., bacterial meningitis)
- Seizures
- High unexplained fevers

- Ototoxic drugs
- Hyperbilirubinemia (if preterm)
- No history (adopted child)
- Colds, ear infections, allergies
- Treatment of ear problems
- Visual difficulties
- Exposure to excessive noise (e.g., monitor alarms, gunshot)

Hearing
- Parental concerns regarding hearing loss (what cues, at what age)
- Response to name calling, loud noises, sounds of different frequencies (crinkling paper, whisper, bell, rattle)
- Results of previous audiometric testing

Speech development
- Age of babbling, first meaningful words, phrases
- Intelligibility of speech
- Present vocabulary

Motor development
- Age of sitting, standing, and walking
- Level of independence in self-care, feeding, toileting, and grooming

Adaptive behavior
- Play activities
- Socialization with other children
- Behaviors: temper tantrums, stubbornness, self-vexation, vibratory stimulus
- Educational achievement
- Recent behavioral and/or personality changes

# Clues for Detecting Hearing Impairment

Orientation response
- Lack of startle reflex or blink reflex to a loud sound
- Persistence of Moro reflex beyond 4 months of age (associated with mental retardation)
- Failure to be awakened by loud environmental noises during early infancy
- Failure to localize a source of sound by 6 months of age
- General indifference to sound
- Lack of response to the spoken word; failure to follow verbal directions
- Response to loud noises as opposed to the voice

Vocalizations and sound production
- Monotone quality, unintelligible speech, lessened laughter
- Normal quality in central auditory loss
- Lessened experimental sound play and squealing

- Normal use of jargon during early infancy in central auditory loss, with persistent use later
- Absence of babble or inflections in voice by age 7 months
- Failure to develop intelligible speech by age 24 months
- Vocal play, head banging, or foot stamping for vibratory sensation
- Yelling or screeching to express pleasure, annoyance, or need
- Asking to have statements repeated or answering them incorrectly

Visual attention
- Augmented visual alertness and attentiveness
- Responding more to facial expression than to verbal explanation
- Being alert to gestures and movement
- Use of gestures rather than verbalization to express desires, especially after age 15 months
- Marked imitativeness in play

Social rapport and adaptations

- Less interest and involvement in vocal nursery games
- Intense preoccupation with things rather than persons
- Avoidance of social interactions; often puzzled and unhappy in such situations
- Inquiring, sometimes confused facial expression
- Suspicious alertness, sometimes interpreted as paranoia, alternating with cooperation
- Marked reactivity to praise, attention, and physical affection
- Shows less interest than peers in casual conversation

- Is often inattentive unless the environment is quiet and the speaker is close to the child
- Is more responsive to movement than to sound
- Intently observes the speaker's face, responding more to facial expression than verbalization
- Often asks to have statements repeated
- May not follow directions exactly

Emotional behavior

- Use of tantrums to call attention to self or needs
- Frequently stubborn because of lack of comprehension
- Irritable at not making self understood
- Shy, timid, and withdrawn
- Often appears dreamy, in a world of his or her own, or markedly inattentive

# Summary of Growth and Development

This summary of growth and development offers a broad overview of the significant physical, psychosocial, and mental achievements during childhood. It begins with a comparison of cognitive and personality development throughout the life span according to different theorists. Following are summaries of the specific developmental milestones associated with each major age-group of children.

## Personality, Moral, and Cognitive Development

| Stage and Age | Psychosexual Stages (Freud) | Psychosocial Stages (Erikson) | Cognitive Stages (Piaget) | Moral Judgment Stages (Kohlberg) |
|---|---|---|---|---|
| I Infancy (Birth-1 year) | Oral sensory | Trust vs mistrust | Sensorimotor (birth to 18 months) | |
| II Toddlerhood (1-3 years) | Anal-urethral | Autonomy vs shame and doubt | Preoperational thought, preconceptual phase (transductive reasoning; e.g., specific to specific) (2-4 years) | Preconventional (premoral) level Punishment and obedience orientation |
| III Early Childhood (3-6 years) | Phallic-locomotion | Initiative vs guilt | Preoperational thought, intuitive phase (transductive reasoning) (4-7 years) | Preconventional (premoral) level Naïve instrumental orientation |
| IV Middle Childhood (6-12 years) | Latency | Industry vs inferiority | Concrete operations (inductive reasoning and beginning logic) | Conventional level Good-boy, nice-girl orientation Law-and-order orientation |
| V Adolescence (13-18 years) | Genitality | Identity and repudiation vs identity confusion | Formal operations (deductive and abstract reasoning) | Postconventional or principled level Social-contract orientation Universal ethical principle orientation (no longer included in revised theory) |
| VI Early Adulthood | | Intimacy and solidarity vs isolation | | |
| VII Young and Middle Adulthood | | Generativity vs self-absorption | | |
| VIII Later Adulthood | | Ego integrity vs despair | | |

## Growth and Development During Infancy

| Physical | Gross Motor | Fine Motor |
|---|---|---|
| **1 Month** | | |
| Weight gain of 150-210 g (5-7 ounces) weekly for first 6 months<br>Height gain of 2.5 cm (1 inch) monthly for first 6 months<br>Head circumference increases by 2 cm (0.75 inch) monthly for first 3 months<br>Primitive reflexes present and strong<br>Doll's eye reflex and dance reflex fading<br>Obligatory nose breathing (most infants) | Assumes flexed position with pelvis high but knees not under abdomen when prone (at birth, knees flexed under abdomen)*<br>Can turn head from side to side when prone; lifts head momentarily from bed*<br>Has marked head lag, especially when pulled from lying to sitting position<br>Holds head momentarily parallel and in midline when suspended in prone position<br>Assumes asymmetric tonic neck reflex position when supine<br>When infant is held in standing position, body limp at knees and hips<br>In sitting position back is uniformly rounded, head control is absent | Hands predominantly closed<br>Grasp reflex strong<br>Hand clenches on contact with rattle |
| **2 Months** | | |
| Posterior fontanel closed<br>Crawling reflex disappears | Assumes less flexed position when prone—hips flat, legs extended, arms flexed, head to side*<br>Less head lag when pulled to sitting position<br>Can maintain head in same plane as rest of body when held in ventral suspension<br>When infant is prone, can lift head almost 45 degrees off table<br>When infant is held in sitting position, head is held up but bobs forward<br>Assumes asymmetric tonic neck reflex position intermittently | Hands frequently open<br>Grasp reflex fading |
| **3 Months** | | |
| Primitive reflexes fading | Able to hold head more erect when sitting but still bobs forward<br>Has only slight head lag when pulled to sitting position<br>Assumes symmetric body positioning<br>Able to raise head and shoulders from prone position to a 45- to 90-degree angle from table; bears weight on forearms<br>When infant is held in standing position, able to bear slight fraction of weight on legs<br>Regards own hand | Actively holds rattle but will not reach for it*<br>Grasp reflex absent<br>Hands kept loosely open<br>Clutches own hand; pulls at blankets and clothes |
| **4 Months** | | |
| Drooling begins<br>Moro, tonic neck, and rooting reflexes have disappeared* | Has almost no head lag when pulled to sitting position*<br>Balances head well in sitting position*<br>Back less rounded, curved only in lumbar area<br>Able to sit erect if propped up<br>Able to raise head and chest off surface to angle of 90 degrees<br>Assumes predominant symmetric position<br>Rolls from back to side* | Inspects and plays with hands; pulls clothing or blanket over face in play*<br>Tries to reach object with hand but overshoots<br>Grasps object with both hands<br>Plays with rattle placed in hand, shakes it, but cannot pick it up if dropped<br>Can carry objects to mouth |

*Milestones that represent essential integrative aspects of development that lay the foundation for the achievement of more advanced skills.
†Degree of visual acuity varies according to vision measurement procedure used.

| Sensory | Vocalization | Socialization and Cognition |
|---|---|---|
| Able to fixate on moving object in range of 45 degrees when held at a distance of 20-25 cm (8-10 inches)<br>Visual acuity approaches 20/100†<br>Follows light to midline<br>Quiets when hears a voice | Cries to express displeasure<br>Makes small, throaty sounds<br>Makes comfort sounds during feeding | Is in sensorimotor phase—stage I, use of reflexes (birth-1 month), and stage II, primary circular reactions (1-4 months)<br>Watches parent's face intently as she or he talks to infant |
| Binocular fixation and convergence to near objects beginning<br>When infant is supine, follows dangling toy from side to point beyond midline<br>Visually searches to locate sounds<br>Turns head to side when sound is made at level of ear | Vocalizes, distinct from crying*<br>Crying becomes differentiated<br>Coos<br>Vocalizes to familiar voice | Demonstrates social smile in response to various stimuli* |
| Follows object to periphery (180 degrees)<br>Locates sound by turning head to side and looking in same direction*<br>Begins to have ability to coordinate stimuli from various sense organs | Squeals to show pleasure*<br>Coos, babbles, chuckles<br>Vocalizes when smiling "Talks" a great deal when spoken to<br>Less crying during periods of wakefulness | Displays considerable interest in surroundings<br>Ceases crying when parent enters room<br>Can recognize familiar faces and objects, such as feeding bottle<br>Shows awareness of strange situations |
| Able to accommodate to near objects<br>Binocular vision fairly well established<br>Can focus on a 1.25-cm (½-inch) block<br>Beginning eye-hand coordination | Makes consonant sounds *n, k, g, p,* and *b*<br>Laughs aloud*<br>Vocalization changes according to mood | Is in stage III, secondary circular reactions<br>Demands attention by fussing; becomes bored if left alone<br>Enjoys social interaction with people<br>Anticipates feeding when sees bottle or mother if breast-feeding<br>Shows excitement with whole body, squeals, breathes heavily<br>Shows interest in strange stimuli<br>Begins to show memory |

*Continued*

## Growth and Development During Infancy—cont'd

| Physical | Gross Motor | Fine Motor |
|---|---|---|
| **5 Months** | | |
| Beginning signs of tooth eruption<br>Birth weight doubles | No head lag when pulled to sitting position<br>When infant is sitting, able to hold head erect and steady<br>Able to sit for longer periods when back is well supported<br>Back straight<br>When infant is prone, assumes symmetric positioning with arms extended<br>Can turn over from abdomen to back*<br>When infant is supine, puts feet to mouth | Able to grasp objects voluntarily*<br>Uses palmar grasp, bidextrous approach<br>Plays with toes<br>Takes objects directly to mouth<br>Holds one cube while regarding a second one |
| **6 Months** | | |
| Growth rate may begin to decline<br>Weight gain of 90-150 g (3-5 ounces) weekly for next 6 months<br>Height gain of 1.25 cm (0.5 inch) monthly for next 6 months<br>Teething may begin with eruption of two lower central incisors*<br>Chewing and biting occur* | When infant is prone, can lift chest and upper abdomen off table, bearing weight on hands<br>When infant is about to be pulled to a sitting position, lifts head<br>Sits in highchair with back straight<br>Rolls from back to abdomen<br>When infant is held in standing position, bears almost all of weight<br>Hand regard absent | Resecures a dropped object<br>Drops one cube when another is given<br>Grasps and manipulates small objects<br>Holds bottle<br>Grasps feet and pulls to mouth |
| **7 Months** | | |
| Eruption of lower central incisors<br>Parachute reflex appears | When infant is supine, spontaneously lifts head off table<br>Sits, leaning forward on hands*<br>When infant is prone, bears weight on one hand<br>Sits erect momentarily<br>Bears full weight on feet<br>When infant is held in standing position, bounces actively | Transfers objects from one hand to the other*<br>Has unidextrous approach and grasp<br>Holds two cubes more than momentarily<br>Bangs cube on table<br>Rakes at a small object |
| **8 Months** | | |
| Begins to show regular patterns in bladder and bowel elimination | Sits steadily unsupported*<br>Readily bears weight on legs when supported; may stand holding on to furniture<br>Adjusts posture to reach an object | Has beginning pincer grasp using index, fourth, and fifth fingers against lower part of thumb<br>Releases objects at will<br>Rings bell purposely<br>Retains two cubes while regarding third cube<br>Secures an object by pulling on a string<br>Reaches persistently for toys out of reach |

*Milestones that represent essential integrative aspects of development that lay the foundation for the achievement of more advanced skills.

| Sensory | Vocalization | Socialization and Cognition |
| --- | --- | --- |
| Visually pursues a dropped object<br>Is able to sustain visual inspection of an object<br>Can localize sounds made below the ear | Squeals<br>Makes vowel cooing sounds interspersed with consonant sounds (e.g., ah-goo) | Smiles at mirror image<br>Pats bottle or breast with both hands<br>More enthusiastically playful but may have rapid mood swings<br>Is able to discriminate strangers from family<br>Vocalizes displeasure when object is taken away<br>Discovers parts of body |
| Adjusts posture to see an object<br>Prefers more complex visual stimuli<br>Can localize sounds made above the ear<br>Will turn head to the side, then look up or down | Begins to imitate sounds*<br>Babbling resembles one-syllable utterances—*ma, mu, da, di, hi*\*<br>Vocalizes to toys, mirror image<br>Takes pleasure in hearing own sounds (self-reinforcement) | Recognizes parents; begins to fear strangers<br>Holds arms out to be picked up<br>Has definite likes and dislikes<br>Begins to imitate (cough, protrusion of tongue)<br>Excites on hearing footsteps<br>Laughs when head is hidden in a towel<br>Briefly searches for a dropped object (object permanence beginning)*<br>Frequent mood swings—From crying to laughing with little or no provocation |
| Can fixate on very small objects*<br>Responds to own name<br>Localizes sound by turning head in an arc<br>Beginning awareness of depth and space<br>Has taste preferences | Produces vowel sounds and chained syllables—*baba, dada, kaka*\*<br>Vocalizes four distinct vowel sounds"Talks" when others are talking | Increasing fear of strangers; shows signs of fretfulness when parent disappears*<br>Imitates simple acts and noises<br>Tries to attract attention by coughing or snorting<br>Plays peek-a-boo<br>Demonstrates dislike of food by keeping lips closed<br>Exhibits oral aggressiveness in biting and mouthing<br>Demonstrates expectation in response to repetition of stimuli |
| | Makes consonant sounds *t, d,* and *w*<br>Listens selectively to familiar words<br>Utterances signal emphasis and emotion<br>Combines syllables, such as *dada,* but does not ascribe meaning to them | Increasing anxiety over loss of parent, particularly mother, and fear of strangers<br>Responds to word "no"<br>Dislikes dressing, diaper change |

*Continued*

## Growth and Development During Infancy—cont'd

| Physical | Gross Motor | Fine Motor |
|---|---|---|
| **9 Months** | | |
| Eruption of upper central incisors may begin | Creeps on hands and knees<br>Sits steadily on floor for prolonged time (10 minutes)<br>Recovers balance when leans forward but cannot do so when leaning sideways<br>Pulls self to standing position and stands holding on to furniture* | Uses thumb and index finger in crude pincer grasp*<br>Preference for use of dominant hand now evident<br>Grasps third cube<br>Compares two cubes by bringing them together |
| **10 Months** | | |
| Labyrinth-righting reflex is strongest—infant in prone or supine position is able to raise head | Can change from prone to sitting position<br>Stands while holding on to furniture, sits by falling down<br>Recovers balance easily while sitting<br>While child is standing, lifts one foot to take a step | Crude release of an object beginning<br>Grasps bell by handle |
| **11 Months** | | |
| Eruption of lower lateral incisors may begin | When child is sitting, pivots to reach toward back to pick up an object<br>Cruises or walks holding on to furniture or with both hands held* | Explores objects more thoroughly (e.g., clapper inside bell)<br>Has neat pincer grasp<br>Drops object deliberately for it to be picked up<br>Puts one object after another into a container (sequential play)<br>Able to manipulate an object to remove it from tight-fitting enclosure |
| **12 Months** | | |
| Birth weight tripled*<br>Birth length increased by 50%*<br>Head and chest circumference equal (head circumference 46 cm [18 inches])<br>Has total of six to eight deciduous teeth<br>Anterior fontanel almost closed<br>Landau reflex fading<br>Babinski reflex disappears<br>Lumbar curve develops; lordosis evident during walking | Walks with one hand held*<br>Cruises well<br>May attempt to stand alone momentarily; may attempt first step alone*<br>Can sit down from standing position without help | Releases cube in cup<br>Attempts to build two-block tower but fails<br>Tries to insert a pellet into a narrow-necked bottle but fails<br>Can turn pages in a book, many at a time |

*Milestones that represent essential integrative aspects of development that lay the foundation for the achievement of more advanced skills.

| Sensory | Vocalization | Socialization and Cognition |
|---|---|---|
| Localizes sounds by turning head diagonally and directly toward sound<br>Depth perception increasing | Responds to simple verbal commands<br>Comprehends "no-no" | Parent (usually mother) is increasingly important for own sake<br>Shows increasing interest in pleasing parent<br>Begins to show fears of going to bed and being left alone<br>Puts arms in front of face to avoid having it washed |
| | Says "dada," "mama" with meaning<br>Comprehends "bye-bye"<br>May say one word (e.g., "hi," "bye," "no") | Inhibits behavior to verbal command of "no-no" or own name<br>Imitates facial expressions; waves bye-bye<br>Extends toy to another person but will not release it<br>Develops object permanence*<br>Repeats actions that attract attention and cause laughter<br>Pulls clothes of another to attract attention<br>Plays interactive games such as pat-a-cake<br>Reacts to adult anger; cries when scolded<br>Demonstrates independence in dressing, feeding, locomotive skills, and testing of parents<br>Looks at and follows pictures in a book |
| | Imitates definite speech sounds | Experiences joy and satisfaction when a task is mastered<br>Reacts to restrictions with frustration<br>Rolls ball to another on request<br>Anticipates body gestures when a familiar nursery rhyme or story is being told (e.g., holds toes and feet in response to "This little piggy went to market")<br>Plays games such as up-down, so big, or peek-a-boo<br>Shakes head for "no" |
| Discriminates simple geometric forms (e.g., circle)<br>Amblyopia may develop with lack of binocularity<br>Can follow rapidly moving object<br>Controls and adjusts response to sound; listens for sound to recur | Says three to five words besides "dada," "mama"*<br>Comprehends meaning of several words (comprehension always precedes verbalization)<br>Recognizes objects by name<br>Imitates animal sounds<br>Understands simple verbal commands (e.g., "Give it to me," "Show me your eyes") | Shows emotions such as jealousy, affection (may give hug or kiss on request), anger, fear<br>Enjoys familiar surroundings and explores away from parent<br>Is fearful in strange situation; clings to parent<br>May develop habit of security blanket or favorite toy<br>Has increasing determination to practice locomotion skills<br>Searches for an object even if it has not been hidden, but searches only where object was last seen* |

## Growth and Development During Toddler Years

| Physical | Gross Motor | Fine Motor |
|---|---|---|
| **15 Months** | | |
| Steady growth in height and weight<br>Head circumference 48 cm (19 inches)<br>Weight 11 kg (24 pounds)<br>Height 78.7 cm (31 inches) | Walks without help (usually since age 13 months)<br>Creeps up stairs<br>Kneels without support<br>Cannot walk around corners or stop suddenly without losing balance<br>Assumes standing position without support<br>Cannot throw ball without falling | Constantly casting objects to floor<br>Builds tower of two cubes<br>Holds two cubes in one hand<br>Releases a pellet into a narrow-necked bottle<br>Scribbles spontaneously<br>Uses cup with lid well, but rotates spoon |
| **18 Months** | | |
| Physiologic anorexia from decreased growth needs<br>Anterior fontanel closed<br>Physiologically able to control sphincters | Runs clumsily, falls often<br>Walks up stairs with one hand held<br>Pulls and pushes toys<br>Jumps in place with both feet<br>Seats self on chair<br>Throws ball overhand without falling | Builds tower of three or four cubes<br>Release, prehension, and reach well developed<br>Turns pages in a book two or three at a time<br>In drawing, makes stroke imitatively<br>Manages spoon without rotation |
| **24 Months** | | |
| Head circumference 49-50 cm (19.5-20 inches)<br>Chest circumference exceeds head circumference.<br>Lateral diameter of chest exceeds anteroposterior diameter.<br>Usual weight gain of 1.8-2.7 kg (4-6 pounds)<br>Usual gain in height of 10-12.5 cm (4-5 inches)<br>Adult height approximately double height at 2 years<br>May have achieved readiness for beginning daytime control of bowel and bladder<br>Primary dentition of 16 teeth | Goes up and down stairs alone with 2 feet on each step<br>Runs fairly well, with wide stance<br>Picks up object without falling<br>Kicks ball forward without overbalancing | Builds tower of six or seven cubes<br>Aligns two or more cubes like a train<br>Turns pages of book one at a time<br>In drawing, imitates vertical and circular strokes<br>Turns doorknob, unscrews lid |
| **30 Months** | | |
| Birth weight quadrupled<br>Primary dentition (20 teeth) completed<br>May have daytime bowel and bladder control | Jumps with both feet<br>Jumps from chair or step<br>Stands on one foot momentarily<br>Takes a few steps on tiptoe | Builds tower of eight cubes<br>Adds chimney to train of cubes<br>Good hand-finger coordination; holds crayon with fingers rather than fist<br>Moves fingers independently<br>In drawing, imitates vertical and horizontal strokes, makes two or more strokes for cross |

| Sensory | Vocalization | Socialization |
|---|---|---|
| Identifies geometric forms; places round object into appropriate hole<br>Binocular vision well developed<br>Displays an intense and prolonged interest in pictures | Uses expressive jargon<br>Says four to six words, including names<br>Asks for objects by pointing<br>Understands simple commands<br>May use head-shaking gesture to denote "no"<br>Uses "no" even while agreeing to the request | Tolerates some separation from parent<br>Less likely to fear strangers<br>Beginning to imitate parents, such as cleaning house (sweeping, dusting), folding clothes, mowing lawn<br>Feeds self using covered cup with little spilling<br>May discard bottle<br>Manages spoon, but rotates it near mouth<br>Kisses and hugs parents, may kiss pictures in a book<br>Expressive of emotions, has temper tantrums |
| | Says 10 or more words<br>Points to a common object, such as shoe or ball, and to two or three body parts | Great imitator (domestic mimicry)<br>Manages spoon well<br>Takes off gloves, socks, and shoes and unzips<br>Temper tantrums may be more evident<br>Beginning awareness of ownership ("my toy")<br>May develop dependency on transitional objects, such as security blanket |
| Accommodation well developed<br>In geometric discrimination, able to insert square block into oblong space | Has vocabulary of approximately 300 words<br>Uses two- to three-word phrases<br>Uses pronouns "I," "me," "you"<br>Understands directional commands<br>Gives first name; refers to self by name<br>Verbalizes need for toileting, food, or drink<br>Talks incessantly | Stage of parallel play<br>Has sustained attention span<br>Temper tantrums decreasing<br>Pulls people to show them something<br>Increased independence from mother<br>Dresses self in simple clothing |
| | Gives first and last names<br>Refers to self by appropriate pronoun<br>Uses plurals<br>Names one color | Separates more easily from mother<br>In play, helps put things away, can carry breakable objects, pushes with good steering<br>Begins to note gender differences; knows own gender<br>May attend to toilet needs without help, except for wiping |

# Growth and Development During Preschool Years

| Physical | Gross Motor | Fine Motor | Language |
|---|---|---|---|
| **3 Years** | | | |
| Usual weight gain of 1.8-2.7 kg (4-6 pounds)<br>Average weight of 14.6 kg (32 pounds)<br>Usual gain in height of 6.75-7.5 cm (2.5-3 inches)<br>Average height of 95 cm (37.25 inches)<br>May have achieved nighttime control of bowel and bladder | Rides tricycle<br>Jumps off bottom step<br>Stands on one foot for a few seconds<br>Goes up stairs using alternate feet, may still come down using both feet on step<br>Broad jumps<br>May try to dance, but balance may not be adequate | Builds tower of 9 or 10 cubes<br>Builds bridge with three cubes<br>Adeptly places small pellets in narrow-necked bottle<br>In drawing, copies a circle, imitates a cross, names what has been drawn, cannot draw stick figure but may make circle with facial features | Has vocabulary of about 900 words<br>Uses primarily "telegraphic" speech<br>Uses complete sentences of three or four words<br>Talks incessantly regardless of whether anyone is paying attention<br>Repeats sentence of six syllables<br>Asks many questions<br>Begins to sing songs |
| **4 Years** | | | |
| Average weight of 16.7 kg (36.75 pounds)<br>Average height of 103 cm (40.5 inches)<br>Length at birth is doubled<br>Maximum potential for development of amblyopia | Skips and hops on one foot<br>Catches ball reliably<br>Throws ball overhand<br>Walks down stairs using alternate footing | Uses scissors successfully to cut out picture following outline<br>Can lace shoes but may not be able to tie bow<br>In drawing, copies a square, traces a cross and diamond, adds three parts to stick figure | Has vocabulary of 1500 words or more<br>Uses sentences of four or five words<br>Questioning is at peak<br>Tells exaggerated stories<br>Knows simple songs<br>May be mildly profane if associates with older children<br>Obeys prepositional phrases, such as "under," "on top of," "beside," "in back of," or "in front of"<br>Names one or more colors<br>Comprehends analogies, such as, "If ice is cold, fire is_____" |
| **5 Years** | | | |
| Average weight of 18.7 kg (41.25 pounds)<br>Average height of 110 cm (43.25 inches)<br>Eruption of permanent dentition may begin<br>Handedness is established (about 90% are right handed) | Skips and hops on alternate feet<br>Throws and catches ball well<br>Jumps rope<br>Skates with good balance<br>Walks backward with heel to toe<br>Balances on alternate feet with eyes closed | Ties shoelaces<br>Uses scissors, simple tools, or pencil very well<br>In drawing, copies a diamond and triangle; adds seven to nine parts to stick figure; prints a few letters, numbers, or words, such as first name | Has vocabulary of about 2100 words<br>Uses sentences of six to eight words, with all parts of speech<br>Names coins (e.g., nickel, dime)<br>Names four or more colors<br>Describes drawing or comment and enumeration<br>Knows names of days of week, months, and other time-associated words<br>Knows composition of articles, such as, "A shoe is made of ____"<br>Can follow three commands in succession |

| Socialization | Cognition | Family Relationships |
|---|---|---|
| Dresses self almost completely if helped with back buttons and told which shoe is right or left | Is in preconceptual phase | Attempts to please parents and conform to their expectations |
| Has increased attention span | Is egocentric in thought and behavior | Is less jealous of younger sibling; may be opportune time for birth of additional sibling |
| Feeds self completely | Has beginning understanding of time; uses many time-oriented expressions; talks about past and future as much as about present; pretends to tell time | Is aware of family relationships and gender-role functions |
| Can prepare simple meals, such as cold cereal and milk | Has improved concept of space as demonstrated in understanding of prepositions and ability to follow directional command | Boys tend to identify more with father or other male figure |
| Can help set table; can dry dishes without breaking any | Has beginning ability to view concepts from another perspective | Has increased ability to separate easily and comfortably from parents for short periods |
| May have fears, especially of dark and of going to bed | | |
| Knows own gender and gender of others | | |
| Play is parallel and associative; begins to learn simple games but often follows own rules; begins to share | | |
| Very independent | Is in phase of intuitive thought | Rebels if parents expect too much, such as impeccable table manners |
| Tends to be selfish and impatient | Causality is still related to proximity of events | Takes aggression and frustration out on parents or siblings |
| Aggressive physically as well as verbally | Understands time better, especially in terms of sequence of daily events | Dos and don'ts become important |
| Takes pride in accomplishments | Judges everything according to one dimension, such as height, width, or order | May have rivalry with older or younger siblings; may resent older sibling's privileges and younger sibling's invasion of privacy and possessions |
| Has mood swings | Immediate perceptual clues dominate judgment | May "run away" from home |
| Shows off dramatically, enjoys entertaining others | Is beginning to develop less egocentrism and more social awareness | Identifies strongly with parent of opposite gender |
| Tells family tales to others with no restraint | May count correctly but has poor mathematic concept of numbers | Is able to run simple errands outside the home |
| Still has many fears | Obeys because parents have set limits, not because of understanding of right and wrong | |
| Play is associative: Imaginary playmates are common | | |
| Uses dramatic, imaginative, and imitative devices Sexual exploration and curiosity demonstrated through play, such as being "doctor" or "nurse" | | |
| Less rebellious and quarrelsome than at age 4 years | Begins to question what parents think by comparing them with age-mates and other adults | Gets along well with parents |
| More settled and eager to get down to business | May note prejudice and bias in outside world | May seek out parent more often than at age 4 years for reassurance and security, especially when entering school |
| Not as open and accessible in thoughts and behavior as in earlier years | Is more able to view another's perspective but tolerates differences rather than understanding them | Begins to question parents' thinking and principles |
| Independent but trustworthy; not foolhardy; more responsible | May begin to show understanding of conservation of numbers through counting objects regardless of arrangement | Strongly identifies with parent of same gender, especially boys with their fathers |
| Has fewer fears; relies on outer authority to control world | Uses time-oriented words with increased understanding | Enjoys activities such as sports, cooking, shopping with parent of same gender |
| Eager to do things right and to please; tries to "live by the rules" | Very curious about factual information regarding world | |
| Has better manners | | |
| Cares for self totally except for teeth; occasionally needs supervision in dress or hygiene | | |
| Not ready for concentrated close work or small print because of slight farsightedness and still unrefined eye-hand coordination | | |
| Play is associative; tries to follow rules but may cheat to avoid losing | | |

# Growth and Development During School-Age Years

| Physical and Motor | Mental | Adaptive | Personal-Social |
|---|---|---|---|
| **6 Years** | | | |
| Growth and weight gain continue slowly | Develops concept of numbers | At table, uses knife to spread butter or jam on bread | Can share and cooperate better |
| Weight: 16-23.6 kg (35.5-53 pounds); height: 106.6-123.5 cm (42-48 inches) | Counts 13 pennies | At play, cuts, folds, and pastes paper toys, sews crudely if needle is threaded | Has great need for children of own age |
| Central mandibular incisors erupt | Knows whether it is morning or afternoon | | Will cheat to win |
| Loses first tooth | Defines common objects such as fork and chair in terms of their use | Takes bath without supervision; performs bedtime activities alone | Often engages in rough play |
| Gradual increase in dexterity | Obeys triple commands in succession | Reads from memory; enjoys oral spelling game | Often jealous of younger brother or sister |
| Active age; constant activity | Knows right and left hands | Likes table games, checkers, simple card games | Does what adults are seen doing |
| Often returns to finger feeding | Says which is pretty and which is ugly of a series of drawings of faces | Giggles a lot | May have occasional temper tantrums |
| More aware of hand as a tool | Describes the objects in a picture rather than simply enumerating them | Sometimes steals money or attractive items | Is a boaster |
| Likes to draw, print, and color | Attends first grade | Has difficulty owning up to misdeeds | Is more independent, probably influence of school |
| Vision reaches maturity | | Tries out own abilities | Has own way of doing things |
| | | | Increases socialization |
| **7 Years** | | | |
| Begins to grow at least 5 cm (2 inches) a year | Notes that certain parts are missing from pictures | Uses table knife for cutting meat; may need help with tough or difficult pieces | Is becoming a real member of the family group |
| Weight: 17.7-30 kg (39-66.5 pounds); height: 111.8-129.7 cm (44-51 inches) | Can copy a diamond | Brushes and combs hair acceptably without help | Takes part in group play |
| Maxillary central incisors and lateral mandibular incisors erupt | Repeats three numbers backward | May steal | Boys prefer playing with boys; girls prefer playing with girls |
| Jaw begins to expand to accommodate permanent teeth | Develops concept of time; reads ordinary clock or watch correctly to nearest quarter hour; uses clock for practical purposes | Likes to help and have a choice | Spends a lot of time alone; does not require a lot of companionship |
| More cautious in approaches to new performances | Attends second grade | Is less resistant and stubborn | |
| Repeats performances to master them | More mechanical in reading; often does not stop at the end of a sentence, skips words such as "it," "the," and "he" | | |
| **8 to 9 Years** | | | |
| Continues to grow at least 5 cm (2 inches) a year | Gives similarities and differences between two things from memory | Makes use of common tools such as hammer, saw, or screwdriver | Is easy to get along with at home |
| Weight: 19.6-39.6 kg (43-87 pounds); height: 117-141.8 cm (46-56 inches) | Counts backward from 20 to 1; understands concept of reversibility | Uses household and sewing utensils | Likes the reward system |
| Lateral incisors (maxillary) and mandibular cuspids erupt | Repeats days of the week and months in order; knows the date | Helps with routine household tasks such as dusting, sweeping | Dramatizes |
| Movement fluid, often graceful and poised | Describes common objects in detail, not merely their use | Assumes responsibility for share of household chores | Is more sociable |
| Always on the go; jumps, chases, skips | | Looks after all of own needs at table | Is better behaved |
| | | | Is interested in boy-girl relationships but will not admit it |
| | | | Goes about home and community freely, alone, or with friends |

## Growth and Development During School-Age Years—cont'd

| Physical and Motor | Mental | Adaptive | Personal-Social |
|---|---|---|---|
| **8 to 9 Years—cont'd** | | | |
| Increased smoothness and speed in fine motor control; uses cursive writing<br>Dresses self completely<br>Likely to overdo; hard to quiet down after recess<br>More limber; bones grow faster than ligaments | Makes change out of a quarter<br>Attends third and fourth grades<br>Reads more; may plan to wake up early just to read<br>Reads classic books but also enjoys comics<br>More aware of time; can be relied on to get to school on time<br>Can grasp concepts of parts and whole (fractions)<br>Understands concepts of space, cause and effect, nesting (puzzles), and conservation (permanence of mass and volume)<br>Classifies objects by more than one quality; has collections<br>Produces simple paintings or drawings | Buys useful articles; exercises some choice in making purchases<br>Runs useful errands<br>Likes pictorial magazines<br>Likes school; wants to answer all the questions<br>Is afraid of failing a grade; is ashamed of bad grades<br>Is more critical of self<br>Takes music and sport lessons | Likes to compete and play games<br>Shows preference in friends and groups<br>Plays mostly with groups of own gender but is beginning to mix<br>Develops modesty<br>Compares self with others<br>Enjoys Scouts, group sports |
| **10 to 12 Years** | | | |
| Boys: Slow growth in height and rapid weight gain; may become obese in this period<br>Girls: Pubescent changes may begin to appear; body lines soften and round out<br>Weight: 24.3-58 kg (54-128 pounds); height: 127.5-162.3 cm (50-64 inches)<br>Posture is more similar to an adult's; will overcome lordosis<br>Remainder of teeth will erupt and tend toward full development (except wisdom teeth) | Writes brief stories<br>Attends fifth to seventh grades<br>Writes occasional short letters to friends or relatives on own initiative<br>Uses telephone for practical purposes<br>Responds to magazine, radio, or other advertising<br>Reads for practical information or own enjoyment—Stories or library books of adventure or romance, or animal stories | Makes useful articles or does easy repair work<br>Cooks or sews in small way<br>Raises pets<br>Washes and dries own hair<br>Is responsible for a thorough job of cleaning hair but may need reminding to do so<br>Is sometimes left alone at home for an hour or so<br>Is successful in looking after own needs or those of other children left in his or her care | Loves friends; talks about them constantly<br>Chooses friends more selectively; may have a best friend<br>Enjoys conversation<br>Develops beginning interest in opposite gender<br>Is more diplomatic<br>Likes family; family really has meaning<br>Likes mother and wants to please her in many ways<br>Demonstrates affection<br>Likes father, who is adored and idolized<br>Respects parents |

# Growth and Development During Adolescence

| Early Adolescence (11-14 years) | Middle Adolescence (14-17 years) | Late Adolescence (17-20 years) |
| --- | --- | --- |
| **Growth** | | |
| Rapidly accelerating growth<br>Reaches peak velocity<br>Secondary sex characteristics appear | Growth decelerating in girls<br>Stature reaches 95% of adult height<br>Secondary sex characteristics well advanced | Physically mature<br>Structure and reproductive growth almost complete |
| **Cognition** | | |
| Explores newfound ability for limited abstract thought<br>Clumsy groping for new values and energies<br>Comparison of "normality" with peers of same gender | Developing capacity for abstract thinking<br>Enjoys intellectual powers, often in idealistic terms<br>Concern with philosophic, political, and social problems | Established abstract thought<br>Can perceive and act on long-range operations<br>Able to view problems comprehensively<br>Intellectual and functional identity established |
| **Identity** | | |
| Preoccupied with rapid bodily changes<br>Trying out of various roles<br>Measurement of attractiveness by acceptance or rejection of peers<br>Conformity to group norms | Modifies bodily image<br>Very self-centered; increased narcissism<br>Tendency toward inner experience and self-discovery<br>Has a rich fantasy life<br>Idealistic<br>Able to perceive future implications of current behavior and decisions; variable application | Bodily image and gender role definition nearly secured<br>Mature sexual identity<br>Phase of consolidation of identity<br>Stability of self-esteem<br>Comfortable with physical growth<br>Social roles defined and articulated |
| **Relationships with Parents** | | |
| Defining independence-dependence boundaries<br>Strong desire to remain dependent on parents while trying to detach<br>No major conflicts over parental control | Major conflicts over independence and control<br>Low point in parent-child relationship<br>Greatest push for emancipation; disengagement<br>Final and irreversible emotional detachment from parents; mourning | Emotional and physical separation from parents completed<br>Independence from family with less conflict<br>Emancipation nearly secured |
| **Relationships with Peers** | | |
| Seeks peer affiliations to counter instability generated by rapid change<br>Upsurge of close idealized friendships with members of the same gender<br>Struggle for mastery takes place within peer group | Strong need for identity to affirm self-image<br>Behavioral standards set by peer group<br>Acceptance by peers extremely important—Fear of rejection<br>Exploration of ability to attract the opposite gender | Peer group recedes in importance in favor of individual friendship.<br>Testing of male-female relationships against possibility of permanent alliance<br>Relationships characterized by giving and sharing |
| **Sexuality** | | |
| Self-exploration and evaluation<br>Limited dating, usually group<br>Limited intimacy | Multiple plural relationships<br>Decisive turn toward heterosexuality (if homosexual, knows by this time)<br>Exploration of "self appeal"<br>Feeling of "being in love"<br>Tentative establishment of relationships | Forms stable relationships and attachment to another<br>Growing capacity for mutuality and reciprocity<br>Dating as a male-female pair<br>Intimacy involves commitment rather than exploration and romanticism. |

## Growth and Development During Adolescence—cont'd

| Early Adolescence (11-14 years) | Middle Adolescence (14-17 years) | Late Adolescence (17-20 years) |
| --- | --- | --- |
| **Psychologic Health** | | |
| Wide mood swings | Tendency toward inner experiences; more introspective | More constancy of emotion |
| Intense daydreaming | Tendency to withdraw when upset or feelings are hurt | Anger more apt to be concealed |
| Anger outwardly expressed with moodiness, temper outbursts, and verbal insults and name calling | Vacillation of emotions in time and range | |
| | Feelings of inadequacy common; difficulty in asking for help | |

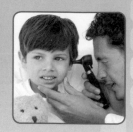
# Health Promotion

**e**volve WEBSITE

Symbol ▶ indicates material that may be photocopied and distributed to families.

- Giving medications to children
- Giving nasogastric tube feedings
- Giving nose drops
- Giving oral medications
- Giving rectal medications—suppositories
- Giving subcutaneous (Sub Q) injections
- Infant cardiopulmonary resuscitation for the layperson
- Interpreting peak expiratory flow rates
- Measuring oxygen saturation with pulse oximetry
- Measuring your child's temperature
- Minimizing pain of blood glucose monitoring
- Monitoring peak expiratory flow
- Obtaining a stool sample
- Obtaining a urine sample
- Oral rehydration guidelines
- Performing clean intermittent bladder catheterization
- Preventing eye injuries
- Preventing spread of HIV and hepatitis B virus infections
- Safe disposal of needles and lancets
- Suctioning the nose and mouth
- Toilet training readiness

# Nutrition

## Dietary Reference Intakes

The Institute of Medicine (IOM) has developed guidelines for nutritional intake that encompass the Recommended Dietary Allowances (RDAs) yet extend their scope to include additional parameters related to nutritional intake. The Dietary Reference Intakes (DRIs)* are composed of four categories. These include estimated average requirements (EARs) for age and gender categories, tolerable upper-limit (UL) nutrient intakes that are associated with a low risk of adverse effects, adequate intakes (AIs) of nutrients, and new standard RDAs. The new guidelines present information about lifestyle factors that may affect nutrient function, such as caffeine intake and exercise, and about how the nutrient may be related to chronic disease (Table 2-1).

## Dietary Guidelines for Children (American Heart Association)

The American Heart Association dietary guidelines (Table 2-2) may also be used to encourage healthy dietary intakes designed to decrease obesity and cardiovascular risk factors and subsequent cardiovascular disease, which is now known to occur in young children as well as adults. For more information on healthy dietary habits and child nutrition, visit the American Heart Association website, available at *http://www.heart.org/HEARTORG/GettingHealthy/NutritionCenter/Dietary-Recommendations-for-Healthy-Children_UCM_303886_Article.jsp*.

## MyPlate for Kids

In 2011 the United States Department of Agriculture replaced the Food Guide Pyramid (MyPyramid) with MyPlate (http://www.choosemyplate.gov/) (Figure 2-1). This colorful plate shows the 5 main food groups—fruits, grains, vegetables, protein, and dairy—with the intended purpose to involve children and their families in making appropriate food choices for meals and decrease the incidence of overweight and obesity in the United States. MyPlate provides an online interactive feature that allows the individual to select (click on) an individual food group and see choices for foods in that group. Approximate serving sizes are suggested and vegetarian substitutions are also provided.

**COMMUNITY FOCUS**

### Fluoride Supplementation*

| Age | Fluoride Concentration in Local Water Supply (ppm) | | |
|---|---|---|---|
| | <0.3 | 0.3-0.6 | >0.6 |
| Birth to 6 mo | 0 | 0 | 0 |
| 6 mo to 3 yr | 0.25[†] | 0 | 0 |
| 3 to 6 yr | 0.50 | 0.25 | 0 |
| 6 to at least 16 yr | 1 | 0.50 | 0 |

From American Academy of Pediatric Dentistry: Reference manual 2009-2010: *Guideline on fluoride therapy,* Chicago, 2010, The Academy, pp 128-130. Accessed June 24, 2010, from *www.aapd.org/media/Policies_Guidelines/G_FluorideTherapy.pdf.*
*Must know fluoride concentration in patient's drinking water before prescribing fluoride supplements.
[†]All values are milligrams of fluoride supplement per day.

---

*For information on DRIs, visit the IOM website *(www.iom.edu)* and either use the site's search engine for DRIs or go to the IOM site map: Ongoing Studies—Dietary Reference Intakes, or call 202-334-1732.

| TABLE 2-1 | Dietary Reference Intakes (DRIs) | | | |
|---|---|---|---|---|
| **DRI Populations and Life Stage Groups** | **Recommended Dietary Allowance (RDA)** | **Estimated Average Requirements (EARS)** | **Adequate Intake (AI)** | **Tolerable Upper Intake Level (UL)** |
| • Pregnancy and lactation<br>• Birth to 6 months<br>• 7-12 mo<br>• 1-3 yr<br>• 4-8 yr<br>• 9-13 yr<br>• 14-18 yr<br>• 19-30 yr<br>• 31-50 yr<br>• 51-70 yr<br>• >70 yr | Average daily dietary intake level sufficient to meet the nutrient requirement of most healthy individuals in a given life stage or gender group. May be used to evaluate nutrient intake of a given population (e.g., vegetarian). | Daily nutrient intake value estimated to meet the requirement of half the healthy persons in a given life stage or gender group (used to assess dietary adequacy and is the basis for RDAs). | Recommended intake value based on observed or experimentally determined approximations of nutrient intake by a group of healthy persons, which are assumed to be adequate when an RDA cannot be determined. In healthy breastfed infants (0-6 mo), AI is the mean intake. | Highest level of daily nutrient intake likely to pose no risk of adverse effects for most individuals in the general population. Risk increases as intake above the UL increases. May be used to set limits on nutrient supplementation, especially for vitamins and minerals that could be harmful. |
| **Clinical Applications** | | | | |
| ***Folate***<br>• Pregnant 19- to 30-year-old women | 600 mcg/d | 520 mcg/d | 400 mcg/d* | 1000 mcg/d |
| ***Iron***<br>• 4- to 8-year-old boys | 10 mg/d | 4.1 mg/d | 10 mg/d | 40 mg/d |
| ***Vitamin C***<br>• 16-year-old girls | 65 mg/d | 56 mg/d | 65 mg/d | 1800 mg/d |

Portions adapted from Dietary Reference Intakes (DRIs): Food and Nutrition Board, Institute of Medicine, National Academy of Sciences, 2004. Available at *www.nap.edu;* and *Dietary Reference Intakes: An Update,* International Food Information Council Foundation, 2005. Available at *http://ific.org.* See also Unit 1 for select DRI values.
*Women of childbearing age and with expectation of becoming pregnant should consume 400 mcg/d from supplements or fortified foods, or both, in addition to intake of folate from a varied diet.

---

### COMMUNITY FOCUS

#### Nutrition: Iron Absorption

To ensure that children receive an adequate supply of iron from foods, consider the following factors that may *increase* or *decrease* iron absorption:

**Increase**

Acidity (low pH)—Administer iron between meals (gastric hydrochloric acid)
Ascorbic acid (vitamin C)—Administer iron with juice, fruit, or multivitamin preparation
Vitamin A
Calcium
Tissue need
Meat, fish, poultry
Cooking in cast iron pots

**Decrease**

Alkalinity (high pH)—Avoid antacid preparations.
Phosphates—Milk is unfavorable vehicle for iron administration.
Phytates—Found in cereals
Oxalates—Found in many fruits and vegetables (e.g., plums, currants, green beans, spinach, sweet potatoes, and tomatoes)
Tannins—Found in tea, coffee
Tissue saturation
Malabsorptive disorders
Disturbances that cause diarrhea or steatorrhea
Infection

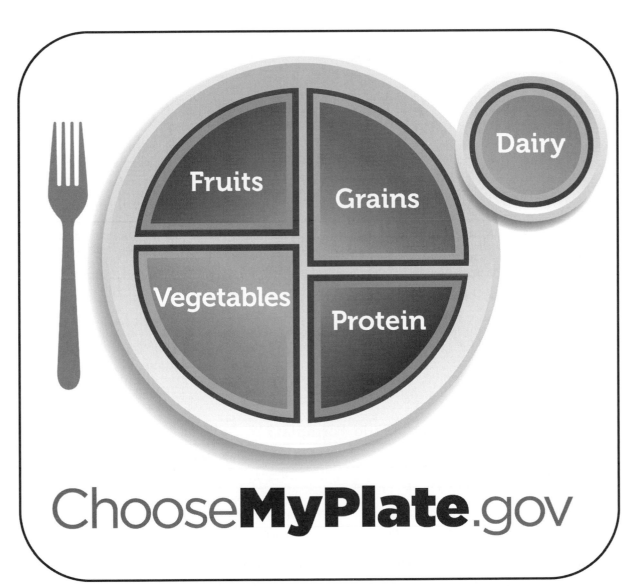

FIGURE **2-1**   MyPlate. MyPlate advocates building a healthy plate by making half of your plate fruits and vegetables and the other half grains and protein. Avoiding oversized portions, making half your grains whole grains, and drinking fat-free or low-fat (1%) milk are additional recommendations for a healthy diet. (From U.S. Department of Agriculture: MyPlate, Washington, DC, June 2011, The Service, available online at *www.choosemyplate.gov.*)

| TABLE 2-2 | Daily Estimated Calories and Recommended Servings for Grains, Fruits, Vegetables, and Dairy Products by Age and Gender | | | | |
|---|---|---|---|---|---|
| | **1 Year** | **2-3 Years** | **4-8 Years** | **9-13 Years** | **14-18 Years** |
| Kilocalories* | | | | | |
| Female | 900 kcal | 1000 kcal | 1200 kcal | 1600 kcal | 1800 kcal |
| Male | 900 kcal | 1000 kcal | 1400 kcal | 1800 kcal | 2200 kcal |
| Fat (% of total kcal) | 30%-40% | 30%-35% | 25%-35% | 25%-35% | 25%-35% |
| Milk or dairy† | 2 cups‡ | 2 cups | 2 cups | 3 cups | 3 cups |
| Lean meat or beans | | | | | |
| Female | 1½ oz | 2 oz | 3 oz | 5 oz | 5 oz |
| Male | 1½ oz | 2 oz | 4 oz | 5 oz | 6 oz |
| Fruits§ | | | | | |
| Female | 1 cup | 1 cup | 1½ cups | 1½ cups | 1½ cups |
| Male | 1 cup | 1 cup | 1½ cups | 1½ cups | 2 cups |
| Vegetables§ | | | | | |
| Female | ¾ cup | 1 cup | 1 cup | 2 cups | 2½ cups |
| Male | ¾ cup | 1 cup | 1½ cups | 2½ cups | 3 cups |
| Grains¶ | | | | | |
| Female | 2 oz | 3 oz | 4 oz | 5 oz | 6 oz |
| Male | 2 oz | 3 oz | 5 oz | 6 oz | 7 oz |

Data from American Heart Association. Available at *www.americanheart.org/presenter.jhtml?identifier53033999*; and American Heart Association, Giddings SS, Dennison BA, and others: Dietary recommendations for children and adolescents: A guide for practitioners, *Pediatrics* 117(2):544-559, 2006. Reprinted with permission *www.heart.org*. Copyright 2011 American Heart Association, Inc.

Estimates are based on sedentary lifestyle. Increased physical activity requires additional calories by 0-200 kcal/day for moderately active children and 200-400 kcal/day for very physically active children.

*For children age 2 years and older. Nutrient and energy contributions from each group are calculated according to the nutrient-dense forms of food in each group (e.g., lean meats and fat-free milk).

†Milk listed is fat-free except for children younger than age 2 years. If 1%, 2%, or whole-fat milk is substituted, this will use, for each cup, 19, 39, or 63 kcal, respectively, of discretionary calories and add 2.6, 5.1, or 9 g, respectively, of fat, of which 1.3, 2.6, or 4.6 g, respectively are saturated fat.

‡For 1-year-old children, calculations are based on 2%-fat milk. If 2 cups of whole milk are substituted, 48 kcal of discretionary calories will be used. The American Academy of Pediatrics recommends that low-fat or reduced-fat milk not be started before age 2 years.

§Serving sizes are ¼ cup for age 1 year, ⅓ cup for ages 2 to 3 years, and ½ cup for age 4 years and older. A variety of vegetables should be selected from each subgroup over the week.

¶Half of all grains should be whole grains.

## Normal and Special Infant and Child Formulas*

| Formula (Manufacturer) | Comments and Nutritional Considerations† |
|---|---|
| **Full-Term Infant Nutrition** | |
| Similac Advance (Abbott) | Contains prebiotics (galactooligosaccharides), antioxidants, DHA, AA, and nucleotides |
| Enfamil Premium Newborn (Mead Johnson); Premium Infant | Contains sources of DHA and AA; iron fortified; prebiotics added; contains vitamin D (400 IU in 27 fl oz) |
| Enfamil AR for Spit Up with Lipil (Mead Johnson) | For mild gastroesophageal reflux; contains rice starch; iron fortified; contains AA and DHA |
| Gerber® Good Start Gentle Plus (Nestlé) & Gerber® Good Start Protect Plus | Contains sources of DHA and AA; Protect Plus contains *Bifidus* BL™ |
| Similac PM 60/40 (Abbott) | Powder only; low solute load; for infants with impaired renal, digestive, and cardiovascular function; lower calcium, potassium, and phosphorus content |
| Enfamil Gentlease (Mead Johnson) | Added DHA, ARA; decreased lactose content (20%) |
| Enfamil RestFull (Mead Johnson) | Rice carbohydrate (not rice cereal) |
| Similac Sensitive for Spit Up (Abbott) | Contains rice starch; Decreased lactose content; contains prebiotics, antioxidants, and nucleotides |

*AA,* Arachidonic acid; *DHA,* docosahexaenoic acid.

*Major retail companies manufacture their own brands of term infant formulas that comply with the Food and Drug Administration guidelines for infant formula composition; these are often less expensive than brand name formulas and contain the same ingredients.

## Normal and Special Infant and Child Formulas—cont'd

| Formula (Manufacturer) | Comments and Nutritional Considerations† |
|---|---|
| **Formulas for Cow's Milk Protein–Sensitive and Lactose-Intolerant Infants*** | |
| Similac Soy Isomil (Abbott) | Soy protein; for infants with lactose intolerance and galactosemia; contains prebiotics, antioxidants, and nucleotides |
| Enfamil ProSobee for Sensitive Tummy (Mead Johnson) | Soy protein; lactose-free and sucrose-free formula for infants with lactose intolerance and galactosemia; contains AA and DHA |
| Similac (Abbott) Expert Care for Diarrhea | Soy based, lactose–free; for diarrhea in infants >6 mo; lessens amount and duration of watery stools |
| Gerber® Good Start Soy PLUS (Nestlé) | Milk–free and lactose free formula with DHA and AA |
| **Protein Hydrolysate–Based and Amino Acid–Based Formulas** | |
| Similac Expert Care Alimentum (Abbott) | Liquid; hydrolyzed casein; hypoallergenic; lactose free; nutritionally complete; for infants with gastrointestinal malabsorption and colic |
| Nutramigen AA Lipil (Mead Johnson) | Powder; amino acid based for infants with severe protein allergy; lactose and sucrose free; nutritionally complete; contains AA and DHA |
| Nutramigen Lipil for Colic (Mead Johnson) | Extensively hydrolyzed; for colic |
| Enfamil Pregestimil Lipil (Mead Johnson) | Powder; hydrolyzed casein; lactose and sucrose free; easily digestible; for infants with postoperative bowel resection and malabsorption conditions |
| Neocate (Nutricia North America) | Powder; amino acid–based formula; for children sensitive to soy, cow's milk protein, and hydrolyzed formula; nutritionally complete; high cost is a factor |
| EleCare (Abbott) Unflavored (for less than 1 year of age) | Powder; amino acid–based formula; hypoallergenic; nutritionally complete; iron fortified; for children sensitive to soy, cow's milk protein, and hydrolyzed formula; high cost is a factor |

*AA,* Arachidonic acid; *DHA,* docosahexaenoic acid.

*This is not an exhaustive list of infant formulas. Other formulas with special additives and uses are available, and information may be obtained from formula company representatives.

†All formulas in this table provide 20 kcal/oz.

## Formulas for Infants and Toddlers with Metabolic Conditions*†

| Formula (Manufacturer) | Comments and Nutritional Considerations |
| --- | --- |
| Phenyl-Free 1 (Mead Johnson) | Phenylalanine free; use for infants and toddlers with PKU; iron fortified; powder; phenylalanine from breast milk, infant formula, or other foods required to support growth; lactose free |
| Phenyl-Free 2 (Mead Johnson) | Phenylalanine free; use for children older than age 1 yr and adults with PKU; iron fortified; powder; permits increased supplementation with normal foods; higher protein content than Phenyl-Free 1 |
| Phenex-1 (Abbott) | Phenylalanine free; powder; use for infants and toddlers with PKU |
| Phenex-2 (Abbott) | Phenylalanine free; powder; use for children and adults with PKU |
| Phenyl-Free 2 HP (Mead Johnson) | Phenylalanine free; powder; use for children and adults with PKU; permits increased supplementation with normal foods |
| RCF (Abbott) | Carbohydrate-free soy formula with iron; may be used in children with carbohydrate intolerance, galactosemia, or for those requiring a ketogenic diet |

*PKU,* Phenylketonuria.

*Ross Laboratories and Mead Johnson manufacture several specialty formulas for metabolic disorders for infants. For a comprehensive list of metabolic disease formulas, contact the manufacturers.

†This is not an exhaustive list of metabolic formulas or companies that offer such products. The reader is advised to consult primary care practitioner for additional information and specific guidelines for feeding children with special dietary needs.

## Preterm Infant Formulas, Human Milk Fortifiers, and Caloric Additives (Diet Modifiers)

| Formula (Manufacturer) | Comments and Nutritional Consideration |
| --- | --- |
| Enfamil EnfaCare (Mead Johnson) | 22 kcal/fluid oz; iron fortified; contains nucleotides, AA and DHA; liquid |
| Similac Expert Care NeoSure (Abbott) | 22 kcal/fluid oz; iron fortified; contains nucleotides; liquid; contains DHA and AA |
| Enfamil Premature with Iron (Mead Johnson) | Available in 24 kcal/fluid oz; contains AA and DHA; liquid |
| Similac Special Care 24 (Abbott); High Protein | 24 kcal/fluid oz; iron fortified; liquid |
| Similac Special Care 20, 24, and Special Care 30 (Abbott) | 20, 24 and 30 kcal/fluid oz; liquid; contains DHA and AA; iron fortified |
| Enfamil Human Milk Fortifier (Mead Johnson) | Powder; add to human milk—do not use as separate formula |
| Similac Human Milk Fortifier (Abbott) | Powder; add to human milk—do not use as separate formula; fortification in excess of 1 package per 25 ml human milk not recommended |
| Polycose (Abbott) | Powder used to augment caloric intake in formulas; 1 tsp powder = 8 kcal; glucose polymer; lactose- and gluten-free; infant formula additive only |
| Portagen (Mead Johnson) | Powder; 87% fat from MCT oil; *not recommended as infant formula;* indicated for use in children with defective mucosal fat absorption, decreased bile salts, and pancreatic lipase; long-term use not recommended; abdominal discomfort and diarrhea possible with initial use if not introduced gradually |

*AA,* Arachidonic acid; *DHA,* docosahexaenoic acid; *MCT,* medium-chain triglyceride.

## Guidelines for Feeding During the First Year

### Birth to 6 Months (Breast- or Bottle-Feeding)
#### *Breast-Feeding*

Most desirable complete diet for first half-year*

May require supplements of fluoride (0.25 mg) after age 6 months

May require iron by age 4 to 6 months (1 mg/kg/day recommended by 4 mos until iron fortified foods are being taken)

Requires vitamin D supplements (400 International units/day) beginning during the first few weeks of life

Exclusively breastfed infants may require supplemental iron (1 mg/kg/day) beginning at age 4 mos if iron-containing complementary foods are not being consumed (American Academy of Pediatrics, 2010)

#### *Formula*

Iron-fortified commercial formula is a complete food for the first half-year.*

Requires fluoride supplements (0.25 mg) after age 6 months when the concentration of fluoride in the local water supply is below 0.3 parts per million (ppm)

Evaporated milk formula requires supplements of vitamin C, iron, and fluoride (in accordance with the fluoride content of the local water supply) after age 6 months.

### Six to 12 Months (Solid Foods)

May begin to add solids by age 4 to 6 months

First foods are strained, pureed, or finely mashed.

Finger foods such as teething crackers and raw fruit or vegetables can be introduced by age 6 to 7 months.

Chopped/cut table food or commercially prepared junior foods can be started by age 9 to 12 months.

With the exception of cereal, the order of introducing foods is variable; a recommended sequence is weekly introduction of other foods, beginning with vegetables, then fruits, and then meat.

As the quantity of solids increases, the amount of formula should be limited to approximately 900 ml (30 ounces) daily and fruit juice to less than 120 ml (4 ounces) daily.

#### *Method of Introduction*

Introduce solids when infant is hungry.

Begin spoon-feeding by pushing food to back of tongue because of infant's natural tendency to thrust tongue forward.

Use small spoon with straight handle; begin with 1 or 2 teaspoons of food; gradually increase to 2 to 3 tablespoons per feeding.

Introduce one food at a time, usually at intervals of 4 to 7 days, to identify food allergies.

As the amount of solid food increases, decrease the quantity of milk to prevent overfeeding.

Avoid introducing foods by mixing them with the formula in the bottle.

#### Cereal

Introduce commercially prepared, iron-fortified infant cereals, and give daily until age 18 months.

Rice cereal usually introduced first because of its low allergenic potential

May discontinue supplemental iron once iron-fortified cereal is given

#### Fruits and Vegetables

Applesauce, bananas, and pears are usually well tolerated.

Avoid fruits and vegetables marketed in cans that are not specifically designed for infants because of variable and sometimes high lead content and addition of salt, sugar, and/or preservatives.

Offer fruit juice only from a cup, not a bottle, to reduce the development of early childhood caries. Limit fruit juice to no more than 4 to 6 oz daily.

#### Meat, Fish, and Poultry

Avoid fatty meats. Offer lean or low fat meats. The following may be substituted for 1 oz meat, fish, or poultry: 1 egg, 2 tbsp peanut butter, or 4 tbsp cooked dry beans or peas (American Academy of Pediatrics, 2009).

Prepare meats by baking, broiling, steaming, or poaching.

Include organ meats such as liver, which has a high iron, vitamin A, and vitamin B complex content.

If soup is given, be sure all ingredients are familiar to child's diet.

Avoid commercial meat and vegetable combinations because protein is low.

#### Eggs and Cheese

Serve egg yolk hard boiled and mashed, soft cooked, or poached.

Introduce egg white in small quantities (1 teaspoon) after the first year of age to detect an allergy.

Use cheese as a substitute for meat and as a finger food.

---

*Breast-feeding or commercial formula–feeding is recommended up to age 12 months. After 1 year, whole cow's milk can be given.
This section may be photocopied and distributed to families.

Source: Wilson D, Hockenberry MJ: *Wong's clinical manual of pediatric nursing,* ed 8, St Louis, 2012, Mosby.

## Developmental Milestones Associated with Feeding

| Age (Months) | Development |
| --- | --- |
| Birth | Has sucking, rooting, and swallowing reflexes |
| | Feels hunger and indicates desire for food by crying; expresses satiety by falling asleep |
| 1 | Has strong extrusion reflex |
| 3-4 | Extrusion reflex fading |
| | Begins to develop hand-eye coordination |
| 4-5 | Can approximate lips to the rim of a cup |
| 5-6 | Can use fingers to feed self a cracker |
| 6-7 | Chews and bites |
| | May hold own bottle but may not drink from it (prefers for it to be held) |
| 7-9 | Refuses food by keeping lips closed; has taste preferences |
| | Holds a spoon and plays with it during feeding |
| | May drink from a straw |
| | Drinks from a cup with assistance |
| 9-12 | Picks up small morsels of food (finger foods) and feeds self |
| | Holds own bottle and drinks from it |
| | Drinks from a household cup without assistance but spills some |
| | Uses spoon with much spilling |
| 12-18 | Drools less |
| | Drinks well from a household cup but may drop it when finished |
| | Holds cup with both hands |
| | Begins to use a spoon but turns it before reaching mouth |
| 24 | Uses straw |
| | Chews food with mouth closed and shifts food in mouth |
| | Distinguishes between finger foods and spoon foods |
| | Holds small cup in one hand; replaces cup without dropping |
| | Uses spoon correctly but with some spilling |
| 36 | Spills small amount from spoon |
| | Begins to use fork; holds it in fist |
| | Uses adult pattern of chewing, which involves rotary action of jaw |
| 48 | Rarely spills when using spoon |
| | Serves self finger foods |
| | Eats with fork; held with fingers |
| 54 | Uses fork in preference to spoon |
| 72 | Spreads with knife |

# Immunizations

## Keeping Current on Vaccine Recommendations

It is much easier to keep current if you know where to look for the official recommendations of the American Academy of Pediatrics and the Centers for Disease Control and Prevention's Advisory Committee on Immunization Practices (ACIP). The primary sources are publications and the Internet. You can also contact each organization at the following addresses to request information:

American Academy of Pediatrics

141 Northwest Point Blvd.

Elk Grove Village, IL 60007

Phone: 847-434-4000

Fax: 847-434-8000

Website: *www.aap.org*

Centers for Disease Control and Prevention

1600 Clifton Road

Atlanta, GA 30333

Phone: 800-232-4636

Website: *www.cdc.gov*

Vaccine and immunization information

*www.cdc.gov/vaccines*

The American Academy of Pediatrics' *Report of the Committee on Infectious Diseases,* known as the *Red Book,* is an authoritative source of information on vaccines and other important pediatric infectious diseases. However, it lacks an in-depth review and reference list of controversial issues. The recommendations in the *Red Book* first appear in the journal *Pediatrics* and/or the *AAP News.* Typically, the most recent immunization schedule appears in the January or February issue of the journal.

The Centers for Disease Control and Prevention now offer a valuable online resource tool for parents and clinicians. The tool prints out an individualized vaccination schedule with dates associated with each vaccination based on the child's date of birth. Clinicians can use this tool for children under age 6 years to serve as a reminder for parents. Nurses should note that the personalized tool is based on the current immunization schedule and may need to be adjusted with the yearly updates from the American Academy of Pediatrics and the ACIP. The tool is available at *www2a.cdc.gov/nip/kidstuff/newscheduler_le.*

A publication of the Centers for Disease Control, *Morbidity and Mortality Weekly Report (MMWR),* contains comprehensive reviews of the literature and important background data regarding vaccine efficacy and side effects. To receive an electronic copy, send an e-mail message to *listserv@listserv.cdc.gov.* The body content should read: SUBscribe mmwr-toc. Electronic copy also is available from the centers' website at *www.cdc.gov* or from the centers' file transfer protocol server at *ftp.cdc.gov.*

Vaccine information statements (VISs) are available by calling your state or local health department. They can also be downloaded from the Immunization Action Coalition's website at *www.immunize.org/vis* or Centers for Disease Control and Prevention's website at *www.cdc.gov/vaccines/pubs/vis/default.htm.* Some translations are available.

Another resource to keep up to date on vaccines that are licensed and commercially available is the U.S. Food and Drug Administration's Center for Biologics Evaluation and Research report for each year, which is available at *www.fda.gov/BiologicsBloodVaccines/Vaccines/default.htm.*

The Immunization Action Coalition also provides a wide variety of immunization information and resources for the public and health professionals. The IAC website is *http://www.immunize.org/.*

## Licensed Vaccines and Toxoids Available in the United States and Recommended Routes of Administration

| Vaccine[a] | Route |
|---|---|
| Adenovirus[b] | Oral |
| Anthrax[b] | Subcutaneous |
| Bacillus of Calmette and Guérin (BCG) | Intradermal or subcutaneous |
| Cholera | Subcutaneous, intramuscular, or intradermal[c] |
| Diphtheria-tetanus–acellular pertussis (DTaP) | Intramuscular |
| Diphtheria-tetanus-pertussis (DTP) | Intramuscular |
| DTaP-Hib conjugate[d] | Intramuscular |
| *Haemophilus influenzae* type b conjugate (Hib)[d] | Intramuscular |
| Hepatitis A | Intramuscular |
| Hepatitis B | Intramuscular[e] |
| Hib conjugate–hepatitis B | Intramuscular |
| Human papillomavirus (HPV$_4$, HPV$_2$) | Intramuscular |
| Influenza-TIV (same route for H1N1[TIV]) | Intramuscular |
| Influenza LAIV (same route for H1N1[LAIV]) | Nasal Mist |
| Japanese encephalitis | Subcutaneous |
| Measles | Subcutaneous |
| Measles-mumps-rubella (MMR) | Subcutaneous |
| Measles-mumps-rubella & varicella (MMRV) | Subcutaneous |
| Measles-rubella | Subcutaneous |
| Meningococcal | Intramuscular (MCV4); subcutaneous (MPSV4) |
| Mumps | Subcutaneous |
| Pertussis | Intramuscular |
| Pneumococcal (polysaccharide; PPV) | Intramuscular or subcutaneous |
| Pneumococcal (polysaccharide-protein conjugate; PCV) | Intramuscular |
| Poliovirus vaccine, inactivated (IPV) | Subcutaneous |
| Rabies | Intramuscular or intradermal[f] |
| Rotavirus | Oral |
| Rubella | Subcutaneous |
| Tetanus | Intramuscular |
| Tetanus-diphtheria (Td or DT) | Intramuscular |
| Tetanus and diphtheria toxoids and acellular pertussis (Tdap) | Intramuscular |
| Typhoid (parenteral) | Subcutaneous[g] |
| Typhoid (Ty21a) | Oral |
| Varicella | Subcutaneous |
| Yellow fever | Subcutaneous |
| Zoster | Subcutaneous |

Modified from American Academy of Pediatrics: Active and passive immunization. In Pickering LK, editor: 2009 *Red book: Report of the Committee on Infectious Diseases,* ed 28, Elk Grove Village, Ill, 2009, The Academy.

[a]Additional vaccines that are licensed but not available to the general public include oral poliovirus and smallpox vaccinia. For a list of currently licensed vaccines, see Food and Drug Administration website: *www.fda.gov/cber/vaccine/licvacc.htm.*

[b]Available only to U.S. Armed Forces.

[c]Intradermal dose is lower than subcutaneous dose.

[d]May be administered in combination products or as reconstituted products with DTP or DTaP if approved by the Food and Drug Administration for the child's age and if administration of other vaccine is justified.

[e]Not administered in dorsogluteal muscle (buttock) because of possible reduced immunologic response.

[f]Intradermal dose of rabies vaccine, human diploid cell (HDCV), is lower than intramuscular dose and is used only for preexposure vaccination. Rabies vaccine, adsorbed (RVA), should not be used intradermally. Another rabies vaccine, PCEC (purified chicken embryo cell culture), RabAvert, may be given by intramuscular route only for preexposure or postexposure prophylaxis in persons who are sensitive to the other rabies vaccines.

[g]Booster doses may be administered intradermally unless vaccine that is acetone killed and dried is used.

# Recommended Immunization Schedule for Persons Ages 0 to 6 Years—United States, 2011

## Recommended Immunization Schedule for Persons Aged 0 Through 6 Years—United States • 2011

| Vaccine ▼ Age ► | Birth | 1 month | 2 months | 4 months | 6 months | 12 months | 15 months | 18 months | 19–23 months | 2–3 years | 4–6 years |
|---|---|---|---|---|---|---|---|---|---|---|---|
| Hepatitis B[1] | HepB | HepB | | | | HepB | | | | | |
| Rotavirus[2] | | | RV | RV | RV[2] | | | | | | |
| Diphtheria, Tetanus, Pertussis[3] | | | DTaP | DTaP | DTaP | see footnote[3] | DTaP | | | | DTaP |
| *Haemophilus influenzae* type b[4] | | | Hib | Hib | Hib[4] | Hib | | | | | |
| Pneumococcal[5] | | | PCV | PCV | PCV | PCV | | | | PPSV | |
| Inactivated Poliovirus[6] | | | IPV | IPV | | IPV | | | | | IPV |
| Influenza[7] | | | | | | Influenza (Yearly) | | | | | |
| Measles, Mumps, Rubella[8] | | | | | | MMR | | see footnote[8] | | | MMR |
| Varicella[9] | | | | | | Varicella | | see footnote[9] | | | Varicella |
| Hepatitis A[10] | | | | | | HepA (2 doses) | | | | HepA Series | |
| Meningococcal[11] | | | | | | | | | | MCV4 | |

Range of recommended ages for all children

Range of recommended ages for certain high-risk groups

2 - HEALTH PROMOTION

This schedule includes recommendations in effect as of December 21, 2010. Any dose not administered at the recommended age should be administered at a subsequent visit, when indicated and feasible. The use of a combination vaccine generally is preferred over separate injections of its equivalent component vaccines. Considerations should include provider assessment, patient preference, and the potential for adverse events. Providers should consult the relevant Advisory Committee on Immunization Practices statement for detailed recommendations: **http://www.cdc.gov/vaccines/ pubs/acip-list.htm**. Clinically significant adverse events that follow immunization should be reported to the Vaccine Adverse Event Reporting System (VAERS) at **http://www.vaers.hhs.gov** or by telephone, **800-822-7967**. Use of trade names and commercial sources is for identification only and does not imply endorsement by the U.S. Department of Health and Human Services.

1. **Hepatitis B vaccine (HepB).** (Minimum age: birth)
   **At birth:**
   • Administer monovalent HepB to all newborns before hospital discharge.
   • If mother is hepatitis B surface antigen (HBsAg)-positive, administer HepB and 0.5 mL of hepatitis B immune globulin (HBIG) within 12 hours of birth.
   • If mother's HBsAg status is unknown, administer HepB within 12 hours of birth. Determine mother's HBsAg status as soon as possible and, if HBsAg-positive, administer HBIG (no later than age 1 week).
   **Doses following the birth dose:**
   • The second dose should be administered at age 1 or 2 months. Monovalent HepB should be used for doses administered before age 6 weeks.
   • Infants born to HBsAg-positive mothers should be tested for HBsAg and antibody to HBsAg 1 to 2 months after completion of at least 3 doses of the HepB series, at age 9 through 18 months (generally at the next well-child visit).
   • Administration of 4 doses of HepB to infants is permissible when a combination vaccine containing HepB is administered after the birth dose.
   • Infants who did not receive a birth dose should receive 3 doses of HepB on a schedule of 0, 1, and 6 months.
   • The final (3rd or 4th) dose in the HepB series should be administered no earlier than age 24 weeks.
2. **Rotavirus vaccine (RV).** (Minimum age: 6 weeks)
   • Administer the first dose at age 6 through 14 weeks (maximum age: 14 weeks 6 days). Vaccination should not be initiated for infants aged 15 weeks 0 days or older.
   • The maximum age for the final dose in the series is 8 months 0 days
   • If Rotarix is administered at ages 2 and 4 months, a dose at 6 months is not indicated.
3. **Diphtheria and tetanus toxoids and acellular pertussis vaccine (DTaP).** (Minimum age: 6 weeks)
   • The fourth dose may be administered as early as age 12 months, provided at least 6 months have elapsed since the third dose.
4. ***Haemophilus influenzae* type b conjugate vaccine (Hib).** (Minimum age: 6 weeks)
   • If PRP-OMP (PedvaxHIB or Comvax [HepB-Hib]) is administered at ages 2 and 4 months, a dose at age 6 months is not indicated.
   • Hiberix should not be used for doses at ages 2, 4, or 6 months for the primary series but can be used as the final dose in children aged 12 months through 4 years.
5. **Pneumococcal vaccine.** (Minimum age: 6 weeks for pneumococcal conjugate vaccine [PCV]; 2 years for pneumococcal polysaccharide vaccine [PPSV])
   • PCV is recommended for all children aged younger than 5 years. Administer 1 dose of PCV to all healthy children aged 24 through 59 months who are not completely vaccinated for their age.
   • A PCV series begun with 7-valent PCV (PCV7) should be completed with 13-valent PCV (PCV13).
   • A single supplemental dose of PCV13 is recommended for all children aged 14 through 59 months who have received an age-appropriate series of PCV7.
   • A single supplemental dose of PCV13 is recommended for all children aged 60 through 71 months with underlying medical conditions who have received an age-appropriate series of PCV7.

   • The supplemental dose of PCV13 should be administered at least 8 weeks after the previous dose of PCV7. See *MMWR* 2010:59(No. RR-11).
   • Administer PPSV at least 8 weeks after last dose of PCV to children aged 2 years or older with certain underlying medical conditions, including a cochlear implant.
6. **Inactivated poliovirus vaccine (IPV).** (Minimum age: 6 weeks)
   • If 4 or more doses are administered prior to age 4 years an additional dose should be administered at age 4 through 6 years.
   • The final dose in the series should be administered on or after the fourth birthday and at least 6 months following the previous dose.
7. **Influenza vaccine (seasonal).** (Minimum age: 6 months for trivalent inactivated influenza vaccine [TIV]; 2 years for live, attenuated influenza vaccine [LAIV])
   • For healthy children aged 2 years and older (i.e., those who do not have underlying medical conditions that predispose them to influenza complications), either LAIV or TIV may be used, except LAIV should not be given to children aged 2 through 4 years who have had wheezing in the past 12 months.
   • Administer 2 doses (separated by at least 4 weeks) to children aged 6 months through 8 years who are receiving seasonal influenza vaccine for the first time or who were vaccinated for the first time during the previous influenza season but only received 1 dose.
   • Children aged 6 months through 8 years who received no doses of monovalent 2009 H1N1 vaccine should receive 2 doses of 2010–2011 seasonal influenza vaccine. See *MMWR* 2010;59(No. RR-8):33–34.
8. **Measles, mumps, and rubella vaccine (MMR).** (Minimum age: 12 months)
   • The second dose may be administered before age 4 years, provided at least 4 weeks have elapsed since the first dose.
9. **Varicella vaccine.** (Minimum age: 12 months)
   • The second dose may be administered before age 4 years, provided at least 3 months have elapsed since the first dose.
   • For children aged 12 months through 12 years the recommended minimum interval between doses is 3 months. However, if the second dose was administered at least 4 weeks after the first dose, it can be accepted as valid.
10. **Hepatitis A vaccine (HepA).** (Minimum age: 12 months)
    • Administer 2 doses at least 6 months apart.
    • HepA is recommended for children aged older than 23 months who live in areas where vaccination programs target older children, who are at increased risk for infection, or for whom immunity against hepatitis A is desired.
11. **Meningococcal conjugate vaccine, quadrivalent (MCV4).** (Minimum age: 2 years)
    • Administer 2 doses of MCV4 at least 8 weeks apart to children aged 2 through 10 years with persistent complement component deficiency and anatomic or functional asplenia, and 1 dose every 5 years thereafter.
    • Persons with human immunodeficiency virus (HIV) infection who are vaccinated with MCV4 should receive 2 doses at least 8 weeks apart.
    • Administer 1 dose of MCV4 to children aged 2 through 10 years who travel to countries with highly endemic or epidemic disease and during outbreaks caused by a vaccine serogroup.
    • Administer MCV4 to children at continued risk for meningococcal disease who were previously vaccinated with MCV4 or meningococcal polysaccharide vaccine after 3 years if the first dose was administered at age 2 through 6 years.

For children who fall behind or start late see the catch up schedule at http://www.cdc.gov/vaccines/recs/schedules/downloads/child/catchup-schedule-bw.pdf

From Centers for Disease Control and Prevention: Recommended immunization schedules for persons aged 0 through 18 years—United States, 2011, *MMWR* 60(5):1-4, 2011.

Website for 2011 charts available at *http://www.cdc.gov/vaccines/recs/schedules/child-schedule.htm.*

# Recommended Immunization Schedule for Persons Ages 7 to 18 Years—United States, 2011

## Recommended Immunization Schedule for Persons Aged 7 Through 18 Years—United States • 2011

| Vaccine ▼        Age ► | 7–10 years | 11–12 years | 13–18 years |
|---|---|---|---|
| Tetanus, Diphtheria, Pertussis[1] | | Tdap | Tdap |
| Human Papillomavirus[2] | see footnote [2] | HPV (3 doses)(females) | HPV Series |
| Meningococcal[3] | MCV4 | MCV4 | MCV4 |
| Influenza[4] | Influenza (Yearly) | | |
| Pneumococcal[5] | Pneumococcal | | |
| Hepatitis A[6] | HepA Series | | |
| Hepatitis B[7] | Hep B Series | | |
| Inactivated Poliovirus[8] | IPV Series | | |
| Measles, Mumps, Rubella[9] | MMR Series | | |
| Varicella[10] | Varicella Series | | |

Range of recommended ages for all children

Range of recommended ages for catch-up immunization

Range of recommended ages for certain high-risk groups

This schedule includes recommendations in effect as of December 21, 2010. Any dose not administered at the recommended age should be administered at a subsequent visit, when indicated and feasible. The use of a combination vaccine generally is preferred over separate injections of its equivalent component vaccines. Considerations should include provider assessment, patient preference, and the potential for adverse events. Providers should consult the relevant Advisory Committee on Immunization Practices statement for detailed recommendations: **http://www.cdc.gov/vaccines/pubs/acip-list.htm** Clinically significant adverse events that follow immunization should be reported to the Vaccine Adverse Event Reporting System (VAERS) at **http://www.vaers.hhs.gov** or by telephone, **800-822-7967.**

1. **Tetanus and diphtheria toxoids and acellular pertussis vaccine (Tdap).**
   (Minimum age: 10 years for Boostrix and 11 years for Adacel)
   - Persons aged 11 through 18 years who have not received Tdap should receive a dose followed by Td booster doses every 10 years thereafter.
   - Persons aged 7 through 10 years who are not fully immunized against pertussis (including those never vaccinated or with unknown pertussis vaccination status) should receive a single dose of Tdap. Refer to the catch-up schedule if additional doses of tetanus and diphtheria toxoid–containing vaccine are needed.
   - Tdap can be administered regardless of the interval since the last tetanus and diphtheria toxoid–containing vaccine.
2. **Human papillomavirus vaccine (HPV).** (Minimum age: 9 years)
   - Quadrivalent HPV vaccine (HPV4) or bivalent HPV vaccine (HPV2) is recommended for the prevention of cervical precancers and cancers in females.
   - HPV4 is recommended for prevention of cervical precancers, cancers, and genital warts in females.
   - HPV4 may be administered in a 3-dose series to males aged 9 through 18 years to reduce their likelihood of genital warts.
   - Administer the second dose 1 to 2 months after the first dose and the third dose 6 months after the first dose (at least 24 weeks after the first dose).
3. **Meningococcal conjugate vaccine, quadrivalent (MCV4).** (Minimum age: 2 years)
   - Administer MCV4 at age 11 through 12 years with a booster dose at age 16 years.
   - Administer 1 dose at age 13 through 18 years if not previously vaccinated.
   - Persons who received their first dose at age 13 through 15 years should receive a booster dose at age 16 through 18 years.
   - Administer 1 dose to previously unvaccinated college freshmen living in a dormitory.
   - Administer 2 doses at least 8 weeks apart to children aged 2 through 10 years with persistent complement component deficiency and anatomic or functional asplenia, and 1 dose every 5 years thereafter.
   - Persons with HIV infection who are vaccinated with MCV4 should receive 2 doses at least 8 weeks apart.
   - Administer 1 dose of MCV4 to children aged 2 through 10 years who travel to countries with highly endemic or epidemic disease and during outbreaks caused by a vaccine serogroup.
   - Administer MCV4 to children at continued risk for meningococcal disease who were previously vaccinated with MCV4 or meningococcal polysaccharide vaccine after 3 years (if first dose administered at age 2 through 6 years) or after 5 years (if first dose administered at age 7 years or older).
4. **Influenza vaccine (seasonal).**
   - For healthy nonpregnant persons aged 7 through 18 years (i.e., those who do not have underlying medical conditions that predispose them to influenza complications), either LAIV or TIV may be used.
   - Administer 2 doses (separated by at least 4 weeks) to children aged 6 months through 8 years who are receiving seasonal influenza vaccine for the first

time or who were vaccinated for the first time during the previous influenza season but only received 1 dose.
   - Children 6 months through 8 years of age who received no doses of monovalent 2009 H1N1 vaccine should receive 2 doses of 2010-2011 seasonal influenza vaccine. See *MMWR* 2010;59(No. RR-8):33–34.
5. **Pneumococcal vaccines.**
   - A single dose of 13-valent pneumococcal conjugate vaccine (PCV13) may be administered to children aged 6 through 18 years who have functional or anatomic asplenia, HIV infection or other immunocompromising condition, cochlear implant or CSF leak. See *MMWR* 2010;59(No. RR-11).
   - The dose of PCV13 should be administered at least 8 weeks after the previous dose of PCV7.
   - Administer pneumococcal polysaccharide vaccine at least 8 weeks after the last dose of PCV to children aged 2 years or older with certain underlying medical conditions, including a cochlear implant. A single revaccination should be administered after 5 years to children with functional or anatomic asplenia or an immunocompromising condition.
6. **Hepatitis A vaccine (HepA).**
   - Administer 2 doses at least 6 months apart.
   - HepA is recommended for children aged older than 23 months who live in areas where vaccination programs target older children, or who are at increased risk for infection, or for whom immunity against hepatitis A is desired.
7. **Hepatitis B vaccine (HepB).**
   - Administer the 3-dose series to those not previously vaccinated. For those with incomplete vaccination, follow the catch-up schedule.
   - A 2-dose series (separated by at least 4 months) of adult formulation Recombivax HB is licensed for children aged 11 through 15 years.
8. **Inactivated poliovirus vaccine (IPV).**
   - The final dose in the series should be administered on or after the fourth birthday and at least 6 months following the previous dose.
   - If both OPV and IPV were administered as part of a series, a total of 4 doses should be administered, regardless of the child's current age.
9. **Measles, mumps, and rubella vaccine (MMR).**
   - The minimum interval between the 2 doses of MMR is 4 weeks.
10. **Varicella vaccine.**
   - For persons aged 7 through 18 years without evidence of immunity (see *MMWR* 2007;56[No. RR-4]), administer 2 doses if not previously vaccinated or the second dose if only 1 dose has been administered.
   - For persons aged 7 through 12 years, the recommended minimum interval between doses is 3 months. However, if the second dose was administered at least 4 weeks after the first dose, it can be accepted as valid.
   - For persons aged 13 years and older, the minimum interval between doses is 4 weeks.

From Centers for Disease Control and Prevention: Recommended immunization schedules for persons aged 0 through 18 years—United States, 2011, *MMWR* 60(5):1-4, 2011.
Website for 2011 charts available at *http://www.cdc.gov/vaccines/recs/schedules/child-schedule.htm.*
NOTE: A recommended catch-up schedule for children who fall behind or start late is available at the Centers for Disease Control and Prevention website *http://www.cdc.gov/vaccines/recs/schedules/downloads/child/catchup-schedule-bw.pdf.*

2 - HEALTH PROMOTION

## Possible Side Effects of Recommended Childhood Immunizations and Nursing Responsibilities

| Immunization | Reaction | Nursing Responsibilities |
|---|---|---|
| Hepatitis B virus | Well tolerated, few side effects | Explain to parents the reason for this immunization. Consider that cost for three injections may be a factor. |
| Diphtheria | Fever usually within 24-48 hours<br>Soreness, redness, and swelling at injection site<br>Behavioral changes: drowsiness, fretfulness, anorexia, prolonged or unusual crying | Nursing responsibilities for DTP/DTaP/Tdap apply to immunizations for diphtheria, tetanus, and pertussis.<br>Instruction for DTP/DTaP/Tdap: Advise parents of possible side effects. |
| Tetanus | Same as for diphtheria but may include urticaria and malaise<br>All may have delayed onset and last several days<br>Lump at injection site may last for weeks, even months, but gradually disappears | Acetaminophen is recommend for prophylactic use at time of DTP/DTaP or Tdap immunization and every 4-6 hours for a total of three doses.<br>Advise parents to notify practitioner immediately of any unusual side effects, such as fever (temperature at or above 40.5° C [105° F]) within 48 hr after vaccination; collapse or shocklike state within 48 hr after receiving dose of DTaP or DTP; seizures within 3 days of receiving dose of DTaP or DTP; Guillain-Barré syndrome within 6 weeks after receiving dose; or persistent, inconsolable crying lasting ≥3 hr within 48 hr after receiving dose of DTaP or DTP |
| Pertussis | Same as for tetanus but may include loss of consciousness, convulsions, persistent inconsolable crying episodes, generalized or focal neurologic signs, fever (temperature at or above 40.5° C [105° F]), systemic allergic reaction | Before administering next dose of DTP/DTaP, or Tdap inquire about reactions, especially those listed above for tetanus. |
| *Haemophilus influenzae* type b | Mild local reactions (erythema, pain) at injection site<br>Low-grade fever | Advise parents of possible mild side effects. |
| Poliovirus (IPV) | No serious adverse effects have been associated with the currently available product<br>Rare reactions possible<br>Trace amounts of neomycin, streptomycin, and polymyxin B may be present in IPV | Advise parents of safety of IPV (i.e., no vaccine-associated polio paralysis with inactivated virus). |
| Measles | Anorexia, malaise, rash, and fever may occur 7 to 10 days after immunization<br>Rarely (estimated risk 1:1 million doses) encephalitis may occur. | Advise parents of more common side effects, and recommend use of antipyretics (acetaminophen) for fever.<br>If persistent fever with other obvious signs of illness occurs, have parents notify physician immediately. |
| Mumps | Essentially no side effects other than a brief, mild fever | See general comment to parents.* |
| Rubella | Fever, lymphadenopathy, or mild rash that lasts 1 or 2 days within a few days after immunization<br>Arthralgia, arthritis, or paresthesia of the hands and fingers may occur approximately 2 weeks after vaccination; more common in older children and adults. | Advise parents of side effects, especially of time delay before joint swelling and pain; assure them that these symptoms will disappear. |

Modified from American Academy of Pediatrics, Committee on Infectious Diseases, Pickering L, editor: 2009 *Red book: Report of the Committee on Infectious Diseases,* ed 28, Elk Grove Village, Ill, 2009, The Academy and Centers for Disease Control and Prevention: General recommendations on immunizations: Recommendations of the Advisory Committee on Immunization Practices (ACIP), MMWR Recommendations and reports 60(2):1-61, 2011. Accessed on March 8, 2011 at *http://www.cdc.gov/mmwr/pdf/rr/rr6002.pdf.*

*DTaP,* Diphtheria-tetanus–acellular pertussis; *DTP,* diphtheria-tetanus-pertussis; *MMR,* measles-mumps-rubella vaccine; *Tdap,* tetanus toxoid, reduced diphtheria toxoid, and acellular pertussis (booster); *TIV,* trivalent inactivated influenza vaccine.

*General comment to parents regarding each immunization: Benefit of being protected by immunization is believed to greatly outweigh risk from the disease.

*Continued*

2 - HEALTH PROMOTION

## Possible Side Effects of Recommended Childhood Immunizations and Nursing Responsibilities—cont'd

| Immunization | Reaction | Nursing Responsibilities |
|---|---|---|
| Varicella | Pain, tenderness, or redness at injection site<br>Mild, vaccine-associated maculopapular or varicelliform rash at injection site or elsewhere | Advise parents of possible side effects.<br>If necessary, recommend use of acetaminophen for pain. |
| Hepatitis A | No severe reactions have been reported.<br>Local erythema may occur in some cases. | Explain to parents and teens rationale for immunization.<br>Encourage parents in high-risk areas to immunize children, especially teens and preteens. |
| Pneumococcal (PCV and PPV) | Fever, fussiness, decreased appetite, drowsiness, local erythema, interrupted sleep, diarrhea, vomiting, and hives | Explain to parents benefits and rationale for vaccination in children younger than age 2 years and older than age 2 years if in high-risk category. |
| Meningococcal | MCV4—Pain at injection site, fever, headache, fatigue, malaise, chills, anorexia, vomiting, diarrhea, rash<br>MPSV4—Pain and redness at injection site, transient fever, urticaria, wheezing, and rash (extremely rare)<br>MCV4/MPSV4—Allergy to vaccine components including diphtheria toxoid and possible reaction to latex; history of GBS. | Explain to parents benefits and rationale for immunization, especially in adolescents and in small children at higher risk for meningococcal disease. |
| Influenza | TIV (trivalent inactivated vaccine)—Fever and local reactions: fever possible in children <24 mo, local reactions occur primarily in children >13 yr<br>Live-attenuated influenza vaccine (LAIV)—Fever, rhinitis, nasal congestion<br>Same reactions may occur with H1N1 vaccines<br>NOTE: Children with severe anaphylactic reaction to chicken or egg protein should not receive the inactivated influenza vaccine. | Explain to parents and adolescents rationale for vaccine; explain that the vaccine will not give the child a mild case of influenza. |
| Human papillomavirus (HPV 2 and HPV 4) | Localized pain, swelling and erythema, fever<br>Syncope in adolescents | Explain to parents and adolescent benefit and rationale for immunization and necessity of completing vaccination series.<br>Observe for 15 minutes after vaccine administration<br>Vaccines should not be given to pregnant female, but may be given to lactating female<br>HPV4 contains baker's yeast.† |
| Rotavirus (RV1 [Rotarix] and RV5 [RotaTeq]) | Diarrhea, vomiting, runny nose and sore throat, ear infection, wheezing and coughing. RV1 oral applicator contains latex—avoid use in children with latex sensitivity. Children with known immunocompetence should be carefully evaluated for risk and benefits before administration of rotavirus vaccine.‡ | Explain to parents rationale for immunization.<br>Assess for latex exposure and allergy (e.g., infants with spina bifida), presence of acute moderate-to-severe gastroenteritis at time of administration; preterm infants should receive age-appropriate dose of rotavirus vaccine prior to discharge from NICU or nursery.‡ |

---

†From Centers for Disease Control and Prevention: FDA licensure of bivalent human papillomavirus vaccine (HPV2, Cervarix) for use in females and updated HPV vaccination recommendations from the Advisory Committee on Immunization Practices (ACIP), *MMWR Weekly* 59(20): 626-629, 2010.

‡American Academy of Pediatrics: Prevention of rotavirus disease: Updated guidelines for use of rotavirus vaccine, *Pediatrics* 123(5):1412-1420, 2009.

# Safety and Injury Prevention

## Child Safety Home Checklist

### Safety: Fire, Electrical, Burns

☐ Guards in front of or around any heating appliance, fireplace, or furnace (including floor furnace)*

☐ Electrical wires hidden or out of reach*

☐ No frayed or broken wires; no overloaded sockets

☐ Plastic guards or caps over electrical outlets or furniture in front of outlets*

☐ Hanging tablecloths out of reach, away from open fires*

☐ Smoke and carbon monoxide detectors tested and operating properly

☐ Matches and other lighters (such as butane) stored out of child's reach*

☐ Large, deep ashtrays throughout house (if used)

☐ Small stoves, heaters, and other hot objects (cigarettes, candles, coffee pots, slow cookers) placed where they cannot be tipped over or reached by children

☐ Hot water heater set at 48.9° C or lower

☐ Pot handles turned toward back of stove or toward center of table

☐ No loose clothing worn near stove

☐ No cooking or eating hot foods or liquids with child standing nearby or sitting in lap

☐ All small appliances, such as iron, turned off, disconnected, and placed out of reach when not in use

☐ Cool, not hot, mist vaporizer used

☐ Fire extinguisher available on each floor and checked periodically

☐ Electrical fuse box and gas shutoff accessible

☐ Family escape plan in case of fire practiced periodically; fire escape ladder available on upper-level floors

☐ Telephone number of fire or rescue squad and address of home with nearest cross street posted near phone

### Safety: Suffocation and Aspiration

☐ Small objects stored out of reach*

☐ Toys inspected for small, removable parts or long strings*

☐ Hanging crib toys and mobiles placed out of reach

☐ Plastic bags stored away from young child's reach; large plastic garment bags discarded after tying in knots*

☐ Mattress or pillow should not be covered with plastic or in such a way that is accessible to child*

☐ Crib designed according to federal regulations (crib slats less than 2⅜ inches [6 cm] apart) with snug-fitting mattress**

☐ Crib positioned away from other furniture or windows*

☐ Portable playpen gates up at all times while in use*

☐ Accordion-style gates not used*

☐ Bathroom doors kept closed, and toilet seats down or toilet lid fasteners used*

☐ Faucets turned off firmly*

☐ Pool fenced with locked gate

☐ Proper safety equipment at poolside

☐ Electric garage door openers stored safely and garage door adjusted to rise when door strikes object

☐ Doors of ovens, trunks, dishwashers, refrigerators, and front-loading clothes washers and dryers kept closed*

☐ Unused appliances such as refrigerators securely closed with lock or doors removed*

☐ Food served in small, noncylindric pieces*

☐ Toy chests without lids or with lids that securely lock in open position*

☐ Buckets and wading pools kept empty when not in use*

☐ Clothesline above head level

☐ At least one member of household trained in basic life support (CPR) including first aid for choking ⊖‡

### Safety: Poisoning

☐ Telephone number of local poison control center and address of home with nearest cross street posted near phone

☐ Toxic substances, including batteries, placed on a high shelf, preferably in a locked cabinet

☐ Toxic plants hung or placed out of reach*

☐ Excess quantities of cleaning fluid, paints, pesticides, drugs, and other toxic substances not stored in home

☐ Used containers of poisonous substances discarded where child cannot obtain access

☐ Medicines clearly labeled in childproof containers and stored out of reach

☐ Household cleaners, disinfectants, and insecticides kept in their original containers, separate from food and out of reach

☐ Smoking only allowed in areas away from children

☐ Cosmetics kept out of children's reach

### Safety: Falls

☐ Nonskid mats, strips, or surfaces in tubs and showers

☐ Exits, halls, and passageways in rooms kept clear of toys, furniture, boxes, and other items that could be obstructive

---

This section may be photocopied and distributed to families.

Source: Wilson D, Hockenberry MJ: *Wong's clinical manual of pediatric nursing,* ed 8, St Louis, 2012, Mosby.

*Safety measures are specific for homes with young children. All safety measures should be implemented in homes where children reside and in homes they visit frequently, such as those of grandparents or babysitters.

**Federal regulations are available from the U.S. Consumer Product Safety Commission, 800-638-CPSC (*www.cpsc.gov*).

‡For patient and family education instructions for infant cardiopulmonary resuscitation and infant and child choking, see Evolve.

2 - HEALTH PROMOTION

Patient and Family Education, Spanish Translations–Infant Cardiopulmonary Resuscitation for the Layperson

- ☐ Stairs and halls well lit, with switches at both top and bottom
- ☐ Sturdy handrails for all steps and stairways
- ☐ Nothing stored on stairways
- ☐ Treads, risers, and carpeting in good repair
- ☐ Glass doors and walls marked with decals
- ☐ Safety glass used in doors, windows, and walls
- ☐ Gates on top and bottom of staircases and elevated areas, such as porch or fire escape*
- ☐ Guardrails on upstairs windows with locks that limit height of window opening and access to areas such as fire escape*
- ☐ Avoid use of drop-side baby cribs. Maintain fixed crib side rails raised to full height; mattress lowered as child grows. Immobilization kits are available on the Internet. Avoid use of tape, wire or other temporary device to immobilize drop-side rail.*
- ☐ Restraints used in high chairs, walkers, or other baby furniture; preferably wheeled walkers not used*

- ☐ Scatter rugs secured in place or used with nonskid backing
- ☐ Walks, patios, and driveways in good repair

## Safety: Bodily Injury

- ☐ Knives, power tools, and <u>unloaded</u> firearms stored safely or placed in locked cabinet
- ☐ Adult supervision for firearm and crossbow or bow-and-arrow use.
- ☐ Use of go carts, ATVs, dirt bikes, and other motorized vehicles with protective equipment and under adult supervision.
- ☐ Age-appropriate use of ATVs (state laws differ, but avoid use in children under age 16 years).
- ☐ Garden tools returned to storage racks after use
- ☐ Pets properly restrained and immunized for rabies
- ☐ Swings, slides, and other outdoor play equipment kept in safe condition
- ☐ Yard free of broken glass, nail-studded boards, and other litter
- ☐ Cement birdbaths positioned and secured so young child cannot tip them over*

## Injury Prevention During Infancy

| Major Developmental Accomplishments | Injury Prevention |
|---|---|
| **Age: Birth to 4 Months** | |
| Involuntary reflexes, such as the crawling reflex, may propel infant forward or backward, and the startle reflex may cause the body to jerk. | *Aspiration* |
| | Not as great a danger in this age-group but should begin practicing safeguards early (see Age: 4 to 7 Months). |
| May roll over | Never shake baby powder directly on infant; place powder in hand and then on infant's skin; store container closed and out of infant's reach. |
| Has increasing eye-hand coordination and voluntary grasp reflex | Hold infant for feeding; do not prop bottle. |
| NOTE: Infants are prone to injury as a result of increasing curiosity about their environment, developing and uncoordinated mobilization skills, increasing skill in handling objects, desire to place objects in mouth or on face, and inability to protect self from potential dangers such as falls from heights (no cognitive basis for cause-effect reasoning). | Know emergency procedures for choking.** |
| | Use pacifier with one-piece construction and loop handle. |
| | *Suffocation and Drowning* |
| | Keep all plastic bags stored out of infant's reach; discard large plastic garment bags after tying in a knot. |
| | Do not cover mattress with plastic that is accessible to infant. Use zippered plastic mattress cover. |
| | Use a firm mattress and loose blankets; no pillows. |
| | Make sure crib design follows federal regulations—crib slats less than $2\frac{3}{8}$ (6 cm) apart—and mattress fits snugly. Avoid drop-side crib rails.† |
| | Position crib away from other furniture, windows, and radiators. |
| | Do not tie pacifier on a string around infant's neck. |
| | Remove bibs at bedtime. |
| | Never leave infant alone in bath, regardless of the depth of the water. |
| | Do not leave infant under 12 months alone on adult or youth mattress. |
| | Avoid placing infant to sleep on couch or day bed; place in crib or bassinet. |
| | Place infant to sleep on back. |

This section may be photocopied and distributed to families.

Source: Wilson D, Hockenberry MJ: *Wong's clinical manual of pediatric nursing,* ed 8, St Louis, 2012, Mosby.

*Safety measures are specific for homes with young children. All safety measures should be implemented in homes where children reside and in homes they visit frequently, such as those of grandparents or babysitters.

**For patient and family education instructions for care of the choking infant, see p. 169; for use of child safety seats, see p. 173.

†The CPSC has recently issued a recommendation against the use of drop-side cribs because of an association with strangulation and asphyxia related to their use. (US Consumer Product Safety Commission: CPSA issues warning on drop-side cribs: 32 fatalities in drop-side cribs in last 9 years, Release #10-225, May 7, 2010. USCPSC, Washington, D.C.; Accessed online July 5, 2010, at *www.cpsc.gov/cpscpub/prerel/prhtml10/10225.html*; The CPSC issued a ban on drop-side cribs in the United States in late 2010.

## Injury Prevention During Infancy—cont'd

| Major Developmental Accomplishments | Injury Prevention |
|---|---|

### Age: Birth to 4 Months—cont'd

*Falls*

Always maintain crib rails at a level above the standing infant's head.

Never leave infant unguarded on a raised surface.

When in doubt as to where to place child, use the floor.

Restrain infant in infant seat, and never leave infant unattended while the seat is resting on a raised surface.

Avoid using a high chair until infant can sit well with support.

Avoid drop-side crib rails.

*Poisoning*

Not as great a danger in this age-group but should begin practicing safeguards early (see Age: 4 to 7 Months).

*Burns*

Install smoke detectors in home.

Use caution when warming formula in microwave oven; always check temperature of liquid before feeding.

Check temperature of bath water before placing infant in water.

Do not pour hot liquids when infant is close by, such as sitting on lap.

Beware of cigarette ashes that may fall on infant.

Do not leave infant in the sun for more than a few minutes; keep exposed skin covered. Use at least a 30 SPF sunscreen.

Wash flame-retardant clothes according to label directions.

Use cool-mist vaporizers.

Do not leave child in parked car.

Check surface heat of restraint before placing child in car seat.

*Motor Vehicles*

Transport infant in federally approved, rear-facing car seat,* preferably in back seat.

Do not place infant on seat or in lap.

Do not place child in a carriage or stroller behind a parked car.

Do not place infant or child in front passenger seat with an air bag (unless it can be deactivated).

*Bodily Damage*

Avoid sharp, jagged objects.

Keep diaper pins closed and away from infant.

### Age: 4 to 7 Months

| Major Developmental Accomplishments | Injury Prevention |
|---|---|

Rolls over

Sits momentarily

Grasps and manipulates small objects

Resecures a dropped object

Has well-developed eye-hand coordination

Can focus on and locate very small objects

Mouthing is very prominent (places objects in mouth)

Can push up on hands and knees

Crawls backward

*Aspiration*

Keep buttons, beads, syringe caps, and other small objects out of infant's reach.

Keep floor free of any small objects.

Do not feed infant hard candy, nuts, food with pits or seeds, or whole or cylindric pieces of hot dog.

Exercise caution when giving teething biscuits because large chunks may be broken off and aspirated.

Do not feed while infant is lying down.

Inspect toys for removable parts.

Keep baby powder, if used, out of reach.

Avoid storing large quantities of cleaning fluid, paints, pesticides, and other toxic substances in home.

Discard used containers of poisonous substances.

Do not store toxic substances in food containers.

Discard used button-sized batteries; store new batteries in safe area.

---

*For patient and family education instructions for use of child safety seats, see p. 173.

*Continued*

## Injury Prevention During Infancy—cont'd

| Major Developmental Accomplishments | Injury Prevention |
|---|---|
| **Age: 4 to 7 Months—cont'd** | |

*Suffocation*

Keep latex balloons out of reach.

Remove all crib toys that are strung across crib or playpen when child begins to push up on hands or knees.

*Falls*

Restrain in a high chair.

Keep crib rails raised to full height.

Avoid drop-side crib rails.

*Poisoning*

Make sure that paint on walls, furniture, windowsills, and toys does not contain lead.

Place toxic substances on a high shelf or in a locked cabinet.

Hang plants, or place them out of reach.

Know telephone number of local poison control center (usually listed in front of telephone directory), and post near phone.

*Burns*

Place hot objects (e.g., cigarettes, candles, incense) on high surface.

Limit exposure to sun; apply sunscreen.

*Motor Vehicles*

See Age: Birth to 4 Months.

*Bodily Damage*

Give toys that are smooth and rounded, preferably made of wood or plastic; avoid long, pointed objects as toys.

Avoid toys that are excessively loud.

Keep sharp objects out of infant's reach.

**Age: 8 to 12 Months**

Crawls and creeps

Stands, holding on to furniture

Stands alone

Cruises around furniture

Walks

Climbs

Pulls on objects

Throws objects

Is able to pick up small objects; has pincer grasp

Explores by putting objects in mouth

Dislikes being restrained

Explores away from parent

Has increasing understanding of simple words and phrases

*Aspiration*

Keep lint and small objects off floor, off furniture, and out of reach of children.

Take care in feeding solid table food to ensure that very small pieces are given.

Do not use beanbag toys or allow child to play with dried beans.

(See Age: 4 to 7 Months.)

*Suffocation and Drowning*

Keep doors of ovens, dishwashers, refrigerators, coolers, and front-loading clothes washers and dryers closed at all times.

If storing an unused appliance, such as a refrigerator, remove the door.

Supervise contact with inflated balloons; immediately discard popped balloons and keep uninflated balloons out of reach.

Fence swimming pools; keep gate locked.

Always supervise when near any source of water, such as buckets, drainage areas, and toilets.

Keep bathroom doors closed.

Eliminate unnecessary pools of water.

Keep one hand on child at all times when child is in bathtub.

## Injury Prevention During Infancy—cont'd

| Major Developmental Accomplishments | Injury Prevention |
|---|---|

### Age: 8 to 12 Months—cont'd

*Falls*

Avoid mobile (wheeled) walkers, especially near stairs, decks, or porches with drop-off surface.‡

Fence stairways at top and bottom if child has access to either end.

Dress infant in safe shoes and clothing (e.g., soles that do not "catch" on floor, tied shoelaces, pant legs that do not touch floor).

Ensure that furniture is sturdy enough for child to pull self to standing position and cruise.

Avoid drop-side crib rails.

*Poisoning*

Do not describe medications as a candy.

Do not administer medications unless prescribed by a practitioner.

Put away medications and poisons immediately after use; replace child-protector caps properly.

Keep cosmetics and facial cleansers out of child's reach—especially purses.

*Burns*

Place guards in front of or around any heating appliances, fireplaces, or furnace.

Keep electrical wires hidden or out of reach.

Place plastic guards over electrical outlets; place furniture in front of outlets.

Keep hanging tablecloths out of reach (child may pull down hot liquids or heavy or sharp objects).

## Injury Prevention During Early Childhood (Ages 1 to 5 Years)

| Developmental Abilities Related to Risk of Injury | Injury Prevention |
|---|---|
| Walks, runs, and climbs<br>Able to open doors and gates<br>Can ride tricycle<br>Can throw ball and other objects | *Motor Vehicles*<br>Use federally approved car restraint.<br>Supervise child while playing outside.<br>Do not allow child to play on curb or behind a parked car.<br>Do not permit child to play in piles of leaves, snow, or large cardboard container in trafficked areas.<br>Supervise tricycle (or any two- or three-wheeled riding cycle) riding.<br>Lock fences and doors if children not directly supervised.<br>Provide close adult supervision, and teach child to obey pedestrian safety rules:<br>• Obey traffic regulations; walk only in crosswalks and when traffic signal indicates it is safe to cross.<br>• Stand back a step from curb until it is time to cross.<br>• Look left, right, and left again, and check for turning cars before crossing street.<br>• Use sidewalks; when there is no sidewalk, walk on left, facing traffic.<br>• At night, wear clothing in light colors and with fluorescent material. |

This section may be photocopied and distributed to families.

Source: Wilson D, Hockenberry MJ: *Wong's clinical manual of pediatric nursing,* ed 8, St Louis, 2012, Mosby.

‡Because there is considerable risk of major and minor injuries and even death from the use of wheeled walkers, and because there is no clear benefit from their use, the AAP recommends a ban on the manufacture and sale of mobile infant walkers in the United States. The particular risk of walkers in households with stairs is falls. (American Academy of Pediatrics, Committee on Injury and Poison Prevention: Injuries associated with infant walkers, *Pediatrics* 95(5):778-780, 1995.)

*Continued*

## Injury Prevention During Early Childhood (Ages 1 to 5 Years)—cont'd

| Developmental Abilities Related to Risk of Injury | Injury Prevention |
|---|---|
| Able to explore if left unsupervised<br>Has great curiosity<br>Helpless in water, unaware of its danger; depth of water has no significance | ***Drowning***<br>Supervise closely when near any source of water, including buckets, inflatable pools, and bathtubs.<br>Keep bathroom door and lid on toilet closed.<br>Have fence around swimming pool; lock gate, and ensure lock is not accessible to small children. Above-ground inflatable pools should be fenced or completely deflated when not in use to prevent accidental drowning.<br>Teach swimming and water safety (not a substitute for protection).* |
| Able to reach heights by climbing, stretching, standing on toes, and using objects as a ladder<br>Pulls objects<br>Explores any holes or openings<br>Can open drawers and closets<br>Unaware of potential sources of heat or fire<br>Plays with mechanical objects | ***Burns***<br>Place electric appliances, such as coffee maker, frying pan, and popcorn popper, toward back of counter.<br>Place guardrails in front of radiators, fireplaces, or other heating elements.<br>Store matches and cigarette lighters in locked or inaccessible area; discard carefully.<br>Turn pot handles toward back of stove.<br>Place burning candles, incense, hot foods, ashes, embers, and cigarettes out of reach.<br>Do not let tablecloth hang within child's reach.<br>Do not let electrical cord from iron or other appliance hang within child's reach.<br>Cover electrical outlets with protective devices.<br>Keep electrical wires hidden or out of reach.<br>Keep electric hair-styling appliances out of child's reach.<br>Do not allow child to play with electrical appliances, wires, or lighters.<br>Stress danger of open flames; explain what "hot" means.<br>Always check bath water temperature; set hot water heater at 48.9° C (120° F) or lower; do not allow children to play with faucets.<br>Apply a sunscreen with sun protection factor (SPF) 15 or higher when child is exposed to sunlight. |
| Explores by putting objects in mouth<br>Can open drawers, closets, and most containers<br>Climbs<br>Cannot read warning labels<br>Does not know safe dose or amount | ***Poisoning***<br>Place all potentially toxic agents (including plants) in a locked cabinet or out of reach.<br>Replace medications and poisons immediately in a safe place out of child's reach; replace child-resistant caps properly.<br>Keep cosmetics out of child's reach (often found in purse within child's reach).<br>Do not refer to medications as candy.<br>Do not store large supplies of toxic agents.<br>Promptly discard empty poison containers; never reuse to store a food item.<br>Teach child not to play in trash containers.<br>Never remove labels from containers of toxic substances.<br>Keep number and location of nearest poison control center (1-800-222-1222), and post near phone.† |

*The American Academy of Pediatrics recommends teaching swimming and water safety to children ages 4 and above who have no physical or developmental disabilities; in addition, studies suggest that teaching swimming to 1 to 4 year olds may decrease the incidence of drowning; however at the time of this writing the AAP will not issue a recommendation for all 1 to 4 year olds to receive swimming lessons (American Academy of Pediatrics: Technical report—prevention of drowning, *Pediatrics* 126(1):e253-e262, 2010).

†Poison prevention brochures that can be downloaded and printed in 12 different languages are available at *www.aapcc.org* (American Association of Poison Control Centers).

2 - HEALTH PROMOTION

## Injury Prevention During Early Childhood (Ages 1 to 5 Years)—cont'd

| Developmental Abilities Related to Risk of Injury | Injury Prevention |
|---|---|
| Able to open doors and some windows<br>Goes up and down stairs<br>Depth perception unrefined<br>Gait is unsteady (toddler)<br>Climbs on objects<br>Unaware of potential danger from objects, situations | ***Falls***<br>Keep screen in window, fasten securely, and use guardrail.<br>Place gates at top and bottom of stairs.<br>Keep doors locked, or use child-resistant doorknob covers at entry to stairs, high porch, or other elevated area, such as laundry chute.<br>Remove unsecured or scatter rugs.<br>Apply nonskid mats in bathtubs or showers.<br>Keep fixed-side crib rails fully raised and mattress at lowest level.<br>Keep large toys and bumper pads out of crib or playpen (child can use these as "stairs" to climb out); move to youth bed when child is able to crawl out of crib.<br>Avoid using walkers with wheels, especially near stairs.<br>Dress in safe clothing (e.g., soles that do not "catch" on floor, tied shoelaces, pant legs that do not touch floor).<br>Keep child restrained in vehicles; never leave unattended in shopping cart or stroller.<br>Supervise at playgrounds; select play areas with soft ground cover and safe equipment. |
| Puts things in mouth<br>May swallow hard or inedible pieces of food<br>Explores places and things (natural curiosity) | ***Choking and Suffocation***<br>Avoid large, round chunks of meat, such as whole hot dogs (slice lengthwise, then into short pieces).<br>Avoid fruit with pits, fish with bones, dried beans, hard candy, chewing gum, nuts, popcorn, grapes, and marshmallows.<br>Choose large, sturdy toys without sharp edges or small removable parts.<br>Discard old refrigerators, ovens, and other appliances; if storing old appliance, remove doors.<br>Keep automatic garage door opener in inaccessible place.<br>Select toy boxes or chests without heavy, hinged lids.<br>Keep window blind cords out of child's reach.<br>Remove drawstrings from clothing. |
| Still clumsy in many skills<br>Easily distracted from tasks<br>Unaware of potential danger from situations and strangers or other people | ***Bodily Damage***<br>Avoid giving sharp or pointed objects (e.g., knives, scissors, toothpicks), especially when walking or running.<br>Do not allow lollipops or similar objects in mouth when walking or running.<br>Teach safety precautions (e.g., to carry fork or scissors with pointed ends away from face).<br>Store all dangerous tools, garden equipment, and firearms in locked cabinets.<br>Be alert to danger from animals, including household pets.<br>Use safety glass and decals on large glassed areas, such as sliding glass doors.<br>Teach personal safety:<br>• Teach name, address, and phone number and to ask for help from appropriate people (cashier, security guard, police officer) if lost; have identification on child (e.g., sewn in clothes or inside shoe).<br>• Avoid letting child wear personalized clothing in public places.<br>• Teach child to never go with a stranger.<br>• Teach child to tell parents if anyone makes child feel uncomfortable in any way.<br>• Always listen to child's concerns regarding behavior of others.<br>• Teach child to say "no" when confronted with uncomfortable situations. |

2 - HEALTH PROMOTION

## Injury Prevention During School-Age Years

| Developmental Abilities Related to Risk of Injury | Injury Prevention |
|---|---|
| Is increasingly involved in activities away from home<br>Is excited by speed and motion<br>Is easily distracted by environment<br>Can be reasoned with | *Motor Vehicles*<br>Educate child regarding proper use of seat belts while riding in a vehicle.<br>Maintain discipline while in a vehicle (e.g., children must keep arms inside, must not lean against doors, must not interfere with driver).<br>Remind parents and children that no one should ride in the bed of a pickup truck.<br>Emphasize safe pedestrian behavior.<br>Insist on wearing safety apparel (e.g., a helmet) when applicable, such as when riding a bicycle, motorcycle, moped, water craft, or all-terrain vehicle.<br>Provide adult supervision for motorized vehicles such as those listed above. |
| Is apt to overdo; has poorly defined awareness of own limitations/boundaries<br>May work hard to perfect a skill<br>Has cautious, but not fearful, gross motor actions<br>Likes swimming | *Drowning*<br>Teach child to swim.<br>Teach basic rules of water safety.<br>Select safe and supervised places to swim.<br>Check sufficient water depth for diving.<br>Teach child to swim with a companion.<br>Make sure child wears an approved personal flotation device in water or while boating.<br>Advocate for legislation requiring fencing around pools.<br>⊜ Learn basic cardiopulmonary resuscitation (CPR). |
| Has increasing independence<br>Is adventuresome<br>Enjoys trying new things | *Burns*<br>Make sure smoke detectors are in home.<br>Set hot-water heater temperature at 48.9° C (120° F) to avoid scald burns.<br>Instruct child in behavior involving contact with potential burn hazards (e.g., gasoline, matches, bonfires or barbecues, lighter fluid, firecrackers/fireworks, cigarette lighters, cooking utensils, chemistry sets) and to avoid climbing or flying kites around high-tension wires.<br>Instruct child in proper behavior in the event of fire (e.g., fire drills at home and school).<br>Teach child safe cooking methods (use low heat; avoid frying; be careful of steam burns, scalds, or exploding food, especially from microwaving).<br>Apply a sunscreen with SPF 15 or higher when child is exposed to sunlight. |
| Adheres to group rules<br>May be easily influenced by peers<br>Has strong allegiance to friends | *Poisoning*<br>Educate child regarding hazards of taking nonprescription and prescription drugs and chemicals, including aspirin and alcohol.<br>Teach child to refuse offered illegal or dangerous drugs or alcohol. Explain danger of prescription drugs used without medical supervision.<br>Keep potentially dangerous products in properly labeled receptacles—preferably locked and out of reach. |

This section may be photocopied and distributed to families.

Source: Wilson D, Hockenberry MJ: *Wong's clinical manual of pediatric nursing,* ed 8, St Louis, 2012, Mosby.

## Injury Prevention During School-Age Years—cont'd

| Developmental Abilities Related to Risk of Injury | Injury Prevention |
|---|---|
| Has increased physical skills | ***Bodily Damage*** |
| Needs strenuous physical activity | Help provide facilities for supervised activities. |
| Is interested in acquiring new skills and in perfecting attained skills | Encourage playing in safe places. |
| Is daring and adventurous, especially with peers | Keep firearms safely locked up except during adult supervision. |
| Frequently plays in hazardous places | Teach proper care of, use of, and respect for devices with potential danger (e.g., power tools, firecrackers/fireworks). |
| Confidence often exceeds physical capacity | Teach children animal safety. |
| Desires group loyalty and has strong need for friends' approval | Stress eye, ear, and mouth protection when using potentially hazardous objects or devices or when engaged in potentially hazardous sports (e.g., baseball, football). |
| Attempts hazardous feats | Teach safety regarding use of corrective devices (glasses); if child wears contact lenses, monitor duration of wear to prevent corneal damage. |
| Accompanies friends to potentially hazardous facilities | Stress careful selection, use, and maintenance of sports and recreation equipment such as skateboards and in-line skates. |
| Is likely to overdo | Emphasize proper conditioning, safe practices, and use of safety equipment for sports or recreational activities. |
| Growth in height exceeds muscular growth and coordination. | Caution against engaging in hazardous sports, such as those involving trampolines. |
| | Use safety glass and decals on large glassed areas, such as sliding glass doors. |
| | Use window guards to prevent falls. |
| | Teach name, address, and phone number and how to ask for help from appropriate people (cashier, security guard, police officer) if lost; have identification on child (e.g., sewn in clothes or inside shoe). |
| | Teach stranger safety: |
| | • Do not let child wear personalized clothing in public places. |
| | • Caution child to never go with a stranger. |
| | • Have child tell parents if anyone makes child feel uncomfortable in any way. |
| | • Always listen to child's concerns regarding behavior of others. |
| | • Teach child to say "no" when confronted with uncomfortable situations. |

2 - HEALTH PROMOTION

## Injury Prevention During Adolescence

| Development Abilities Related to Risk of Injury | Injury Prevention |
|---|---|
| Need for independence and freedom<br>Testing independence<br>Age permitted to drive a motor vehicle (varies)<br>Inclination for risk taking<br>Feeling of indestructibility<br>Need for discharging energy, often at expense of logical thinking and other control mechanisms<br>Strong need for peer approval<br>May attempt hazardous feats<br>Peak incidence for practice and participation in sports<br>Access to more complex tools, objects, and locations<br>Can assume responsibility for own actions<br>Personal disregard for safety (e.g, in association with depression) | ***Motor and Nonmotor Vehicles***<br>*Pedestrian*—Emphasize and encourage safe pedestrian behavior.<br>At night, walk with a friend, not alone.<br>If someone is following you, go to nearest place with people.<br>Do not walk in secluded areas; take well-traveled walkways.<br>*Passenger*—Promote and encourage appropriate behavior while riding in a motor vehicle.<br>*Driver*—Provide competent driver education; encourage judicious use of vehicle, discourage drag racing, playing chicken; maintain vehicle in proper condition (brakes, tires, etc.).<br>Teach and promote safety and maintenance of recreational motor vehicles such as motorcycles, ATVs; promote and encourage wearing of safety apparel, such as a helmet and long trousers.<br>Reinforce teaching about the dangers of drugs, including alcohol, when operating a motor vehicle of any kind.<br>***Drowning***<br>Teach nonswimmers to swim.<br>Teach basic rules of water safety:<br>• Judicious selection of place to swim.<br>• Sufficient water depth for diving.<br>• Swimming with companion.<br>• Use of personal flotation device on water craft and/or boat<br>***Burns***<br>Reinforce proper behavior involving contact with burn hazards (gasoline, electric wires, fires).<br>Advise regarding excessive exposure to natural or artificial (ultraviolet) light, such as tanning.<br>Discourage cigarette smoking, chewing tobacco, or snuff.<br>Encourage use of sunscreen.<br>***Poisoning***<br>Educate in hazards of nonprescription, prescription, and recreational drug use, including alcohol.<br>***Falls***<br>Teach and encourage general safety measures in all activities.<br>***Bodily Damage***<br>Promote proper instruction in sports and safe use of sports and recreational equipment.<br>Instruct in safe use of and respect for firearms and other devices with potential danger (e.g., power tools, fireworks).<br>Provide and encourage use of protective equipment when using potentially hazardous devices.<br>Promote access to and/or provision of safe facilities for sports and recreation.<br>Be alert for signs of depression (potential suicide).<br>Discourage use and/or availability of hazardous sports equipment (e.g., trampoline, surfboards).<br>Instruct regarding proper use of corrective devices, such as glasses, contact lenses, and hearing aids.<br>Encourage judicious application of safety principles and prevention. |

This section may be photocopied and distributed to families.
Source: Wilson D, Hockenberry MJ: *Wong's clinical manual of pediatric nursing,* ed 8, St Louis, 2012, Mosby.

# Guidelines for Automobile Safety Seats

This important information is provided because motor vehicle crashes cause significant numbers of deaths and injuries in infants and young children. These deaths and injuries are mostly preventable. All states now have laws that require children to be properly secured in motor vehicles.

Remember that the most dangerous place for an infant or child to ride is in the arms or on the lap of another person; or in the bed of a pick -up truck.

Nurses have a responsibility for educating parents regarding the importance of car restraints and their proper use. Five types of restraints are available: (1) infant-only devices, (2) convertible models for both infants and toddlers, (3) boosters, (4) safety belts, and (5) devices for children with special needs.

The ***infant-only restraint*** is a semireclined seat (45 to 50 degrees) that faces the rear of the car. A rear-facing car seat provides the best protection for the disproportionately heavy head and weak neck of an infant. This position minimizes the stress on the neck by spreading the forces of a frontal crash over the entire back, neck, and head; the spine is supported by the back of the car seat. If the seat were faced forward, the head would whip forward because of the force of the crash, creating enormous stress on the neck. The restraint is anchored to the vehicle with the vehicle's seat belt or LATCH (lower anchors and tethers for children) system, and the restraint has a harness system for securing the infant. The five-point harness system provides the most effective support for infant restraint; the three-point harness system secures only the upper body. Many infant seats have a plastic base that can be left in the car; the seat latches or clicks into the base so that the base does not have to be installed each time the car seat is removed.

The ***convertible restraint*** is suitable for infants and most toddlers in the rear-facing position (Figure 2-2). It is now recommended that all infants and toddlers ride in a rear-facing car safety seat until they have reached the age of 2 years or they reach the highest weight or height recommended by the car seat manufacturer (American Academy of Pediatrics, 2011). Studies indicate that toddlers (up to 24 months of age) are safer riding in convertible seats in the rear-facing position (Bull and Durbin, 2008; Henary, Sherwood, Crandall and others, 2007). A convertible safety seat is positioned semireclined and facing the rear of the car. Once the child has outgrown the rear-facing seat, a forward facing seat with a harness is recommended.

The restraint consists of a molded hard plastic with energy-absorbing padding and a special harness system designed to hold the child firmly in the seat and distribute the forces to body areas that can withstand the impact.

Convertible restraints use different types of harness systems: a *five-point harness* that consists of a strap over each shoulder, one on each side of the pelvis, and one between the legs (all five come together at a common buckle), as well as a *padded overhead shield* that uses shoulder straps attached to a shield that is held in place by a crotch strap. With both the infant and toddler restraints, it is important that extra blankets, head cushions, or padding that did not come as original equipment not be added behind or above the child because these "add-ons" create spaces of air between the child and the restraint and decrease support for the back, head, and neck. Cars with free-sliding latch plates on the lap or shoulder belt require the use of a metal locking clip to keep the belt in a tight-holding position. The locking clip is threaded onto the belt above the latch plate (Figure 2-3, A). Children aged 2 years and older who have reached the maximum recommended height or weight for the rear-facing car seat should ride forward facing in a car safety seat with a harness as long as possible (American Academy of Pediatrics, 2011).

***Booster seats*** are not restraint systems like the convertible devices because they depend on the vehicle belts to hold the child and booster seat in place. Three booster models have been approved by the National Highway Traffic Safety Administration (NHTSA): the high-back belt-positioning seat, which provides head and neck support for the child riding in a vehicle seat without a head rest; the no-back belt-positioning seat, which should be used only if the vehicle seat has a head rest; and a combination seat, which converts from

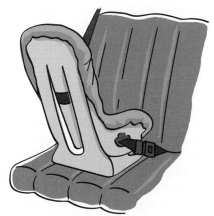

FIGURE **2-2**    Convertible seat in rear-facing position for toddlers.

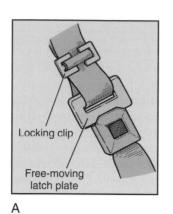

Locking clip

Free-moving
latch plate

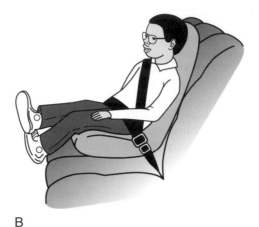

A      B

FIGURE **2-3**   A, Locking clip used with free-sliding lap/shoulder belt to keep the belt in a tight holding position. B, Automobile booster seat. Note placement of shoulder strap (away from neck and face).

a forward-facing toddler seat to a booster seat. This last model is equipped with a harness for use in toddlers; the harness may be removed and a shoulder-lap belt used when the child outgrows the harness. Booster seats are used for children who are less than 145 cm (4 feet, 9 inches) tall and who weigh 15.9 kg to 36.3 kg (35 to 80 lb, depending on the type of booster seat), typically those between 4 and 8 years of age. A booster seat should be used until the child is able to sit against the back of the seat with feet hanging down and legs bent at the knees. The belt-positioning booster model raises a child higher in the seat, moving the shoulder part of the belt off the neck and the lap portion of the belt off the abdomen onto the pelvis (Figure 2-3, B).

Children with special needs may require a restraint system that secures them appropriately in the event of a crash. Examples of such devices include car bed restraints for infants who cannot tolerate a semireclining position and specially adapted molded-plastic chairs for children who have spica casts. The E-Z-On vest is a special safety harness for larger children with poor trunk control. Additional safety restraints and a list of distributors are available at the SafetyBeltSafe U.S.A. website (*www.carseat.org*).

Children should use specially designed car restraints until they are 145 cm (4 feet, 9 inches) in height or are 8 to 12 years old. Children who outgrow the convertible restraint may still be able to ride safely in a booster seat until the midpoint of the head is higher than the vehicle seat back. Shoulder-lap safety belts should be worn low on the hips, snug, and not on the abdominal area. Children should be taught to sit up straight to allow for proper fit. The shoulder belt is used only if it does not cross the child's neck or face. Air bags do not take the place of child safety seats or seat belts and can be lethal to young children.

The LATCH universal child safety seat system was implemented as a requirement starting in 2002 for all new automobiles and child safety seats. This system provides a uniform anchorage consisting of two lower anchorages and one upper anchorage in the rear seat of the vehicle. When used appropriately, the top anchor (tether) strap prevents the child from pitching forward in a crash. If the tether strap is not used, up to 90% of the restraint's protection is lost. Instructions for proper installation of the tether strap and permanent bracket are included with the car restraint. New child safety seats will have a hook, buckle, strap, or other connector that attaches to the anchorage (Figure 2-4). Seat belts will no longer be used to anchor child safety seats to newer vehicles.

The safest area of the car for children of any age is the middle of the back seat. Children should not ride in the front seat of any activated air bag–equipped car, except in emergencies, and then the vehicle seat must be as far back as possible. Many newer model cars are equipped with a "smart" air bag system that allows air bag deactivation when a child is riding in the passenger seat. Parents should remember to turn the air bag switch back on once the child is no longer in the front seat. Also, many newer model vehicles are equipped with side-impact air bags for protection; these air bags are reported to be safe as long as the child is in a proper restraint system. The NHTSA recommends that vehicle owners with side-impact air bags check the manufacturer's recommendations for child safety. The NHTSA (2010) recommends that children not lean on chest-only or head-chest combination side air bags. Because of a large number of adverse events involving serious injuries and even some child fatalities with air bags, some manufacturers designed and installed air bags designed to minimize injury to adults and children at deployment yet still protect the passenger. Because diverse types of air bags continue to be in use, parents are cautioned to continue placing all children younger than age 13 years in the back seat with the proper child restraint system. Built-in seats are available in some cars and vans. They may be used for children who are at least 1 year of age and weigh at least 9 kg (20 lb). Built-in seats

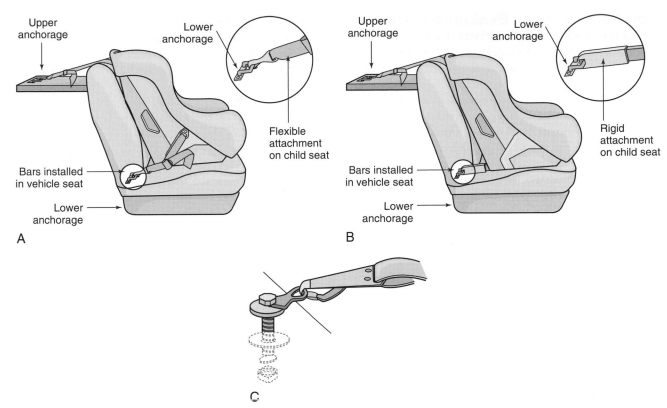

FIGURE **2-4**    Lower anchors and tethers for children (LATCH). A, Flexible two-point attachment with top tether. B, Rigid two-point attachment with top tether. C, Top tether. (Courtesy of U.S. Department of Transportation, National Highway Traffic Safety Administration.)

eliminate installation problems. However, weight and height limits vary. Reinforce that owners must verify with vehicle manufacturers details about built-in seats.

For any restraint to be effective, it must be used consistently and properly. Examples of misuse include misrouting of the vehicle seat belt through the restraint, failing to use the vehicle seat belt through the restraint, failing to use a tether strap, failing to use the restraint's harness system, and incorrectly positioning the child, especially facing infants forward instead of rearward. To address these issues, nurses must stress correct use of car restraints and rules that ensure compliance and can emphasize to parents that children riding in car safety seats are generally better behaved than children left unrestrained. Despite widespread education and publicity regarding seat belt safety restraint and the danger of front seat air bags for children, surveys indicate that children are still placed in potentially lethal situations of either improper seat restraint or no restraint.

---

> **! SAFETY ALERT**
>
> **Parent Resources, Car Seat Safety**
>
> American Academy of Pediatrics
> 141 Northwest Point Blvd.
> Elk Grove Village, IL 60007
> Phone: 847-434-4000
> Website: *www.healthychildren.org/English/safety-prevention/on-the-go/pages/Car-Safety-Seats-Information-for-Families-2011.aspx*
>
> U.S. Department of Transportation
> National Highway Traffic Safety Administration
> 1200 New Jersey Ave, SE, West Building
> Washington, DC 20590
> Phone: 888-327-4236
> Website: *www.nhtsa.gov*
>
> SafeKids USA
> Website: *www.safekids.org*
> Contact your local SafeKids chapter, which sponsors Seat Belt Fit clinics to ensure that seat belt restraint systems being used are adequate protection.
> For children with special needs, the following is an available resource for car restraint information:
>
> **Automotive Safety Program**
> Riley Hospital for Children
> 575 Riley Hospital Drive, Room 004
> Indianapolis, IN 46202
> Phone: 317-944-2977; 800-543-6227
> Website: *www.preventinjury.org*

## Neonatal Car Seat Evaluation: The Preterm and Late-Preterm Infant*

The American Academy of Pediatrics (AAP,1999; Bull, Engle and American Academy of Pediatrics, 2009) recommends that infants born before 37 weeks of gestation be evaluated for apnea, bradycardia, and oxygen desaturation episodes before hospital discharge. The AAP suggests that facilities develop policies for implementing an evaluation program; however, few evidence-based practice recommendations have been published to date delineating specific requirements for such a program. Based on the available literature, suggestions for providing a car seat evaluation of infants born before 37 weeks of gestation and/or weighing less than 2500 grams at birth include the following:

- Use the parents' car seat for the evaluation.
- Perform the evaluation 1 to 7 days before the infant's anticipated discharge.
- Secure the infant in the car seat per guidelines using blanket rolls on side.
- Set pulse oximeter low alarm at 88% (arbitrary).
- Set heart rate low alarm limit at 80 beats/min and apnea alarm at 20 seconds (cardiorespiratory monitor).

- Leave the infant undisturbed in car seat for 90 minutes *or* for the time parents state it takes to arrive at their home (if more than the 90 minutes).
- Document the infant's tolerance to the car seat evaluation.
- An episode of desaturation, bradycardia, or apnea (20 seconds or more) constitutes a failure, and evaluation by the practitioner must occur before discharge.
- Repeat the test after 24 hours once modifications are made to the car seat, car bed, or infant's position in either restraint system.
- It is recommended that a certified car seat technician place the infant in the car seat (or bed) if a failure occurs (see National Highway Traffic Safety Administration website {*www.nhtsa.dot.gov*} for car seat inspection station). The technician will demonstrate appropriate positioning of the infant in the restraint device to the parents and have the parents do a return demonstration.
- Document the interventions, the infant's tolerance, and the parents' return demonstration.

# Parental Guidance

## Guidance During Infancy

### First 6 Months

Teach car safety with use of federally approved car seat, facing rearward, in the middle of the back seat—not in a front seat with an air bag.

Understand each parent's adjustment to newborn, especially mother's postpartal emotional needs.

Teach routine care of infant (feeding, sleep, jaundice, elimination, and skin care); assist parents to understand infant's individual needs and temperament and that the infant expresses wants through crying.

Reassure parents that infant cannot be spoiled by too much attention during the first 4 to 6 months.

Encourage parents to establish a schedule that meets needs of child and themselves.

Help parents understand infant's need for personal, social, and environmental stimulation.

Support parents' pleasure in seeing child's growing friendliness and social responses, especially smiling.

Plan anticipatory guidance for safety, including placing infant on back to sleep.

Stress need for routine immunizations.

Prepare for introduction of solid foods.

Encourage parent to take an infant and child CPR class.

### Second 6 Months

Prepare parents for child's stranger anxiety.

Encourage parents to allow child to cling to them and avoid long separation from either parent.

Guide parents concerning discipline because of infant's increasing mobility.

Encourage use of negative voice and eye contact rather than physical punishment as a means of discipline.

Encourage showing most attention when infant is behaving well, rather than when infant is crying.

Teach injury prevention because of child's advancing motor skills and curiosity.

Encourage parents to leave child with suitable caregiver to allow themselves some free time.

Discuss appropriate feeding, introduction of solid foods, and weaning process.

Explore parents' feelings regarding infant's sleep patterns.

Provide anticipatory guidance for safety.

*Modified from Bull MJ, Engle WA, and American Academy of Pediatrics: Safe transportation of preterm and low birth weight infants at hospital discharge, *Pediatrics* 123(5):1424-1429, 2009; and American Academy of Pediatrics: Transporting children with special health care needs, *Pediatrics* 104(4):988-992, 1999.

# Guidance During Toddler Years

## Ages 12 to 18 Months

Prepare parents for expected behavioral changes of toddler, especially negativism and ritualism.

Assess present feeding habits, and encourage gradual weaning from bottle to cup and increased intake of solid foods.

Stress expected feeding changes of physiologic anorexia, presence of food fads and strong taste preferences, need for scheduled routine at mealtimes, inability to sit through an entire meal, and lack of table manners.

Assess sleep patterns at night, particularly habit of a bedtime bottle, which is a major cause of dental caries, and procrastination behaviors that delay hour of sleep.

Prepare parents for potential dangers of the home, particularly drowning, poisoning, burns, and falling injuries; give appropriate suggestions for childproofing the home.

Discuss need for firm but gentle discipline and ways in which to deal with negativism and temper tantrums; stress positive benefits of appropriate discipline.

Emphasize importance for both child and parents of brief, periodic separations.

Discuss toys that use developing gross and fine motor, language, cognitive, and social skills.

Emphasize need for dental supervision, types of basic dental hygiene at home, and food habits that predispose children to caries; stress importance of supplemental fluoride (if adequate amounts are not in potable water source).

Discuss options for safe day care (in home or outside of home) as required by parents' work status.

Provide anticipatory guidance for safety.

## Ages 18 to 24 Months

Stress importance of peer companionship in play.

Explore need for preparation for additional sibling; stress importance of preparing child for new experiences.

Discuss present discipline methods, their effectiveness, and parents' feelings about child's negativism; stress that negativism is important aspect of developing self-assertion and independence and is not a sign of spoiling.

Discuss signs of readiness for toilet training; emphasize importance of waiting for physical and psychologic readiness.

Discuss development of fears, such as of darkness or loud noises, and of habits, such as security blanket or thumb sucking; stress normalcy of these transient behaviors.

Prepare parents for signs of regression in time of stress.

Assess child's ability to separate easily from parents for brief periods under familiar circumstances.

Allow parents opportunity to express their feelings of weariness, frustration, and exasperation; be aware that it is often difficult to love toddlers at times when they are not asleep!

Point out some of the expected changes of the next year, such as longer attention span, somewhat less negativism, and increased concern for pleasing others.

Provide anticipatory guidance for safety.

## Ages 24 to 36 Months

Discuss importance of imitation and domestic mimicry and need to include child in activities.

Discuss approaches toward toilet training, particularly realistic expectations and attitude toward toileting accidents.

Stress uniqueness of toddlers' thought processes, especially regarding their use of language, poor understanding of time, causal relationships in terms of proximity of events, and inability to see events from another's perspective.

Stress that discipline must still be quite structured and concrete and that relying solely on verbal reasoning and explanations leads to confusion, misunderstanding, and even injuries.

Discuss investigation of preschool or daycare center toward completion of second year.

Provide anticipatory guidance for safety.

# Guidance During Preschool Years

## Age 3 Years

Prepare parents for child's increasing interest in widening relationships.

Discuss and encourage enrollment in preschool.

Emphasize importance of setting limits.

Prepare parents to expect exaggerated tension-reduction behaviors, such as need for security blanket.

Encourage parents to offer choices when child vacillates.

Prepare parents to expect marked changes at $3\frac{1}{2}$ years, when child becomes less coordinated, becomes insecure, and exhibits emotional extremes.

Prepare parents for normal dysfluency in speech, and advise them to avoid focusing on the pattern.

Prepare parents to expect extra demands on their attention as a reflection of child's emotional insecurity and fear of loss of love.

Discuss with parents that equilibrium of 3-year-old will change to the aggressive, out-of-bounds behavior of 4-year-old.

Inform parents to anticipate a more stable appetite with wider food selections.

Stress need for protection and education of child to prevent injury.

## Age 4 Years

Prepare parents for more aggressive behavior, including motor activity and offensive language.

Prepare parents to expect resistance to their authority.

Explore parental feelings regarding child's behavior.

Suggest some type of respite for primary caregivers, such as placing child in preschool for part of the day.

Prepare parents for child's increasing curiosity about genitals and function.

Emphasize importance of realistic limit setting on behavior and appropriate discipline techniques.

Prepare parents for highly imaginative 4-year-old who indulges in tall tales (to be differentiated from lies) and who has imaginary playmates.

Prepare patients to expect nightmares or an increase in nightmares, and suggest that they make sure child is fully awakened from a frightening dream.

Provide reassurance that a period of calm begins at 5 years of age.

Suggest swimming lessons for child as appropriate for child's development.

## Age 5 Years

Inform parents to expect tranquil period at 5 years.

Help parents to prepare child for entrance into school environment.

Make sure immunizations are up-to-date before child enters school.

Suggest that unemployed mothers or fathers consider own activities when child begins school.

# Guidance During School-Age Years

## Age 6 Years

Prepare parents to expect child's strong food preferences and frequent refusals of specific food items.

Inform parents to expect increasing appetite in child.

Prepare parents for emotionality as child experiences erratic mood changes.

Help parents anticipate continued susceptibility to illness.

Teach injury prevention and safety, especially bicycle safety.

Encourage parents to respect child's need for privacy and to provide a separate bedroom for child, if possible.

Prepare parents for child's increasing interests outside the home.

Help parents understand the importance of encouraging child's interactions with peers.

Encourage balanced diet and routine exercise for prevention of obesity, diabetes, and other preventable cardiovascular disorders.

## Ages 7 to 10 Years

Prepare parents to expect improvement in child's health and fewer illnesses, but inform them that allergies may increase or become apparent.

Prepare parents to expect an increase in minor injuries.

Emphasize caution in selecting and maintaining sports equipment, and reemphasize safety.

Prepare parents to expect increased involvement with peers and interest in activities outside the home.

Emphasize the need to encourage independence while maintaining limit setting and discipline.

Prepare mothers to expect more demands when child is 8 years of age.

Prepare fathers to expect increasing admiration at 10 years of age; encourage father-child activities.

Prepare parents for prepubescent changes in girls.

Discuss safety aspects of online usage, and monitor child's involvement in same (see Electronic Communication Safety, p. 179)

## Ages 11 to 12 Years

Help parents prepare child for body changes of pubescence.

Prepare parents to expect a growth spurt in girls.

Make certain child's sex education is adequate with accurate information.

Prepare parents to expect energetic but stormy behavior at 11, to become more even tempered at 12.

Encourage parents to support child's desire to grow up but to allow regressive behavior when needed.

Prepare parents to expect an increase in exploratory sexual activity such as masturbation.

Instruct parents that the amount of rest child needs may increase.

Help parents educate child regarding experimentation with potentially harmful activities.

Encourage keeping immunizations up to date.

## Health Guidance

Help parents understand the importance of regular health and dental care for child.

Encourage parents to teach and model sound health practices, including diet, rest, activity, and exercise.

Stress the need to encourage children to engage in appropriate physical activities.

Emphasize providing a safe physical and emotional environment.

Encourage parents to teach and model safety practices.

## Electronic Communication Safety*

The Internet and electronic media, including mobile (cellular) phones, are an ever-present factor in the lives of children, adolescents, and adults. With the increasing popularity of Internet capabilities with mobile phone technology, children and adolescents may experience a decrease in parental or adult supervision of such activities and an increase in exposure to persons who may want to harm the child. *Cyber bullying* through social media such as the mobile phone is a reality of modern technology. Although direct injury may not occur through the Internet, there is increasing concern about predators who may use such a medium to attract, meet, and harm children and adolescents. Several parent rules may be helpful in providing Internet safety for the child and family:

- Become familiar with the Internet and mobile phone services the child or adolescent uses. Find out what kinds of services the Internet provider provides for home and mobile use and methods to block objectionable or offensive material. If blocking services are available, it is recommended that these be used, especially if children are on the Internet frequently. Such blockers often do not prevent scholarly research.
- Become familiar with materials available to Internet and mobile phone users (even if you never avail yourself of such material).
- Discuss with the adolescent or child the types of services he or she accesses and what types of communication (e-mail, instant messaging) or chatrooms the child or adolescent frequents.
- Discuss the benefits and potential hazards of Internet chatrooms according to the child's developmental age.
- Place the family computer in a public area of the home.
- Understand and encourage discussion of the fact that not all material printed on the Internet is true.
- Never allow the child to meet in person with someone with whom they have chatted on the Internet unless you are present.
- Discourage the child or adolescent from providing anyone on the Internet (other than a close known personal friend) with personal information such as entire name, school name, address, telephone or mobile phone number, personal photo, or credit card number. This applies to anyone, including a representative of the Internet service provider (ISP)—in such cases, a parent should communicate with the company's representative.
- Encourage child to not respond to messages or bulletin boards that include offensive, suggestive, obscene, or threatening information or anything that makes the child or adolescent uncomfortable.
- Help adolescent understand that persons on the Internet may misrepresent themselves for the purpose of committing a crime.
- If pornography, harassing messages, sexually explicit material, or threats are transmitted to your computer or mobile phone by another person, contact the local authorities and your service provider.
- Discuss with adolescent the harm of transmitting sexually explicit photos (sexting) which may appear to some adolescents be a harmless game but which in fact may lead to considerable personal and emotional harm.
- Discuss Internet safety rules with all household members, including young children.
- Be reasonable in setting rules for computer use, and monitor computer use in the home.
- Monitor time spent on the computer and the time of day when most computer access is popular. Excessive computer activities may suggest a potential problem, especially if child or adolescent does not engage in other social activities with peers.
- Know the type of games children and adolescents are involved in via the Internet; some may not be harmless and may contain adult material.
- The best advice from consumer and government agencies is to apply a filter to block objectionable materials to which you prefer your child not have access. Some ISPs provide a filtering service for subscribers; contact them for service and prices. Examples of Internet filters available to the public (at a price) include Yahoo, MSN, KidsNet, SafeEyes, SafeKids, Cyberpatrol, and Cybersitter. Be aware that different filters may only filter as much as 80% of all objectionable materials, whereas others may block research material with objectionable words, phrases, or themes. Parents may also wish to read through the publication *A Parent's Guide to Internet Safety,* available at *www.fbi.gov/publications/pguide/pguidee.htm.*

## Guidance During Adolescence

### Encourage Parents to:

Accept adolescent as a unique individual.

Recognize the influence of adolescent's peer group.

Respect adolescent's ideas, likes and dislikes, and wishes.

Be involved with school functions and attend adolescent's performances, whether they are sporting events or a school play.

Be involved in adolescent's choice of Internet chatrooms, e-mail, Web "surfing," and cellular phone communication options (see Electronic Communication Safety).

Listen and try to be open to adolescent's views, even when they differ from parental views.

Avoid criticism about no-win topics.

*This section may be photocopied and distributed to families.

Provide opportunities for choosing options and to accept the natural consequences of these choices.

Allow adolescent to learn by doing, even when choices and methods differ from those of adults.

Provide adolescent with clear, reasonable limits.

Clarify home rules and the consequences for breaking them.

Let society's rules and the consequences teach responsibility outside the home.

Allow increasing independence within limitations of safety and well-being.

Be available, but avoid pressing adolescent too far.

Respect adolescent's privacy.

Try to share adolescent's feelings of joy or sorrow. Respond to feelings as well as to words.

Be available to answer questions, give information, and provide companionship.

Try to make communication clear.

Avoid comparisons with siblings.

Assist adolescent in setting appropriate career goals and in preparing for adult role.

Welcome adolescent's friends into the home, and treat them with respect.

Provide unconditional love.

Be willing to apologize when mistaken.

Prepare adolescent for and guide him or her in relationships with peers that will carry over into adulthood.

## Be Aware That Adolescents:

Are subject to turbulent, unpredictable behavior.

Are struggling for independence.

Are extremely sensitive to feelings and behaviors that affect them.

May receive a different message than what was sent.

Consider friends extremely important.

Have a strong need to belong.

# Play

## Functions of Play

### Sensorimotor Development

Improves fine motor and gross motor skills and coordination

Enhances development of all the senses

Encourages exploration of the physical nature of the world

Provides for release of surplus energy

Encourages and enhances communication

### Intellectual Development

Provides multiple sources of learning:

- Exploration and manipulation of shapes, sizes, textures, and colors
- Experience with numbers, spatial relationships, and abstract concepts
- Opportunity to practice and expand language skills

Provides opportunity to rehearse past experiences to assimilate them into new perceptions and relationships

Helps children to comprehend the world in which they live and to distinguish between fantasy and reality

### Socialization and Moral Development

Teaches adult roles, including gender role behavior

Provides opportunities for testing relationships

Develops social skills

Encourages interaction and development of positive attitudes toward others

Reinforces approved patterns of behavior and moral standards

### Creativity

Provides an expressive outlet for creative ideas and interests

Allows for fantasy and imagination

Enhances development of special talents and interests

### Self-Awareness

Facilitates the development of self-identity

Encourages regulation of own behavior

Allows for testing of own abilities (self-mastery)

Provides for comparison of own abilities with those of others

Allows opportunities to learn how own behavior affects others

### Therapeutic Value

Provides for release from tension and stress

Allows expression of emotions and release of unacceptable impulses in a socially acceptable fashion

Encourages experimentation and testing of fearful situations in a safe manner

Facilitates nonverbal and indirect verbal communication of needs, fears, and desires

Meets own ongoing developmental needs

### Cultural Value

Allows expression of cultural values and beliefs

## General Trends During Childhood

| Age | Social Character of Play | Content of Play | Most Prevalent Type of Play | Characteristics of Spontaneous Activity | Purpose of Dramatic Play | Development of Ethical Sense |
|---|---|---|---|---|---|---|
| Infant Toddler | Solitary Parallel | Social-affective Imitative | Sensorimotor Body movement | Sense-pleasure Intuitive judgment | Self-identity Learning gender role | Beginning of moral values |
| Preschool | Associative | Imaginative | Fantasy Informal games | Concept formation Reasonably constant ideas | Imitating social life Learning social roles | Developing concern for playmates Learning to share and cooperate |
| School-age | Cooperative | Competitive games and contests Fantasy | Physical activity Group activities Formal games Play acting | Testing concrete situations and problem solving Adding fresh information | Vicarious mastery | Peer loyalty Playing by the rules Hero worship |
| Adolescent | Cooperative | Competitive games and contests Daydreaming | Social interaction | Abstract problem solving | Presenting ideas | Causes and projects |

## Play During Infancy

| Age (Months) | Visual Stimulation | Auditory Stimulation | Tactile Stimulation | Kinetic Stimulation |
|---|---|---|---|---|
| **Suggested Activities** | | | | |
| Birth-1 | Hang bright, shiny object within 20-25 cm (8-10 inches) of infant's face and in midline. Hang mobiles with black-and-white designs and high-contrast colors and designs. | Talk to infant; sing in soft voice. Play music box, radio, or television. Have ticking clock or metronome nearby. | Hold, caress, and cuddle infant. Keep infant warm. Infant may like to be swaddled. | Rock infant; place in cradle. Use stroller or carrier for walks. |
| 2-3 | Provide bright objects. Make room bright with pictures or mirrors. Take infant to various rooms while doing chores. Place in infant seat for vertical view of environment. | Talk to infant. Include in family gatherings. Expose to various environmental noises other than those of home. Use rattles, interactive toys (toys that respond when handled). | Caress infant while bathing and at diaper change. Comb hair with a soft brush. | Use infant swing. Take in car for rides. Exercise body by moving extremities in swimming motion. Use cradle gym. |

This section may be photocopied and distributed to families.
Source: Wilson D, Hockenberry MJ: *Wong's clinical manual of pediatric nursing,* ed 8, St Louis, 2012, Mosby.

*Continued*

2 - HEALTH PROMOTION

## Play During Infancy—cont'd

| Age (Months) | Visual Stimulation | Auditory Stimulation | Tactile Stimulation | Kinetic Stimulation |
|---|---|---|---|---|
| **Suggested Activities—cont'd** | | | | |
| 4-6 | Place infant in front of safety (unbreakable) mirror. Give infant brightly colored toys to hold (small enough to grasp). Give infant books made of cloth, vinyl, or thick cardboard. | Talk to infant; repeat sounds infant makes. Laugh when infant laughs. Call infant by name. Crinkle different papers by infant's ear. Place rattle or bell in hand. Introduce nursery rhymes and songs. | Give infant soft squeeze toys of various textures. Allow infant to splash in bath. Place infant nude on soft, furry rug and move extremities. Provide interactive toys Place infant supine, and provide dangling toys a few inches above that she or he can touch; provide rattling or soft noise toys | Use swing or stroller. Bounce infant in lap while holding in standing position. Support infant in sitting position; let infant lean forward to balance self. Place infant on floor to crawl, roll over, and sit. |
| 6-9 | Give infant large toys with bright colors, movable parts, and noise makers. Place unbreakable mirror where infant can see self. Play peek-a-boo, especially hiding face in a towel. Play hide and seek with toy. Make funny faces to encourage imitation. | Call infant by name. Repeat simple words, such as "dada," "mama," and "bye-bye." Speak clearly. Name parts of body, people, and foods. Tell infant what you are doing. Use "no" only when necessary. Give simple commands. Show how to clap hands, bang a drum. | Let infant play with fabrics of various textures. Have bowl with foods of different sizes and textures to feel. Let infant catch running water. Encourage water play in large bathtub or shallow pool. Give infant a wad of sticky tape to manipulate. | Hold upright to bear weight and bounce. Pick up, and say "up." Put down, and say "down." Place toys out of reach, and encourage infant to get them. Play pat-a-cake. |
| 9-12 | Show infant large pictures in books. Take infant to places where there are animals, many people, and different objects (e.g., shopping center). Play ball by rolling it to infant, and demonstrate throwing it back. Demonstrate building a two-block tower. | Read simple nursery rhymes to infant. Point to body parts and name each one. Imitate sounds of animals. | Give infant finger foods of different textures. Allow infant to mess up and squash food. Allow infant to feel cold (ice cube) or warm (bath water); say what temperature each is. Allow infant to feel a breeze (fan blowing). | Give infant large push-pull toys. Place furniture in a circle to encourage cruising on floor. Turn in different positions. |
| **Suggested Toys** | | | | |
| Birth-6 | Nursery mobiles Books with high-contrast pictures Unbreakable mirrors Contrasting colored sheets | Music boxes Musical mobiles Small-handled clear rattle Infant activity gym (hangs above infant so she or he can touch) | Stuffed animals Soft clothes Soft or furry quilt Soft mobiles | Rocking crib or cradle Weighted or suction toy Infant swing |

## Play During Infancy—cont'd

| Age (Months) | Visual Stimulation | Auditory Stimulation | Tactile Stimulation | Kinetic Stimulation |
|---|---|---|---|---|
| **Suggested Toys—cont'd** | | | | |
| 6-12 | Various colored blocks<br>Nested boxes or cups<br>Books with rhymes and bright pictures<br>Strings of big beads<br>Simple take-apart toys<br>Large ball<br>Cup and spoon<br>Large puzzles<br>Pop-up toys (Jack-in-the-box) | Rattles of different sizes, shapes, tones, and bright colors<br>Squeaky animals and dolls<br>Recordings of light, rhythmic music<br>Rhythmic musical instruments<br>Interactive toys | Soft, different-textured animals and dolls<br>Sponge toys, floating toys<br>Squeeze toys<br>Teething toys<br>Books with textures and objects, such as fur and zippers | Activity box for crib<br>Push-pull toys<br>Wind-up swing |

## Play During Toddlerhood

| Physical Development | Social Development | Mental Development and Creativity |
|---|---|---|
| **Suggested Activities** | | |
| Provide spaces that encourage physical activity.<br>Provide sandbox, swing, and other scaled-down playground equipment. | Provide replicas of adult tools and equipment for imitative play.<br>Permit child to help with adult tasks.<br>Encourage imitative play.<br>Provide toys and activities that allow for expression of feelings.<br>Allow child to play with some actual items used in the adult world; for example, let child help wash dishes or play with pots and pans and other utensils (check for safety). | Provide opportunities for water play.<br>Encourage building, drawing, and coloring.<br>Provide various textures in objects for play.<br>Provide large boxes and other safe containers for imaginative play.<br>Provide books with pictures of animals, cars, trucks, and trains.<br>Read stories appropriate to age.<br>Monitor TV viewing. |
| **Suggested Toys** | | |
| Push-pull toys<br>Rocking horse, stick horse<br>Riding toy<br>Balls (large)<br>Blocks (unpainted)<br>Pounding board<br>Low gym and slide<br>Pail and shovel<br>Containers<br>Play-Doh | CD player or tape recorder<br>Purse<br>Housekeeping toys (broom, dishes)<br>Toy telephone<br>Dishes, stove, table and chairs<br>Mirror<br>Puppets, dolls, stuffed animals (check for safety [e.g., no button eyes]) | Wooden puzzles<br>Cloth or vinyl picture books<br>Paper, finger paint, thick crayons<br>Blocks (wood or plastic)<br>Large beads to string<br>Wooden shoe for lacing<br>Appropriate TV programs, videos, music CDs<br>Shape sorters<br>Cause/effect toys such as pop-ups |

This section may be photocopied and distributed to families.
Source: Wilson D, Hockenberry MJ: *Wong's clinical manual of pediatric nursing,* ed 8, St Louis, 2012, Mosby.

## Play During Preschool Years

| Physical Development | Social Development | Mental Development and Creativity |
|---|---|---|
| **Suggested Activities** | | |
| Provide spaces for the child to run, jump, and climb. | Encourage interactions with neighborhood children. | Encourage creative efforts with raw materials. |
| Teach child to swim. Teach water safety. | Intervene when children become destructive. | Read stories. |
| Teach simple sports and activities. | Enroll child in preschool. | Monitor TV viewing. |
| | | Attend theater and other cultural events appropriate to child's age. |
| | | Take short excursions to park, seashore, museums, zoo. |
| **Suggested Toys** | | |
| Medium-height slide | Child-sized playhouse | Books |
| Adjustable swing | Dolls, stuffed toys | Jigsaw puzzles |
| Vehicles to ride | Dishes, table | Musical toys (xylophone, piano, drum, horns) |
| Tricycle | Ironing board and iron | Picture games |
| Wading pool | Cash register, toy typewriter, computer | Blunt scissors, paper, glue |
| Wheelbarrow | Trucks, cars, trains, airplanes | Newsprint, crayons, poster paint, large brushes, easel, finger paint |
| Sled | Play clothes for dress-up | Flannel board and pieces of felt in colors and shapes |
| Wagon | Doll carriage, bed, high chair | CDs/tapes |
| Roller skates, speed graded to skill | Doctor and nurse kits | Dry erase board |
| | Toy nails, hammer, saw | Sidewalk chalk (different colors) |
| | Grooming aids, play makeup, or shaving kits | Wooden and plastic construction sets |
| | | Magnifying glass, magnets |

# Play During Hospitalization

## Functions of Play in the Hospital

Facilitates mastery over an unfamiliar situation

Provides opportunity for decision making and control

Helps to lessen stress of separation

Provides opportunity to learn about parts of body, their functions, and own disease or disability

Corrects misconceptions about the use and purpose of medical equipment and procedures

Helps children have an age-appropriate understanding of illness and treatment

Aids in assessment and diagnosis

Meets ongoing developmental needs

Provides for continuation of development

Speeds recovery and rehabilitation

Provides diversion and brings about relaxation

Helps the child feel more secure in a strange environment

Provides a means to release tension and express feelings

Encourages interaction and development of positive attitudes toward others

Provides an expressive outlet for creative ideas and interests

Provides a means for accomplishing therapeutic goals

### Therapeutic Play Activities for Hospitalized Children
#### Oral Fluid Intake

Make snow cones or freezer pops using child's favorite juice.

Cut gelatin into fun shapes.

Make game of taking sip when turning page of book or during games such as Simon Says.

Use small medicine cups; decorate the cups.

Color water with food coloring or powdered drink mix.

Have a tea party; pour at small table.

Let child fill an oral medication syringe and squirt it into mouth, or use it to fill small, decorated cups.

Cut straw in half, and place in small container (much easier for child to suck liquid).

This section may be photocopied and distributed to families.

Source: Wilson D, Hockenberry MJ: *Wong's clinical manual of pediatric nursing,* ed 8, St Louis, 2012, Mosby.

Decorate straw; place small sticker on straw.

Use a "crazy" straw.

Make a progress poster; give rewards for drinking a predetermined quantity.

Play "fluid checkers" using medicine cups with different colors of juice; every time someone is "jumped," they must drink some juice.

### Deep Breathing

Blow bubbles with bubble blower.

Blow bubbles with straw (no soap).

Blow on pinwheel, feathers, whistle, harmonica, balloons, toy horns, or party noisemakers.

Practice on band instruments.

Have blowing contest using balloons, boats, cotton balls, feathers, marbles, Ping-Pong balls, or pieces of paper; blow such objects over a tabletop goal line, over water, through an obstacle course, up in the air, against an opponent, or up and down a string.

Move paper or cloth from one container to another using suction from a straw.

Use blow bottles with colored water to transfer water from one side to the other (bubble painting).

Dramatize scenes, such as "I'll huff and puff and blow your house down" from the "Three Little Pigs."

Do straw-blowing painting.

Take a deep breath and "blow out the candles" on a birthday cake.

Use a little paintbrush to paint nails with water, and then blow nails dry.

### Range of Motion and Use of Extremities

Throw beanbags at a fixed or movable target; toss wadded paper into a wastebasket.

Touch or kick Mylar balloons held or hung in different positions (if child is in traction, hang balloon from trapeze). NOTE: Latex balloons and latex gloves inflated into balloons pose a choking hazard and also present the risk of an allergic reaction.

Play tickle toes; have child wiggle them on request.

Play games such as Twister or Simon Says.

Do bed aerobics, shadow dancing.

Engage in puppet play.

Play pretend and guess games (e.g., imitate a bird, butterfly, or horse).

Have tricycle or wheelchair races in a safe area.

Play kickball or throw ball with a soft foam ball in a safe area.

Position bed so that child must turn to view television or doorway.

Have child climb wall with fingers like a spider.

Pretend to teach aerobic dancing or exercise; encourage parents to participate.

Encourage swimming if feasible.

Play video games or pinball (fine motor movement).

Play hide-and-seek game; hide toy somewhere in bed (or room, if ambulatory), and have child find it using specified hand or foot.

Provide clay to mold with fingers.

Have child paint or draw on large sheets of paper placed on floor or wall.

Encourage combing own hair; play beauty shop with "customer" in different positions.

### Tension-Release Activities

Muscle relaxation exercises

Distraction by telling stories or singing

Breathing through party blower or pinwheel

Blowing or watching bubbles

Counting

Pillow punching

Finger painting with shaving cream, pudding, or paint

Water play (water balloon target practice); target squirting with syringes

Make magic glitter wands

Carpentry (pounding or hammering wood pegs)

Finger paint with edible Play-Doh.

Looking at pop-up books

Squeezing Nerf or stress ball

Listening to music

Make imagery scrapbook of pleasant images

Throwing sponge ball at a target on wall or door

Playing handheld games

Make a foil (aluminum) sculpture

Giving detailed explanation of procedure

Soothing touches or hugs

Deep breathing

Building tower blocks and knocking them over to allow acceptable, safe outlet for aggression

Playing with Play-Doh or clay sculptures

Target squirting with syringes

Punching holes in bottom of plastic cup, filling with water, and letting it rain on child

### Injections

Let child handle syringe (without needle), vial, and alcohol swab and pretend to give an injection to doll or stuffed animal.

Use syringes to decorate cookies with frosting, squirt paint, or target shoot into a container.

Draw a "magic circle" on area before injection; draw smiling face in circle after injection (but avoid drawing on puncture site).

Allow child to have a collection of syringes (without needles); make wild creative objects with syringes.

If child is receiving multiple injections or venipunctures, make a progress poster; give rewards for predetermined number of injections.

Have child count to 10 or 15 during injection or "blow the hurt away."

Needle painting with colored sterile water on paper towels (use blunt needle)

### Oral Medication Intake

NOTE: Remember to ask the pharmacist or physician if pill/medication can be crushed, divided in half, or mixed with food or liquid.

Allow child to choose how to take medication (e.g., by spoon, syringe, or medicine cup) to allow sense of control.

Offer a favorite drink as a "chaser" to cover up the taste.

Ask the pharmacist about using a flavor additive to help medication taste better. These do not require a prescription.

Suck on something cold (popsicles or crushed ice) to numb the taste buds on the tongue before giving medication.

Make a reward chart to chart child's progress.

Drip a spoon with chocolate syrup, and place medication on coated spoon. Other flavored syrups such as maple, strawberry, and flavored coffee syrups work well too.

Play "beat the clock."

Keep liquid medication cold. This can make them more palatable. Ask your pharmacist.

Suck on chocolate morsels, or coat tongue with peanut butter before and/or after medication.

Inquire if it is safe to mix liquid medication in juice or food. Only use as much as your child will consume to assure he or she takes the full dosage. Be cautious of the downside of negative association with food or liquid that is mixed with medication (for younger children).

Dip a flavored popsicle (e.g., ice pops) into the liquid medication, and allow child to eat the popsicle.

### Pill Swallowing Tips

Train child in small steps with success at every step (e.g., have child practice with a piece of small cake decoration, mini M&M, or Tic Tac). Practice until child accomplishes the smallest size without a problem, and then move up to something slightly larger.

Place pill or capsule into ice cream, yogurt, applesauce, or pudding, and swallow it all together (avoid this in younger child because of association with food).

Place pill on a spoon of JELLO, and slurp it right down. Little JELLO snack packs work great for this.

Some pills are easier to swallow if cut in half. Ask pharmacist if this is acceptable and if medication does not lose its potency.

Place pill on tongue, and have child drink a glass of water through a straw.

Purchase a "pill cup" (a cup with a little pocket in it that aids pill to float down with liquid when drinking).

Crush medication, and mix with chocolate syrup on spoon.

### Ambulation

Give child something to push:
- Toddler—push-pull toy
- School-age child—wagon or a doll in a stroller or wheelchair
- Adolescent—decorated intravenous (IV) stand

Have a parade; make hats, drum, and so on.

Encourage foot pointing.

Have a treasure hunt or interdepartmental field trip.

Play Simon Says or Red Light/Green Light

### Immobilization or Isolation

Flashlight play—Use flashlights to create designs on wall or ceiling.

Smiling masks—Draw mask to decrease threatening appearance.

Use isolation pen pals or phone pals to provide social experience for confined children.

Play "traction" basketball or volleyball with a soft ball.

Unit scrapbook—View photographs of people and places on unit.

Make bed into a pirate ship or airplane with decorations.

Move patient's bed frequently, especially to playroom, hallway, or outside.

Remote control cars/truck to provide sense of motion

Play fishing game—fishing pole with magnets into a tub or bath basin for prizes.

Velcro darts with string attached for easy retrieval

## REFERENCES

American Academy of Pediatrics, Committee on injury, violence, and poison prevention: Policy statement—Child passenger safety, *Pediatrics* 127(4):788-793, 2011.

American Academy of Pediatrics, Committee on Nutrition: *Pediatric nutrition handbook*, ed 6, Elk Grove Village, Ill, 2009, The Academy.

American Academy of Pediatrics: Clinical report—diagnosis and prevention of iron deficiency and iron-deficiency anemia in infants and young children (0-3 years of age), *Pediatrics* 126(5):1040-1050, 2010.

American Academy of Pediatrics: Transporting children with special health care needs, *Pediatrics* 104(4):988-992, 1999.

Bull MJ, Engle WA, and American Academy of Pediatrics: Safe transportation of preterm and low birth weight infants at hospital discharge, *Pediatrics* 123(5):1424-1429, 2009.

Bull MJ, Durbin DR: rear-facing car safety seats: getting the message right, *Pediatrics* 121(3): 619-620, 2008.

Henary B, Sherwood CP, Crandall JR, and others: Car safety seats for children: Rear facing for best protection, *Inj Prev* 13(6):398-402, 2007.

Kallan MJ, Durbin DR, Arbogast KB, and others: Seating patterns and corresponding risk of injury among 0- to 3-year-old children in child safety seats, *Pediatrics* 121(5):e1342-e1347, 2008.

National Highway Transportation Safety Administration: Air bags: Minimize injury: Parents and caregivers, NHTSA "Safercar.gov"; accessed online July 5, 2010, at *www.safercar.gov/portal/site/safercar/menuitem.13dd5c887c7e1358fefe0a2f35a67789/?vgnextoid=bcbbe66aeee35110VgnVCM1000002fd17898RCRD.*

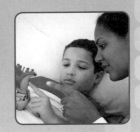

# Pain Assessment and Management

## EVOLVE WEBSITE

# Procedural Sedation and Analgesia

## Children's Response to Pain

Children's ability to describe pain changes as they grow older and as they cognitively and linguistically mature. Three types of measures—behavioral, physiologic, and self-report— have been developed to measure children's pain, and their applicability depends on the child's cognitive and linguistic ability.

## Developmental Characteristics of Children's Responses to Pain

### Preterm Infant
- The preterm infant's response may be behaviorally blunted or absent, however there is sufficient evidence that preterm infants are neurologically capable of experiencing pain.

- Use a preterm infant pain scale.
- Assume that painful procedures in older child and adult are also painful in preterm infant (e.g., venipuncture, lumbar puncture, endotracheal

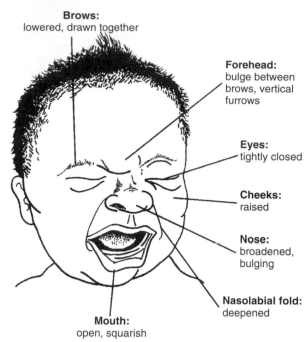

**Brows:** lowered, drawn together

**Forehead:** bulge between brows, vertical furrows

**Eyes:** tightly closed

**Cheeks:** raised

**Nose:** broadened, bulging

**Nasolabial fold:** deepened

**Mouth:** open, squarish

FIGURE **3-1** Facial expression of physical distress is the most consistent behavioral indicator of pain in infants.

intubation, circumcision, chest tube insertion, heel puncture).

## Young Infant

- Generalized body response of rigidity or thrashing, possibly with local reflex withdrawal of stimulated area (Figure 3-1)
- Loud crying
- Facial expression of pain (brows lowered and drawn together, eyes tightly closed, and mouth open and squarish)
- No association demonstrated between approaching stimulus and subsequent pain

## Older Infant

- Localized body response with deliberate withdrawal of stimulated area
- Loud crying
- Facial expression of pain or anger
- Physical resistance, especially pushing the stimulus away after it is applied

## Young Child

- Loud crying, screaming
- Verbal expressions such as "Ow," "Ouch," or "It hurts"
- Thrashing of arms and legs
- Attempts to push stimulus away before it is applied
- Lack of cooperation; need for physical restraint
- Requests termination of procedure
- Clings to parent, nurse, or other significant person
- Requests emotional support, such as hugs or other forms of physical comfort
- May become restless and irritable with continuing pain
- Behaviors occurring in anticipation of actual painful procedure

## School-Age Child

- May see all behaviors of young child, especially during actual painful procedure, but less in anticipatory period
- Stalling behavior, such as "Wait a minute" or "I'm not ready"
- Muscular rigidity, such as clenched fists, white knuckles, gritted teeth, contracted limbs, body stiffness, closed eyes, wrinkled forehead

## Adolescent

- Less vocal protest
- Less motor activity
- More verbal expressions, such as "It hurts" or "You're hurting me"
- Increased muscle tension and body control

---

| TABLE **3-1** | Behavioral Pain Assessment Scales for Infants and Young Children |
|---|---|
| **Ages of Use** | **Instrument** |
| 4 months to 18 years | Objective Pain Score (OPS) (Hannallah and others, 1987) |
| 1 to 5 years | Children's Hospital of Eastern Ontario Pain Scale (CHEOPS) (McGrath and others, 1985) |
| Newborn to 16 years | Nurses Assessment of Pain Inventory (NAPI) (Stevens, 1990) |
| 3 to 36 months | Behavioral Pain Score (BPS) (Robieux and others, 1991) |
| 4 to 6 months | Modified Behavioral Pain Scale (MBPS) (Taddio and others, 1995) |
| <36 months and children with cerebral palsy | Riley Infant Pain Scale (RIPS) (Schade and others, 1996) |
| 2 months to 7 years | FLACC Postoperative Pain Tool (Merkel and others, 1997) |
| 1 to 7 months | Postoperative Pain Score (POPS) (Attia and others, 1987) |
| Average gestational age 33.5 weeks | Neonatal Infant Pain Scale (NIPS) (Lawrence and others, 1993) |
| 27 weeks gestational age to full term | Pain Assessment Tool (PAT) (Hodgkinson and others, 1994) |
| 1 to 36 months | Pain Rating Scale (PRS) (Joyce and others, 1994) |
| 32 to 60 weeks gestational age | CRIES (Krechel, Bildner, 1995) |
| 28 to 40 weeks gestational age | Premature Infant Pain Profile (PIPP) (Stevens and others, 1996) |
| 0 to 28 days | Scale for Use in Newborns (SUN) (Blauer, Gerstmann, 1998) |
| Birth (23 weeks gestational age) and full-term newborns up to 100 days | Neonatal Pain, Agitation, and Sedation Scale (NPASS) (Puchalski, Hummel, 2002) |

| TABLE 3-2 | FLACC Scale | | |
|---|---|---|---|
| | **0** | **1** | **2** |
| Face | No particular expression or smile | Occasional grimace or frown, withdrawn, disinterested | Frequent to constant frown, clenched jaw, quivering chin |
| Legs | Normal position or relaxed | Uneasy, restless, tense | Kicking, or legs drawn up |
| Activity | Lying quietly, normal position, moves easily | Squirming, shifting back and forth, tense | Arched, rigid, or jerking |
| Cry | No cry (awake or asleep) | Moans or whimpers, occasional complaint | Crying steadily, screams or sobs, frequent complaints |
| Consolability | Content, relaxed | Reassured by occasional touching, hugging, or talking to; distractible | Difficult to console or comfort |

From Merkel S and others: The FLACC: A behavioral scale for scoring postoperative pain in young children, *Pediatr Nurs* 23(3):293-297, 1997. Used with permission of Jannetti Publications, Inc., and the University of Michigan Health System. Can be reproduced for clinical and research use.

| TABLE 3-3 | Pain Rating Scales for Children |
|---|---|
| **Pain Scale, Description** | **Recommended Age, Comments** |
| **FACES Pain Rating Scale***<br>Uses six cartoon faces ranging from smiling face for "no pain" to tearful face for "worst pain" | Children as young as 3 years. Use original instructions without affect words, such as *happy* or *sad,* or brief words resulted in same range of pain rating, probably reflecting child's rating of pain intensity. For coding purposes, numbers 0, 2, 4, 6, 8, 10 can be substituted for 0-5 system to accommodate 0-10 system.<br>Provides three scales in one: facial expressions, numbers, and words.<br>Research supports cultural sensitivity of FACES for Caucasian, African-American, Hispanic, Thai, Chinese, and Japanese children. |

| 0 | 1 or 2 | 2 or 4 | 3 or 6 | 4 or 8 | 5 or 10 |
|---|---|---|---|---|---|
| No hurt | Hurts little bit | Hurts little more | Hurts even more | Hurts whole lot | Hurts worst |

| | |
|---|---|
| **Oucher (Beyer, Denyes, and Villarruel, 1992)**<br>Uses six photographs of Caucasian child's face representing "no hurt" to "biggest hurt you could ever have"; also includes vertical scale with numbers from 0 to 100; scales for African-American and Hispanic children have been developed (Villarruel and Denyes, 1991) | Children 3 to 13 years. Use numeric scale if child can count any two numbers, or by tens (Jordan-Marsh and others, 1994).<br>Determine whether child has cognitive ability to use photographic scale; child should be able to rate six geometric shapes from largest to smallest.<br>Determine which ethnic version of Oucher to use. Allow child to select version of Oucher, or use version that most closely matches physical characteristics of child.<br>NOTE: Ethnically similar scale may not be preferred by child when given choice of ethnically neutral cartoon scale (Luffy and Grove, 2003). |
| **Poker Chip Tool (Hester and others, 1998)**<br>Uses four red poker chips placed horizontally in front of child | Children as young as 4 years. Determine whether child has cognitive ability to use numbers by identifying larger of any two numbers. |

*Wong-Baker FACES Pain Rating Scale reference manual describing development and research of the scale is available from City of Hope Pain/Palliative Care Resource Center, 1500 East Duarte Road, Duarte, CA 91010; 626-359-8111, ext. 3829; fax: 626-301-8941; www1.us.elsevierhealth.com/FACES.

*Continued*

TABLE 3-3   Pain Rating Scales for Children—cont'd

| Pain Scale, Description | Recommended Age, Comments |
|---|---|

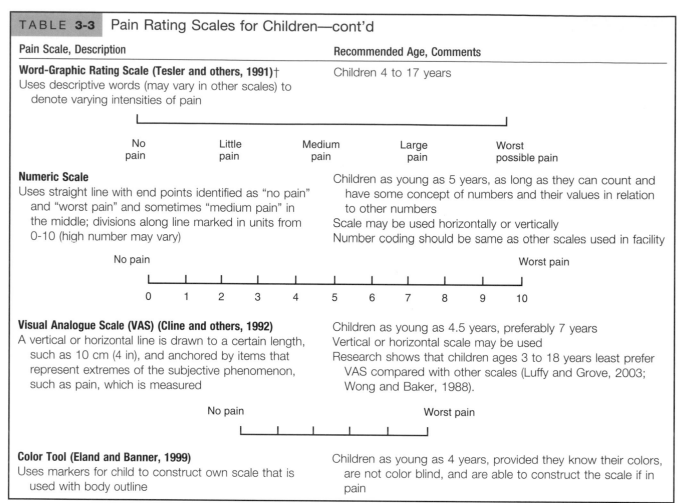

**Word-Graphic Rating Scale (Tesler and others, 1991)†**
Uses descriptive words (may vary in other scales) to denote varying intensities of pain

Children 4 to 17 years

No pain — Little pain — Medium pain — Large pain — Worst possible pain

**Numeric Scale**
Uses straight line with end points identified as "no pain" and "worst pain" and sometimes "medium pain" in the middle; divisions along line marked in units from 0-10 (high number may vary)

Children as young as 5 years, as long as they can count and have some concept of numbers and their values in relation to other numbers
Scale may be used horizontally or vertically
Number coding should be same as other scales used in facility

No pain ... Worst pain
0 1 2 3 4 5 6 7 8 9 10

**Visual Analogue Scale (VAS) (Cline and others, 1992)**
A vertical or horizontal line is drawn to a certain length, such as 10 cm (4 in), and anchored by items that represent extremes of the subjective phenomenon, such as pain, which is measured

Children as young as 4.5 years, preferably 7 years
Vertical or horizontal scale may be used
Research shows that children ages 3 to 18 years least prefer VAS compared with other scales (Luffy and Grove, 2003; Wong and Baker, 1988).

No pain ... Worst pain

**Color Tool (Eland and Banner, 1999)**
Uses markers for child to construct own scale that is used with body outline

Children as young as 4 years, provided they know their colors, are not color blind, and are able to construct the scale if in pain

**References**
Beyer JE, Denyes MJ, Villarruel AM: The creation, validation and continuing development of the Oucher: a measure of pain intensity in children, *J Pediatr Nurs* 7(5):335-346, 1992.
Cline ME, Herman J, Shaw ER, and others: Standardization of the visual analogue scale, *Nurs Res* 41(6):378-380, 1992.
Eland JA, Banner W: Analgesia, sedation, and neuromuscular blockage in pediatric critical care. In Hazinski ME, editor: *Manual of pediatric critical care*, St Louis, 1999, Mosby.
Hester NO, Foster RL, Jordan-Mash M, and others: Putting pain measurement into clinical practice. In Finley GA, McGrath PJ, editors: *Measurement of pain in infants and children*, vol 10, Seattle, 1998, International Association for the Study of Pain Press.
Jordan-Marsh M, Yoder L, Hall D, and others: Alternate Oucher form testing: Gender ethnicity, and age variations, *Res Nurs Health* 17(2):111-118, 1994.
Luffy R, Grove SK: Examining the validity, reliability, and preference of three pediatric pain measurement tools in African-American children, *Pediatr Nurs* 29(1):54-60, 2003.
Tesler MD, Savedra MC, Holzemer WL, and others: The word-graphic rating scale as a measure of children's and adolescents' pain intensity, *Res Nurs Health* 14(5):361-371, 1991.
Villarruel AM, Denyes MJ: Pain assessment in children: Theoretical and empirical validity, *Adv Nurs Sci* 14(2):32-41, 1991.
Wong DL, Baker CM: Pain in children: Comparison of assessment scales, *Pediatr Nurs* 14(1):9-17, 1988.
†Instructions for Word-Graphic Rating Scale from Acute Pain Management Guideline Panel: *Acute pain management in infants, children, and adolescents: operative and medical procedures; quick reference guide for clinicians*, ACHPR Pub. No. 92-0020, Rockville, Md, 1992, Agency for Health Care Research and Quality, US Department of Health and Human Services. Word-Graphic Rating Scale is part of the Adolescent Pediatric Pain Tool and is available from Pediatric Pain Study, University of California, School of Nursing, Department of Family Health Care Nursing, Scan Francisco, CA 94143-0606; 415-476-4040.

TABLE 3-4   CRIES Neonatal Postoperative Pain Scale

| | 0 | 1 | 2 |
|---|---|---|---|
| Crying | No | High pitched | Inconsolable |
| Requires oxygen for saturation >95% | No | <30% | >30% |
| Increased vital signs | Heart rate and blood pressure less than or equal to preoperative state | Heart rate and blood pressure increase <20% of preoperative state | Heart rate and blood pressure increase >20% of preoperative state |
| Expression | None | Grimace | Grimace/grunt |
| Sleepless | No | Wakes at frequent intervals | Constantly awake |

# Nonpharmacologic Strategies for Pain Management

## ⊖ General Strategies

Use nonpharmacologic interventions to supplement, not replace, pharmacologic interventions, and use for mild pain and pain that is reasonably well controlled with analgesics.

Form a trusting relationship with child and family. Express concern regarding their reports of pain, and intervene appropriately.

Use general guidelines to prepare child for procedure.

Prepare child before potentially painful procedures, but avoid "planting" the idea of pain. For example, instead of saying, "This is going to (or may) hurt," say, "Sometimes this feels like pushing, sticking, or pinching, and sometimes it doesn't bother people. Tell me what it feels like to you."

Use "nonpain" descriptors when possible (e.g., "It feels like heat" rather than "It's a burning pain"). This allows for variation in sensory perception, avoids suggesting pain, and gives the child control in describing reactions.

Avoid evaluative statements or descriptions (e.g., "This is a terrible procedure" or "It really will hurt a lot").

Stay with child during a painful procedure.

Allow parents to stay with child if child and parent desire; encourage parent to talk softly to child and to remain near child's head.

Involve parents in learning specific nonpharmacologic strategies and in assisting child with their use.

Educate child about the pain, especially when explanation may lessen anxiety (e.g., that pain may occur after surgery and does not indicate something is wrong); reassure the child that he or she is not responsible for the pain.

For long-term pain control, give child a doll, which represents "the patient," and allow child to do everything to the doll that is done to the child; pain control can be emphasized through the doll by stating, "Dolly feels better after the medicine."

Teach procedures to child and family for later use.

## Specific Strategies

### Distraction

Involve parent and child in identifying strong distracters.

Involve child in play; use radio, tape recorder, CD player, or computer game; have child sing or use rhythmic breathing.

Have child take a deep breath and blow it out until told to stop.

Have child blow bubbles to "blow the hurt away."

Have child concentrate on yelling or saying "ouch," with instructions to "yell as loud or soft as you feel it hurt; that way I know what's happening."

Have child look through kaleidoscope (type with glitter suspended in fluid-filled tube) and encourage him or her to concentrate by asking, "Do you see the different designs?"

Use humor, such as watching cartoons, telling jokes or funny stories, or acting silly with child.

Have child read, play games, or visit with friends.

### Relaxation

With an infant or young child:

Hold in a comfortable, well-supported position, such as vertically against the chest and shoulder.

Rock in a wide, rhythmic arc in a rocking chair or sway back and forth, rather than bouncing child.

With a slightly older child:

Ask child to take a deep breath and "go limp as a rag doll" while exhaling slowly; then ask child to yawn (demonstrate if needed).

Help child assume a comfortable position (e.g., pillow under neck and knees).

Begin progressive relaxation: starting with the toes, systematically instruct child to let each body part "go limp" or "feel heavy"; if child has difficulty relaxing, instruct child to tense or tighten each body part and then relax it.

Allow child to keep eyes open, since children may respond better if eyes are open rather than closed during relaxation.

### Guided Imagery

Have child identify some highly pleasurable real or imaginary experience.

Have child describe details of the event, including as many senses as possible (e.g., "feel the cool breezes," "see the beautiful colors," "hear the pleasant music").

Have child write down or tape-record script.

Encourage child to concentrate only on the pleasurable event during the painful time; enhance the image by recalling specific details through reading the script or playing the tape.

Combine with relaxation and rhythmic breathing.

## Positive Self-Talk

Teach child positive statements to say when in pain (e.g., "I will be feeling better soon," "When I go home, I will feel better, and we will eat ice cream").

## Thought Stopping

Identify positive facts about the painful event (e.g., "It does not last long").

Identify reassuring information (e.g., "If I think about something else, it does not hurt as much").

Condense positive and reassuring facts into a set of brief statements, and have child memorize them (e.g., "Short procedure, good veins, little hurt, nice nurse, go home").

Have child repeat the memorized statements whenever thinking about or experiencing the painful event.

## Behavioral Contracting

Informal—May be used with children as young as four or five years of age:

Use stars, tokens, or cartoon character stickers as rewards.

Give a child who is uncooperative or procrastinating during a procedure a limited time (measured by a visible timer) to complete the procedure.

Proceed as needed if child is unable to comply.

Reinforce cooperation with a reward if the procedure is accomplished within specified time.

Formal—Use written contract, which includes the following:

Realistic (seems possible) goal or desired behavior

Measurable behavior (e.g., agrees not to hit anyone during procedures)

Contract written, dated, and signed by all persons involved in any of the agreements

Identified rewards or consequences that are reinforcing

Goals that can be evaluated

Commitment and compromise requirements for both parties (e.g., while timer is used, nurse will not nag or prod child to complete procedure)

# Analgesic Drug Administration

## Routes and Methods

### Oral

Oral route preferred because of convenience, cost, and relatively steady blood levels

Higher dosages of oral form of opioids required for equivalent parenteral analgesia

Peak drug effect occurs after 1 to 2 hours for most analgesics

Delay in onset a disadvantage when rapid control of severe pain or of fluctuating pain is desired

In young infants, oral sucrose can provide analgesia for painful procedures.

### Sublingual, Buccal, or Transmucosal

Tablet or liquid placed between cheek and gum (buccal) or under tongue (sublingual)

Highly desirable because more rapid onset than oral route

Produces less first-pass effect through liver than oral route, which normally reduces analgesia from oral opioids (unless sublingual or buccal form is swallowed, which occurs often in children)

Few drugs commercially available in this form

Many drugs can be compounded into sublingual troche or lozenge.

### Intravenous (IV) (Bolus)

Preferred for rapid control of severe pain

Provides most rapid onset of effect, usually in about 5 minutes

Advantage for acute pain, procedural pain, and breakthrough pain

Needs to be repeated hourly for continuous pain control

Drugs with short half-life (morphine, fentanyl, hydromorphone) preferable to avoid toxic accumulation of drug

### IV (Continuous)

Preferred over bolus and intramuscular injection for maintaining control of pain

Provides steady blood levels

Easy to titrate dosage

### Subcutaneous (SC) (Continuous)

Used when oral and IV routes not available

Provides equivalent blood levels to continuous IV infusion

Suggested initial bolus dose to equal 2-hour IV dose; total 24-hour dose usually requires concentrated opioid solution to minimize infused volume; use smallest gauge needle that accommodates infusion rate

### Patient-Controlled Analgesia (PCA)

Generally refers to self-administration of drugs, regardless of route

Typically uses programmable infusion pump (IV, epidural, SC) that permits self-administration of boluses of medication at preset dose and time interval (lockout interval is time between doses)

PCA bolus administration often combined with initial bolus and continuous (basal or background) infusion of opioid

Optimum lockout interval not known but must be at least as long as time needed for onset of drug

*Text continued on p. 194.*

## EVIDENCE-BASED PRACTICE

### Reduction of Minor Procedural Pain in Infants

Carol Turnage Carrier

### Ask the Question
**Question**

In newborns and infants, does sucrose provide adequate analgesia during minor painful procedures? Are the effects age dependent?

### Search for the Evidence
**Search Strategies**

Search selection criteria included English publications within past 10 years, research-based articles (level 1 or lower) on neonates or infants undergoing venipuncture or immunizations.

**Databases Used**

PubMed, Cochrane Collaboration, MD Consult, Joanna Briggs Institute, National Guideline Clearinghouse (AHQR), TRIP Database Plus, PedsCCM, BestBETs

### Critically Analyze the Evidence
**Grade criteria:** Evidence quality high; recommendation strong (Guyatt, Oxman, Vist, and others, 2008)

#### *Venipuncture Versus Heel Lance for Blood Sampling*
- Four randomized controlled trials reviewed by the Cochrane Collaboration (Shah and Ohlsson, 2004) compared the efficacy and painfulness of blood sampling by venipuncture or heel lance in full-term neonates. The researchers concluded that venipuncture performed by skilled phlebotomists results in less pain than heel stick for blood sampling. Decreased pain scores, cry duration, and mother's rating of infant's pain demonstrated venipuncture as the preferred method of blood collection. The researchers noted that infants receiving heel stick may also require more than one stick to get enough for the sample, whereas venipuncture reduces the risk of additional sticks.

#### *Glucose Versus EMLA Cream for Venipuncture in Neonates*
- In a randomized control, double-blind study of 201 newborn infants (Gradin, Lenclen, Gajdos, and others, 2002), 99 received EMLA (lidocaine and prilocaine) and oral placebo, and 102 were given 30% oral glucose and placebo on the skin. The 30% glucose group had significantly lower Premature Infant Pain Profile (PIPP) scores and duration of crying than the EMLA group. Significantly fewer patients in the glucose group were scored on the PIPP as having pain or a score above 6 (19.3% compared with 41.7%).

#### *Glucose Compared with EMLA for Venipuncture Pain*
- In a randomized controlled, double-blind study, Lindh, Wiklund, Blomquist, and others (2003) compared the pain response of 90 infants divided equally into EMLA plus 1 ml water by mouth as control placebo with a treatment group given occlusive dressing plus 1 ml oral glucose (300 mg/ml). The combination of EMLA and oral glucose significantly reduced pain response associated with diphtheria-pertussis-tetanus immunizations in 3-month-old infants.

#### *Sucrose for Minor Painful Procedures (Heel Lance and Venipuncture)*
- One hundred fifty full-term newborns were randomly assigned to one of six treatment groups: (1) no treatment, (2) 2 ml sterile water placebo, (3) 2 ml 30% glucose, (4) 2 ml 30% sucrose, (5) 2 ml 30% sucrose with pacifier, and (6) pacifier alone. Results: The pacifier alone was more effective than sweet solutions, sweet solutions and pacifier were significantly more effective than the placebo, and sucrose and glucose were equally effective in lowering pain scores (Carbajal, Chauvet, Couderc, and others, 1999).
- Acharya, Annamali, Taub, and colleagues (2004) studied 28 infants (mean gestation at birth of 30.5 weeks and postnatal age of 27.2 days) who received either 2 ml of a placebo of sterile water or 25% sucrose slowly over 2 minutes into the mouth by syringe 4 minutes before two routine venipunctures. Results: Behavioral state and difficulty and duration of venipuncture were not significantly different between the two liquids. Heart rate, crying times, and neonatal facial coding system scores were significantly lower in the treatment group.
- Abad, Diaz-Gomez, Domenech, and colleagues (2001) compared oral sucrose with EMLA in a prospective randomized trial of 51 full-term newborn infants less than 4 days old receiving venipuncture. The 2 ml of 24% sucrose solution alone was the most effective analgesic compared with placebo (spring water), EMLA, or EMLA combined with 2 ml sucrose. The combination of EMLA and sucrose did not enhance the analgesic effects.
- In the Stevens, Yamada, and Ohlsson (2005) review, 21 randomized, controlled trials met criteria for review, 11 with full-term infants and nine with preterm infants, with one study including both populations (1616 infants; maximum postnatal age of 28 days after reaching 40 weeks corrected age). Heel lance was the most common procedure observed as the painful stimulus; three studies used venipuncture. Sucrose in a wide variety of dosages delivered by syringe or pacifier was found to decrease crying time, heart rate, facial action, and composite pain scores during venipuncture and heel lance. These reviewers recommend the use of sucrose in a range of 0.012 to 0.12 g (0.05 to 0.5 ml) of a 24% solution 2 minutes before a single heel lance or venipuncture for safe and effective pain relief. They also recommend concomitant use of other methods of pain relief, since some studies included use of pacifier, rocking, kangaroo care, or holding along with sucrose intervention.

### Apply the Evidence and Nursing Implications
**Sucrose**
- Sucrose is effective in reducing pain response in infants 6 months and younger undergoing minor acute painful procedures.
- Adverse effects such as hyperglycemia, aspiration, or necrotizing enterocolitis have not been reported with sucrose administered without additives.
- The most effective dose has been 24% solution given at least 2 minutes before a procedure.
- Doses of 50% to 75% have been effective for relieving pain during immunizations in infants up to age 6 months, suggesting that higher concentrations may be required for older infants.
- Effective dose volumes range from 0.05 to 2 ml, with lower volumes used for low-birth-weight infants and larger volumes used for older infants.
- The analgesic effect of sucrose in combination with sucking a bottle or pacifier appears to be enhanced.

*Continued*

3 - PAIN ASSESSMENT AND MANAGEMENT

### Reduction of Minor Procedural Pain in Infants—cont'd

- Studies of older infants have used both increased volume and concentration of sucrose.
- Sucrose in combination with nonpharmacologic support during a procedure may increase the analgesic response for older infants (2 months) even with lower concentrations of sucrose. Interventions include pacifier, holding, swaddling, skin-to-skin contact, and rocking.
- Administration can be by labeled oral syringe, dipped pacifier, or bottle, depending on the infant's ability and age.
- The advantages of minimum wait time, low cost, and decreased risk of adverse effects were significant.
- Effects of repeated dosing over time and dosing of infants younger than 27 weeks are not known.

#### Glucose
- Glucose 30% 1 ml given orally by syringe is more effective than EMLA for venipuncture pain.
- Comparisons between sucrose and glucose have been inconclusive.

#### References

Abad F, Diaz-Gomez NM, Domenech E, and others: Oral sucrose compares favorably with lidocaine-prilocaine cream for pain relief during venepuncture in neonates, *Acta Paediatr* 90(2):160-165, 2001.

Acharya AB, Annamali S, Taub NA, and others: Oral sucrose analgesia for preterm infant venepuncture, *Arch Dis Child Fetal Neonatal Educ* 89(1):F17-F18, 2004.

Carbajal R, Chauvet X, Couderc S, and others: Randomised trial of analgesic effects of sucrose, glucose, and pacifiers in term neonates, *BMJ* 319(7222):1393-1397, 1999.

Gradin M, Lenclen R, Gajdos V, and others: Crossover trial of analgesic efficacy of glucose and pacifier in very preterm neonates during subcutaneous injections, *Pediatrics* 110(6):1053-1057, 2002.

Guyatt GH, Oxman AD, Vist GE, and others: GRADE: An emerging consensus on rating quality of evidence and strength of recommendations, *BMJ* 336(7650):924-926, 2008.

Lindh V, Wiklund U, Blomquist HK, and others: EMLA cream and oral glucose for immunization pain in 3-month old infants, *Pain* 104(1-2):381-388, 2003.

Shah V, Ohlsson A: Venepuncture versus heel lance for blood sampling in term neonates, *Cochrane Database Syst Rev* (4):CD001452.pub2; DOI: 10.1002/14651858.CD001452.pub2, 2004.

Stevens B, Yamada J, Ohlsson A: Sucrose for analgesia in newborn infants undergoing painful procedures (review), 2005. In Cochrane Neonatal Collaboration, available at *www.thecochranelibrary.com* (accessed April 16, 2009).

*Text continued from p. 192.*

Should effectively control pain during movement or procedures

Longer lockout provides larger dose

## Family-Controlled Analgesia

One family member (usually a parent) or other caregiver designated as child's primary pain manager with responsibility for pressing PCA button

Guidelines for selecting a primary pain manager for family-controlled analgesia:

- Spends a significant amount of time with the patient
- Is willing to assume responsibility of being primary pain manager
- Is willing to accept and respect patient's reports of pain (if able to provide) as best indicator of how much pain the patient is experiencing; knows how to use and interpret a pain rating scale
- Understands the purpose and goals of patient's pain management plan
- Understands concept of maintaining a steady analgesic blood level
- Recognizes signs of pain and side effects and adverse reactions to opioid

## Nurse-Activated Analgesia

Child's primary nurse designated as primary pain manager and is only person who presses PCA button during that nurse's shift.

Guidelines for selecting primary pain manager for family-controlled analgesia also applicable to nurse-activated analgesia

May be used in addition to a basal rate to treat breakthrough pain with bolus doses; patients assessed every 30 minutes for the need for a bolus dose

May be used without a basal rate as a means of maintaining analgesia with around-the-clock bolus doses

## Intramuscular

NOTE: Not recommended for pediatric pain control; not current standard of care

## Intranasal

Available commercially as butorphanol (Stadol NS); approved for those age 18 years and older

Should not be used in patient receiving morphine-like drugs because butorphanol is partial antagonist that will reduce analgesia and may cause withdrawal

## Intradermal

Used primarily for skin anesthesia (e.g., before lumbar puncture, bone marrow aspiration, arterial puncture, skin biopsy)

Local anesthetics (e.g., lidocaine) cause stinging, burning sensation

Duration of stinging dependent on type of "caine" used

To avoid stinging sensation associated with lidocaine:

- Buffer the solution by adding 1 part sodium bicarbonate (1 mEq/ml) to 9 to 10 parts 1% or 2% lidocaine with or without epinephrine

## Topical or Transdermal

EMLA (eutectic mixture of local anesthetics [lidocaine and prilocaine]) cream and anesthetic disk or LMX4 (4% lidocaine cream)

- Eliminates or reduces pain from most procedures involving skin puncture
- Must be placed on intact skin over puncture site and covered by occlusive dressing or applied as anesthetic disc for 1 hour or more before procedure

*Text continued on p. 197.*

# EVIDENCE-BASED PRACTICE

## Needle-Free Injection System: J-Tip to Administer Buffered Lidocaine

Terri L. Brown

## Ask the Question
### Question
In pediatrics, are needle-free injection systems (e.g., J-Tip) effective and safe in relieving pain during peripheral intravenous (PIV) cannulation?

## Search for the Evidence
### Search Strategies
English language research-based publications on jet injectors for delivery of lidocaine during PIV cannulation without time limitation were included. Exclusions included dental products, insulin, growth factor, and medications other than lidocaine.

### Databases Used
Cochrane Collaboration Database, Joanna Briggs Institute, National Guideline Clearinghouse (AHRQ), PubMed, SUMSearch, CINAHL, Scopus, UpToDate, BestBETs, manufacturers' or distributors' websites (National Medical Products, Bioject, and Injex)

## Critically Analyze the Evidence
**Grade criteria:** Evidence quality strong; recommendation strong (Guyatt, Oxman, Vist, and others, 2008)

Three randomized controlled trials (RCTs) conducted in children reached favorable conclusions using J-Tip to administer buffered lidocaine for pain prevention during PIV cannulation. Two of the studies found J-Tip superior in pain prevention to LMX (lidocaine cream) or EMLA (a eutectic mix of lidocaine and prilocaine) and no different in the success rate of PIV access on first attempt.

J-Tip with 0.2 ml 1% buffered lidocaine provided greater anesthesia than a 30-minute application of LMX in children ages 8 to 15 years undergoing 22-gauge or 24-gauge PIV catheter insertion (Spanos, Booth, Koenig, and others, 2008). Seventy children in a tertiary care pediatric emergency department self-reported pain using a visual analog scale (VAS) before and after PIV cannulation. Blinded observer VAS scores from videotapes were also assigned for pain at jet injection and PIV catheter insertion. Subject VAS scores were significantly different immediately after PIV catheter insertion (17.3 for J-Tip versus 44.6 for LMX, $p < .001$). Blinded reviewer VAS scores were not statistically significant (21.7 for J-Tip versus 31.9 for LMX, $p = .23$). Researchers also concluded that J-Tip did not alter the insertion site or affect the success of PIV success on first attempt and that multiple injections could be performed if necessary without causing lidocaine toxicity.

J-Tip with 0.25 ml of 1% buffered lidocaine provided greater anesthesia than application of 2.5 g of EMLA in a study of 116 children ages 7 to 19 years undergoing PIV catheter insertion (Jimenez, Bradford, Seidel, and others, 2006). The subjects' self-report median pain ratings of PIV cannulation using a 0 to 10 VAS were 0 for J-Tip and 3 for EMLA ($p = .0001$ for patients receiving EMLA ≥60 minutes before cannulation; and $p = .0013$ for those receiving EMLA <60 minutes before). Additionally, more scores were favorable for the J-Tip application (84% reported no pain at the time of injection) compared with EMLA application (61% reported pain at time of Tegaderm dressing removal; $p = .004$). No significant differences were found in the number of PIV attempts. The cost of the J-Tip ($2.10) was less than the cost of EMLA ($2.80) at the study facility. J-Tip makes a popping sound when activated, and

investigators provided an additional J-Tip for each subject to see and hear how it worked before actual use, if desired.

J-Tip with 0.2 ml of 1% buffered lidocaine was no more effective than jet-delivered placebo (preservative-free normal saline) during PIV cannulation, but may provide superior analgesia compared with no local anesthetic pretreatment (Auerbach, Tunik, and Mojica, 2009). In phase I, 150 children ages 5 to 18 years received either J-Tip (0.2 ml of buffered 1% lidocaine) or jet-delivered placebo (0.2 ml of preservative-free normal saline) 60 seconds before PIV cannulation in an emergency department. Subjects reported pain on injection and on PIV cannulation using a 100-mm color analog scale. In phase II, 47 children described the effect of using the jet device. The mean needle insertion pain score for jet lidocaine (28 mm) was similar to the mean score for placebo (34 mm) and lower than the no device group (52 mm). Most patients reported they would request this device for future PIV access. Providers' ratings of their ability to visualize veins and the patient cooperation were similar in all three groups.

### Cost-Effectiveness
In a decision model on cost-effectiveness of topical and inhalation analgesics during PIV cannulation in the pediatric emergency setting, Porshad, Steinberg, and Waters (2008) concluded that J-Tip had the lowest incremental cost-effectiveness ratio of eight agents. Costs included the cost of the agent plus costs associated with time in the emergency department. Additional variables considered were peak onset time, PIV cannulation success rate, and mean reduction in VAS scores. Additional agents included were intradermal injection of buffered lidocaine, lidocaine iontophoresis, nitrous oxide inhalation analgesia, Synera (lidocaine-tetracaine patch), Sonosite (sonophoresis with lidocaine cream), LMX, and EMLA. Seventeen RCTs involving 1287 children were included in the cost analysis.

## Apply the Evidence: Nursing Implications
- J-Tip with 0.2 ml of buffered lidocaine 1% decreases pain during PIV insertion.
- Wait 1 minute after administration before attempting PIV insertion.
- Do not use in children with a known hypersensitivity to lidocaine or other amide-type local anesthetics such as prilocaine, mepivacaine, bupivacaine, or etidocaine.

## References
Auerbach M, Tunik M, Mojica M: A randomized, double-blind controlled study of jet lidocaine compared to jet placebo for pain relief in children undergoing needle insertion in the emergency department, *Acad Emerg Med* 16(1):1-6, 2009.

Guyatt GH, Oxman AD, Vist GE, and others: GRADE: an emerging consensus on rating quality of evidence and strength of recommendations, *BMJ* 336:924-926, 2008.

Jimenez N, Bradford H, Seidel KD, and others: A comparison of a needle-free injection system for local anesthesia versus EMLA® for intravenous catheter insertion in the pediatric patient, *Anesth Analgesia* 102(2):411-414, 2006.

Pershad J, Steinberg S, Waters T: Cost-effectiveness analysis of anesthetic agents during peripheral intravenous cannulation in the pediatric emergency department, *Arch Pediatr Adolesc Med* 162(20):952-961, 2008.

Spanos S, Booth R, Koenig H, and others: Jet injection of 1% buffered lidocaine versus topical ELA-Max for anesthesia before peripheral intravenous catheterization in children: a randomized controlled trial, *Pediatr Emerg Care* 24(8):511-515, 2008.

**3 - PAIN ASSESSMENT AND MANAGEMENT**

# EVIDENCE-BASED PRACTICE

## Analgesic Patches: Synera to Decrease Pain During Painful Procedures

Terri L. Brown

### Ask the Question
#### Question
Do topical analgesic patches (e.g., lidocaine-tetracaine [Synera, S-Caine]) offer additional advantages (less time, ease of use, lower cost, higher effectiveness, decreased anxiety) in relieving pain during peripheral intravenous (PIV) cannulation in children compared with LMX (lidocaine) cream and buffered lidocaine via injection?

### Search for the Evidence
#### Search Strategies
English research-based publications on lidocaine-tetracaine patches for venipuncture without time limitation were included. Exclusions included epidural use, dermatologic procedures, and S-Caine Peel.

#### Databases Used
Cochrane Collaboration Database, Joanna Briggs Institute, National Guideline Clearinghouse (AHRQ), PubMed, SUMSearch, CINAHL, Scopus, Micromedex, UpToDate, BestBETs, manufacturer's websites (Endo Pharmaceuticals, ZARS Pharma)

### Critically Analyze the Evidence
**Grade criteria:** Evidence quality strong; recommendation strong (Guyatt, Oxman, Vist, and others, 2008)

Two randomized controlled trials (RCTs) in children and two RCTs in adults have demonstrated that Synera is effective in inducing local anesthesia before PIV access. One RCT in adults concluded that Synera was as effective as EMLA in a much shorter timeframe with fewer adverse reactions (Sawyer, Febbraro, Masud, and others, 2009). The manufacturer reports 23 additional clinical trials (including one demonstrating safety in infants as young as 4 months), but these were not found in the search of published literature.

#### Pediatric Studies
Synera reduced PIV cannulation pain and did not alter the success rate in a double-blind, placebo-controlled RCT of 45 children 3 to 17 years old in a suburban emergency center (Singer, Taira, Chisena, and others, 2008). Synera or a placebo patch was placed over the antecubital or hand vein. The median self-reported pain using a visual analog scale (VAS) or Wong-Baker faces scale in the Synera group was significantly lower than in the placebo group ($p = .04$). PIV cannulation success on the first attempt was similar in both groups (90% versus 85%).

In a double-blind, placebo-controlled RCT, a 20-minute application of the S-Caine Patch was effective in lessening pain in 64 children scheduled for vascular access at two centers (Sethna, Verghese, Hannallah, and others, 2005). Synera was developed under the name of S-Caine Patch and renamed at time of U.S. Food and Drug Administration approval. The pain patch significantly reduced pain compared with placebo (median Oucher scores of 0 versus 60; $p < .001$); 59% of children in the pain patch group reported no pain compared with 20% in the placebo group. Investigator estimations of pain and independent observer ratings also favored the S-Caine Patch ($p < .001$). Mild skin erythema (<38%) and edema (<2%) occurred with similar frequencies between the groups.

#### Cost-Effectiveness
In a decision model on cost-effectiveness of topical and inhalation analgesics during PIV cannulation in the pediatric emergency setting, Pershad, Steinberg, and Waters concluded that the lidocaine-tetracaine (S-Caine) patch ranked fifth out of eight agents. Costs included the cost of the agent plus costs associated with time in the emergency department. Additional variables considered were peak onset time, PIV cannulation success rate, and mean reduction in VAS scores. Seventeen RCTs involving 1287 children were included in the cost analysis. Researchers found "the needle-free jet injection of lidocaine device [J-Tip®] had the lowest incremental cost-effectiveness ratio, followed by intradermal injection of buffered lidocaine; lidocaine iontophoresis; nitrous oxide inhalation analgesia; a heated lidocaine and tetracaine patch; sonophoresis with lidocaine cream, 4%; lidocaine cream alone, 4% [LMX®]; and use of a eutectic mixture of lidocaine and prilocaine cream [EMLA®]" (Pershad, Steinberg, and Waters, 2008).

### Apply the Evidence: Nursing Implications
- Synera use during PIV cannulation in children age 3 years and older decreases pain.
- Do not use in children with a sensitivity to lidocaine, tetracaine, para-aminobenzoic acid (PABA), or amide or ester-type anesthetics. Use with caution in patients with hepatic impairment or receiving class I antiarrhythmic drugs (such as tocainide and mexiletine). Do not apply to broken skin.
- Use immediately after opening pouch, since patch begins to heat once removed from pouch. To ensure proper heating without thermal injury, do not cut the patch or remove any layers of the patch, and ensure that the holes on the patch are not covered by clothing.
- Do not keep the patch on longer than 20 to 30 minutes.
- There are limited data to support the safety of applying multiple patches simultaneously or sequentially. Follow the distributor's recommendations to not apply multiple patches.
- As with all transdermal patches containing medication, after use fold adhesive together and dispose of used patches in a location out of the reach of children. Do not use in magnetic resonance imaging suite.

### References
Guyatt GH, Oxman AD, Vist GE, and others: GRADE: An emerging consensus on rating quality of evidence and strength of recommendations, *BMJ* 336(7650): 924-926, 2008.

Pershad J, Steinberg S, Waters T: Cost-effectiveness analysis of anesthetic agents during peripheral intravenous cannulation in the pediatric emergency department, *Arch Pediatr Adolesc Med* 162(20):952-961, 2008.

Sawyer J, Febbraro S, Masud S, and others: Heated lidocaine/tetracaine patch (Synera™, Rapydan™) compared with lidocaine/prilocaine cream (EMLA®) for topical anaesthesia before vascular access, *Br J Anaesthesia* 102(2):210-215, 2009.

Sethna NF, Verghese ST, Hannallah RS, and others: A randomized controlled trial to evaluate S-Caine Patch™ for reducing pain associated with vascular access in children, *Anesthesiology* 102(2):403-408, 2005.

Singer AJ, Taira BR, Chisena EN, and others: Warm lidocaine/tetracaine patch versus placebo before pediatric intravenous cannulation: a randomized controlled trial, *Ann Emerg Med* 52(1):41-47, 2008.

| TABLE 3-5 | Antipyretic and Nonsteroidal Antiinflammatory Drugs (NSAIDs) Approved for Children* |

| Drug | Dosage | Comments |
| --- | --- | --- |
| Acetaminophen (Tylenol)—not an NSAID | 10-15 mg/kg/dose q 4-6 h, not to exceed 5 doses in 24 h or 75 mg/kg/day, orally | Available in numerous preparations<br>Nonprescription<br>Higher dosage range may provide increased analgesia |
| Choline magnesium trisalicylate (Trilisate) | Children <37 kg (81.5 lb): 50 mg/kg/day divided into 2 doses<br>Children >37 kg (81.5 lb): 2250 mg/day divided into 2 doses | Available in suspension, 500 mg/5 ml<br>Prescription |
| Ibuprofen (Children's Motrin, Children's Advil) | Children >6 months: 5-10 mg/kg/dose q 6-8 h, not to exceed 40 mg/kg/day | Available in numerous preparations<br>Available in suspension, 100 mg/5 ml, and drops, 100 mg/2.5 ml<br>Nonprescription |
| Naproxen (Naprosyn) | Children ≥2 years: 5-7 mg/kg/dose q 8-12 h | Available in suspension, 125 mg/5 ml, and several different dosages for tablets<br>Prescription |
| Tolmetin (Tolectin) | Children ≥2 years: 5-7 mg/kg/dose q 6-8 h | Available in 200-mg, 400-mg, and 600-mg tablets<br>Prescription |

Data from Olin BR and others: *Drug facts and comparisons,* St Louis, 2002, Facts and Comparisons.

NOTE: Newer formulations of NSAIDs selectively inhibit one of the enzymes of cyclooxygenase (COX-2, which is responsible for pain transmission) but do not inhibit the other (COX-1). Inhibition of COX-1 decreases prostaglandin production, which is necessary for normal organ function. For example, prostaglandins help maintain gastric mucosal blood flow and barrier protection, regulate blood flow to the liver and kidneys, and facilitate platelet aggregation and clot formation. Theoretically, the COX-2 NSAIDs provide similar analgesic and antiinflammatory benefits with fewer gastric and platelet side effects than the nonselective agents. COX-2 NSAIDs are approved for use in patients older than age 18 years.

*All NSAIDs in this table (except acetaminophen) have significant antiinflammatory, antipyretic, and analgesic actions. Acetaminophen has a weak antiinflammatory action, and its classification as an NSAID is controversial. Patients respond differently to various NSAIDs; therefore changing from one drug to another may be necessary for maximum benefit. Acetylsalicylic acid (aspirin) is also an NSAID but is not recommended for children because of its possible association with Reye's syndrome. The NSAIDs in this table have no known association with Reye's syndrome. However, caution should be exercised in prescribing any salicylate-containing drug (e.g., Trilisate) for children with known or suspected viral infection.
Side effects of ibuprofen, naproxen, and tolmetin include nausea, vomiting, diarrhea, constipation, gastric ulceration, bleeding nephritis, and fluid retention.
Acetaminophen and choline magnesium trisalicylate are well tolerated in the gastrointestinal tract and do not interfere with platelet function. NSAIDs (except acetaminophen) should not be given to patients with allergic reactions to salicylates. All NSAIDs should be used cautiously in patients with renal impairment.

*Text continued from p. 194.*

LAT (lidocaine-adrenaline-tetracaine) or tetracaine-phenylephrine (tetraphen)
- Provides skin anesthesia about 15 minutes after application on nonintact skin

Gel (preferable) or liquid placed on wounds for suturing
Adrenaline not for use on end arterioles (fingers, toes, tip of nose, penis, earlobes) because of vasoconstriction

### Transdermal fentanyl (Duragesic)

Available as patch for continuous pain control
Safety and efficacy not established in children younger than age 12 years
Not appropriate for initial relief of acute pain because of long interval to peak effect (12 to 24 hours); for rapid onset of pain relief, give an immediate-release opioid.
Orders for "rescue doses" of an immediate-release opioid recommended for breakthrough pain, a flare of severe pain that breaks through the medication being administered at regular intervals for persistent pain

Has duration of up to 72 hours for prolonged pain relief
If respiratory depression occurs, possible need for several doses of naloxone

### Vapocoolant

Use of prescription spray coolant, such as Fluori-Methane or ethyl chloride (Pain-Ease); applied to the skin for 10 to 15 seconds immediately before the needle puncture; anesthesia lasts about 15 seconds.
Cold disliked by some children; may be less uncomfortable to spray coolant on a cotton ball and then apply this to the skin
Application of ice to the skin for 30 seconds found to be ineffective.

### Rectal

Alternative to oral or parenteral routes
Variable absorption rate
Generally disliked by children
Many drugs able to be compounded into rectal suppositories*

Data primarily from American Pain Society: *Principles of analgesic use in the treatment of acute pain and chronic cancer pain,* ed 4, Skokie, Ill, 1999, The Society; and McCaffery M, Pasero C: *Pain: a clinical manual,* ed 2, St Louis, 1999, Mosby.
*For further information about compounding drugs in troche or suppository form, contact Professional Compounding Centers of America (PCCA), 9901 S. Wilcrest Drive, Houston, TX 77009; (800) 331-2498; http://www.pccarx.com.

**TABLE 3-6   Dosage of Selected Opioids for Children**

| Drug | Appropriate Equianalgesic | Approximate Equianalgesic Parenteral Dose | RECOMMENDED STARTING DOSE (CHILDREN <50 kg (110 lb) BODY WEIGHT)* | |
|---|---|---|---|---|
| | | | Oral | Parenteral* |
| Morphine | 30 mg every 3-4 hr | 10 mg every 3-4 hr | 0.2-0.4 mg/kg every 3-4 hr<br>0.3-0.6 mg/kg time released every 12 hr | 0.1-0.2 mg/kg IM every 3-4 hr<br>0.02-0.1 mg/kg IV bolus every 2 hr<br>0.015 mg/kg every 8 min PCA<br>0.01-0.02 mg/kg/hr IV infusion (neonates)<br>0.01-0.06 mg/kg/hr IV infusion (child) |
| Fentanyl (Sublimaze) (oral mucosal form [Actiq])† | Not available | 0.1 mg IV | 5-15 mcg/kg; maximum dose 400 mcg | 0.5-1.5 mcg/kg IV bolus every 30 min<br>1-2 mcg/hr IV infusion |
| Codeine‡ | 200 mg every 3-4 hr | 130 mg every 3-4 hr | 1 mg/kg every 3-4 hr | Not recommended |
| Hydromorphone§ (Dilaudid) | 7.5 mg every 3-4 hr | 1.5 mg every 3-4 hr | 0.04-0.1 mg/kg every 3-4 hr | 0.02-0.1 mg/kg every 3-4 hr<br>0.005-0.2 mg/kg IV bolus every 2 hr |
| Hydrocodone and acetaminophen (Lorcet, Lortab, Vicodin, others) | 30 mg every 3-4 hr | Not available | 0.2 mg/kg every 3-4 hr | Not available |
| Levorphanol (Levo-Dromoran) | 4 mg every 6-8 hr | 2 mg every 6-8 hr | 0.04 mg/kg every 6-8 hr | 0.02 mg/kg every 6-8 hr |
| Methadone (Dolophine, others)¶ | 20 mg every 6-8 hr | 10 mg every 6-8 hr | 0.2 mg/kg every 6-8 hr | 0.1 mg/kg/dose q 4 hr for 2-3 doses then q 6-12 h prn, max 10 mg/dose |
| Oxycodone (Roxicodone, OxyContin; also in Percocet, Percodan, Tylox, others) | 20 mg every 3-4 hr | Not available | 2 mg/kg every 3-4 hr# | Not available |

Data from Acute Pain Management Guideline Panel: *Acute pain management: Operative or medical procedures and trauma: Clinical practice guideline,* AHCPR Pub No 92-0032, Rockville, Md, 1992, Agency for Health Care Policy and Research, Public Health Service, US Department of Health and Human Services; Berde C and others: Report of the subcommittee on disease-related pain in childhood cancer, *Pediatrics* 86(5 pt 2):820, 1990.

*IM,* Intramuscular; *IV,* intravenous; *PCA,* patient-controlled analgesia.

Note: Published tables vary in suggested doses that are equianalgesic to morphine. Clinical response is criterion that must be applied for each patient; titration to clinical response is necessary. Because there is no complete cross-tolerance among these drugs, it is usually necessary to use a lower than equianalgesic dose when changing drugs and to retitrate to response.

Caution: Recommended doses do not apply to patients with renal or hepatic insufficiency or other conditions affecting drug metabolism and kinetics.

*Caution: Doses listed for patients with body weight less than 50 kg (110 lb) cannot be used as initial starting doses in infants less than 6 months of age. For nonventilated infants younger than age 6 months, the initial opioid dose should be about ¼ to ⅓ of the dose recommended for older infants and children. For example, morphine could be used at a dose of 0.03 mg/kg instead of the traditional 0.1 mg/kg.

†Actiq is indicated only for management of breakthrough cancer pain in patients with malignancies who are already receiving and are tolerant to opioid therapy, but it can be used for preoperative or preprocedural sedation/analgesia.

‡Caution: Codeine doses above 65 mg often are not appropriate because of diminishing incremental analgesia with increasing doses but continually increasing constipation and other side effects. Dosages are from McCaffery M, Pasero C: *Pain: A clinical manual,* ed 2, St Louis, 1999, Mosby.

§For morphine, hydromorphone, and oxymorphone, rectal administration is an alternate route for patients unable to take oral medications, but equianalgesic doses may differ from oral and parenteral doses because of pharmacokinetic differences.

¶Initial dose is 10% to 25% of equianalgesic morphine dose. Parenteral Dolophine is no longer available in the United States.

#Caution: Doses of aspirin and acetaminophen in combination with opioid or nonsteroidal antiinflammatory drug preparations must also be adjusted to patient's body weight. Daily dose of acetaminophen should not exceed 75 mg/kg, or 4000 mg.

| TABLE 3-7 | Co-analgesic Adjuvant Drugs | | |
|---|---|---|---|
| **Category and Drug** | **Dosage** | **Indication** | **Comments** |
| **Antidepressants** | | | |
| Amitriptyline | 0.2 to 0.5 mg/kg PO hs<br>Titrate upward by 0.25 mg/kg q 5-7 days prn<br>Available in 10-mg and 25-mg tablets<br>Usual starting dose is 10-25 mg | Continuous neuropathic pain with burning, aching, dysthesia with insomnia | Provides analgesia by blocking reuptake of serotonin and norepinephrine, possibly slowing transmission of pain signals |
| Nortriptyline | 0.2 to 1 mg/kg PO AM or bid<br>Titrate up by 0.5 mg q 5-7 days<br>Max 25 mg/dose | Neuropathic pain as above without insomnia | Helps with pain related to insomnia and depression (use nortriptyline if patient is oversedated)<br>Analgesic effects seen earlier than antidepressant effects<br>Side effects include dry mouth, constipation, urinary retention |
| **Anticonvulsants** | | | |
| Gabapentin | 5 mg/kg PO hs<br>Increase to bid on day 2, tid on day 3<br>Max 300 mg/day | Neuropathic pain | Mechanism of action unknown<br>Side effects include sedation, ataxia, nystagmus, dizziness |
| Carbamazepine | <6 years:<br>  2.5-5 mg/kg PO bid initially<br>  Increase weekly prn to optimal response<br>  Max 100 mg bid<br>6 to 12 years:<br>  5 mg/kg PO bid initially<br>  Increase weekly prn to optimal dose<br>  Usual max: 100 mg/dose bid<br>>12 years:<br>  200 mg PO bid initially<br>  Increase weekly prn to optimal response<br>  Max: 1.6-2.4 g/24 hr | Sharp, cutting neuropathic pain<br>Peripheral neuropathies<br>Phantom limb pain | Similar analgesic effect as amitriptyline<br>Monitor blood levels for toxicity only<br>Side effects include decreased blood counts, ataxia, and GI irritation |
| **Anxiolytics** | | | |
| Lorazepam | 0.03-0.1 mg/kg q4-6 h PO or IV; max 2 mg/dose | Muscle spasm<br>Anxiety | May increase sedation in combination with opioids |
| Diazepam | 0.1-0.3 mg/kg q4-6 h PO or IV; max 10 mg/dose | | Can cause depression with prolonged use |
| **Corticosteroids** | | | |
| Dexamethasone | Dose dependent on clinical situation; higher bolus doses in cord compression, then lower daily dose<br>Try to wean to NSAIDs if pain allows<br>Cerebral edema: 1-2 mg/kg load then 1-1.5 mg/kg/day-divided every 6 hr; max 4 mg/dose<br>Antiinflammatory: 0.08-0.3 mg/kg/day divided every 6-12 hr | Pain from increased intracranial pressure<br>Bony metastasis<br>Spinal or nerve compression | Side effects include edema, GI irritation, increased weight, acne<br>Use gastroprotectants such as $H_2$ blockers (e.g., ranitidine) or proton pump inhibitors (e.g., omeprazole) for long-term administration of steroids or NSAIDs in end-stage cancer with bony pain |
| **Others** | | | |
| Clonidine | 2-4 mcg/kg PO q4-6 h<br>May also use a 100-mcg transdermal patch q 7 days for patients >40 kg | Neuropathic pain<br>Cutting, sharp, electrical, shooting pain<br>Phantom limb pain | Alpha-2 adrenoreceptor agonist modulates ascending pain sensations<br>Routes of administration include oral, transdermal, and spinal<br>Manage withdrawal symptoms<br>Monitor for orthostatic hypertension, decreased heart rate<br>Sedation common |

*Continued*

| TABLE 3-7 | Co-analgesic Adjuvant Drugs—cont'd | | |
|---|---|---|---|
| **Category and Drug** | **Dosage** | **Indication** | **Comments** |
| Mexiletine | 2-3 mg/kg/dose PO tid— May titrate 0.5 mg/kg q 2-3 weeks prn Max 300 mg/dose | | Similar to lidocaine, longer acting Stabilizes sodium conduction in nerve cells, reduces neuronal firing Can enhance action of opioids, antidepressants, anticonvulsants Side effects include dizziness, ataxia, nausea, vomiting May measure blood levels for toxicity |

*bid,* Twice daily; *GI,* gastrointestinal; *hs,* at bedtime; *IV,* intravenous; *NSAIDs,* nonsteroidal antiinflammatory drugs; *PO,* by mouth; *prn,* as needed; *tid,* three times a day.

| TABLE 3-8 | Management of Opioid Side Effects | |
|---|---|---|
| **Side Effect** | **Adjuvant Drugs** | **Nonpharmacologic Techniques** |
| Constipation | **Senna and docusate sodium** *Tablet:* 2 to 6 years: Start with ½ tablet once a day; max: 1 tablet twice a day 6 to 12 years: Start with 1 tablet once a day; max: 2 tablets twice a day >12 yr: Start with 2 tablets once a day; max: 4 tablets twice a day *Liquid:* 1 month to 1 year: 1.25-5 ml q hs 1 to 5 years: 2.5-5 ml q hs 5 to 15 years: 5-10 ml q hs >15 years: 10-25 ml q hs **Casanthranol and docusate sodium** *Liquid:* 5-15 ml q hs *Capsules:* 1 cap PO q hs **Bisacodyl: PO or PR** 3 to 12 years: 5 mg/dose/day >12 years: 10-15 mg/dose/day **Lactulose** 7.5 ml/day after breakfast Adult: 15-30 ml/day PO **Mineral oil:** 1-2 tsp/day PO **Magnesium citrate** <6 years: 2-4 ml/kg PO once 6 to 12 years: 100-150 ml PO once >12 years: 150-300 ml PO once **Milk of Magnesia** <2 years: 0.5 ml/kg/dose PO once 2 to 5 years: 5-15 ml/day PO 6 to 12 years: 15-30 ml PO once >12 years: 30-60 ml PO once | Increase water intake Prune juice, bran cereal, vegetables Exercise |
| Sedation | **Caffeine:** single dose of 1-1.5 mg PO **Dextroamphetamine:** 2.5-5 mg PO in AM and early afternoon **Methylphenidate:** 2.5-5 mg PO in AM and early afternoon Consider opioid switch if sedation is persistent | Caffeinated drinks (e.g., Mountain Dew, cola drinks) |
| Nausea, vomiting | **Promethazine:** 0.5 mg/kg q 4-6 hr; max: 25 mg/dose **Ondansetron:** 0.1-0.15 mg/kg IV or PO q 4 hr; max: 8 mg/dose **Granisetron:** 10-40 mcg/kg q 2-4 hr; max: 1 mg/dose **Droperidol:** 0.05-0.06 mg/kg IV q 4-6 hr; can be very sedating | Imagery, relaxation Deep, slow breathing |
| Pruritus | **Diphenhydramine:** 1 mg/kg IV or PO q 4-6 hr prn; max: 25 mg/dose **Hydroxyzine:** 0.6 mg/kg/dose PO q 6 hr; max: 50 mg/dose **Naloxone:** 0.5 mcg/kg q 2 min until pruritus improves (diluted in solution of 0.1 mg of naloxone per 10 ml of saline) **Butorphanol:** 0.3-0.5 mg/kg IV (use cautiously in opioid-tolerant children; may cause withdrawal symptoms); max: 2 mg/dose because mixed agonist-antagonist | Oatmeal baths, good hygiene Exclude other causes of itching Change opioids |

| TABLE 3-8 | Management of Opioid Side Effects—cont'd | |
|---|---|---|
| Side Effect | Adjuvant Drugs | Nonpharmacologic Techniques |
| Respiratory depression: mild to moderate | Hold dose of opioid<br>Reduce subsequent doses by 25% | Arouse gently, give oxygen, encourage to deep breathe |
| Respiratory depression: severe | **Naloxone**<br>*During disease pain management:*<br>0.5 mcg/kg in 2-min increments until breathing improves (American Pain Society, 1999; McCaffery and Pasero, 1999)<br>Reduce opioid dose if possible<br>Consider opioid switch<br>*During sedation for procedures:*<br>5-10 mcg/kg until breathing improves (Yaster,1997)<br>Reduce opioid dose if possible<br>Consider opioid switch | Oxygen, bag and mask if indicated |
| Dysphoria, confusion, hallucinations | Evaluate medications, eliminate adjuvant medications with central nervous system effects as symptoms allow<br>Consider opioid switch if possible<br>**Haloperidol (Haldol):** 0.05-0.15 mg/kg/day divided in 2-3 doses; max: 2-4 mg/day | Rule out other physiologic causes |
| Urinary retention | Evaluate medications, eliminate adjuvant medications with anticholinergic effects (e.g., antihistamines, tricyclic antidepressants)<br>Occurs with spinal analgesia more frequently than with systemic opioid use<br>**Oxybutynin**<br>1 year: 1 mg tid<br>1 to 2 years: 2 mg tid<br>2 to 3 years: 3 mg tid<br>4 to 5 years: 4 mg tid<br>>5 years: 5 mg tid | Rule out other physiologic causes<br>In/out or indwelling urinary catheter |

*hs,* At bedtime; *IV,* intravenous; *PO,* by mouth; *PR,* by rectum; *prn,* as needed; *q,* every; *tid,* three times a day.

# Regional Nerve Block

Use of long-acting local anesthetic (bupivacaine or ropivacaine) injected into nerves to block pain at site

Provides prolonged analgesia postoperatively, such as after inguinal herniorrhaphy

May be used to provide local anesthesia for surgery, such as dorsal penile nerve block for circumcision or for reduction of fractures

# Inhalation

Use of anesthetics, such as nitrous oxide, to produce partial or complete analgesia for painful procedures

Side effects (e.g., headache) possible from occupational exposure to high levels of nitrous oxide

# Epidural or Intrathecal

Involves catheter placed into epidural, caudal, or intrathecal space for continuous infusion or single or intermittent administration of opioid with or without a long-acting local anesthetic (e.g., bupivacaine, ropivacaine)

Analgesia primarily from drug's direct effect on opioid receptors in spinal cord

Respiratory depression rare but may have slow and delayed onset; can be prevented by checking level of sedation and respiratory rate and depth hourly for initial 24 hours and decreasing dose when excessive sedation is detected

Nausea, itching, and urinary retention are common dose-related side effects from the epidural opioid.

Mild hypotension, urinary retention, and temporary motor or sensory deficits are common unwanted effects of epidural local anesthetic.

Catheter for urinary retention inserted during surgery to decrease trauma to child; if inserted when child is awake, anesthetize urethra with lidocaine

3 - PAIN ASSESSMENT AND MANAGEMENT

# Side Effects of Opioids

## General

a. **Constipation (possibly severe)**
b. **Respiratory depression**
c. **Sedation**
d. **Nausea and vomiting**
e. **Agitation, euphoria**
f. **Mental clouding**
g. **Hallucinations**

h. **Orthostatic hypotension**
i. **Pruritus**
j. **Urticaria**
k. **Sweating**
l. **Miosis (may be sign of toxicity)**
m. **Anaphylaxis (rare)**

## Signs of Tolerance

a. Decreasing pain relief
b. Decreasing duration of pain relief

## Signs of Withdrawal Syndrome in Patients with Physical Dependence

1. Initial signs of withdrawal
   a. Lacrimation
   b. Rhinorrhea
   c. Yawning
   d. Sweating

2. Later signs of withdrawal
   a. Restlessness
   b. Irritability
   c. Tremors
   d. Anorexia
   e. Dilated pupils
   f. Gooseflesh
   g. Nausea, vomiting

---

### GUIDELINES

#### Managing Opioid-Induced Respiratory Depression

**If Respirations Are Depressed**

Assess sedation level
Reduce infusion by 25% when possible
Stimulate patient (shake shoulder gently, call by name, ask to breathe)

**If Patient Cannot Be Aroused or Is Apneic**

Administer naloxone (Narcan): Doses may need to be repeated
- For children ≤ 5 years or ≤ 20 kg, 0.1 mg/kg.
- For children > 5 years or > 20 kg, 2 mg/dose.
Administer bolus slow IV push every 2 minutes until effect is obtained.

Closely monitor patient. Naloxone's duration of antagonist action may be shorter than that of opioid, requiring repeated doses of naloxone.

NOTE: Respiratory depression caused by benzodiazepines (e.g., diazepam [Valium] or midazolam [Versed]) can be reversed with flumazenil (Romazicon). Pediatric dosing experience suggests an initial dose 0.01 mg/kg (max 0.2 mg); if no (or inadequate) response after 45 seconds repeat the dose, 0.01 mg/kg dose can be repeated as needed at 60-second intervals for maximum cumulative dose of 0.05 mg/kg or 1 mg, lowest of the two (usual total dose 0.08-1 mg).

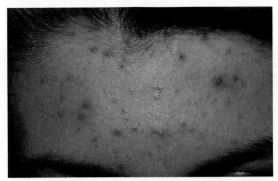

FIGURE **1**    Acne vulgaris. From Weston: *Color textbook of pediatric dermatology*, ed 4, Philadelphia, 2007, Mosby.

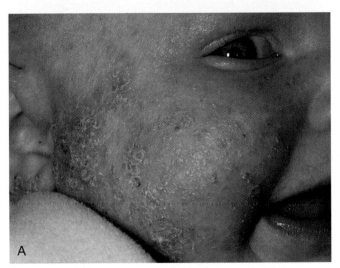

A

FIGURE **2A**    Atopic dermatitis. From Habif T: *Clinical dermatology: A color guide to diagnosis and therapy*, ed 5, Philadelphia, 2010, Mosby.

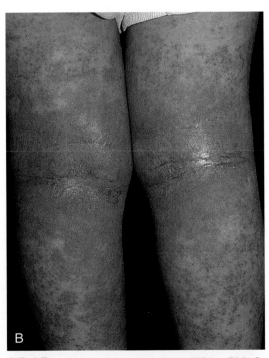

B

FIGURE **2B**    Atopic dermatitis. From White GM, Cox NH: *Diseases of the skin: A color atlas and text*, ed 2, Edinburgh, 2006, Mosby.

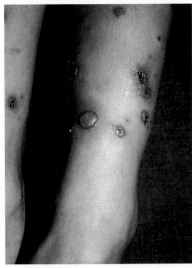

FIGURE **3**    Bullous Impetigo. From James WD, Berger TG, Elston DM: Andrews' diseases of the skin: *Clinical dermatology*, ed 10, Edinburgh, 2006, Saunders.

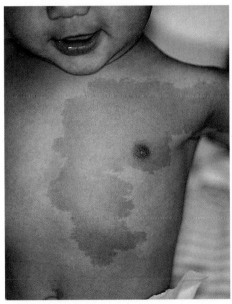

FIGURE **4**    Café-au-lait spots. From Eichenfield LF, Frieden IJ, and Esterly NB: *Neonatal dermatology*, ed 2, Philadelphia, 2008, Saunders.

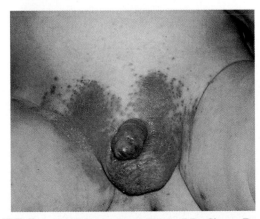

FIGURE **5**    Candidiasis. From Feigin RD, Cherry D, editors: *Textbook of pediatric infectious diseases*, ed 6, Philadelphia, 2009, Saunders.

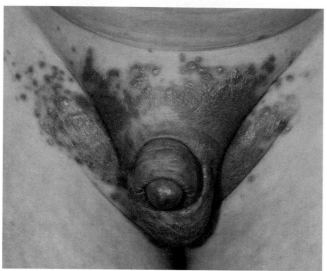

FIGURE **6**   Diaper dermatitis. From Habif T: *Clinical dermatology: A color guide to diagnosis and therapy*, ed 5, Philadelphia, 2010, Mosby.

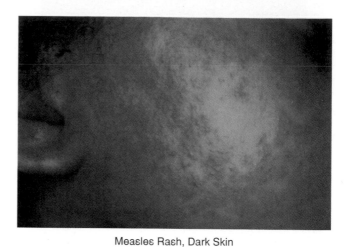

Measles Rash, Dark Skin

FIGURE **9**   Measles. From Feigin RD, Cherry D, editors: *Textbook of pediatric infectious diseases*, ed 6, Philadelphia, 2009, Saunders.

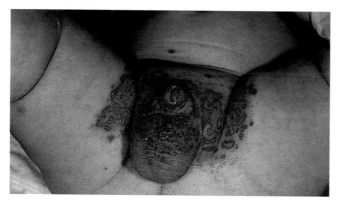

FIGURE **7**   Herpes simplex. From Callen JP, Greer KE, Paller AS, Swinyer LJ: *Color atlas of dermatology*, ed 2, Philadelphia, 2000, Saunders.

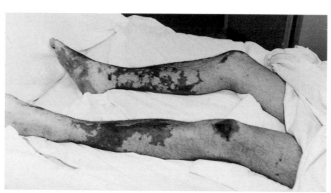

FIGURE **10**   Meningococcemia. From Hockenberry MJ, Wilson D: *Wong's nursing care of infants and children*, ed 9, St Louis, 2010, Mosby.

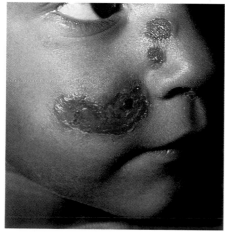

FIGURE **8**   Impetigo. From James WD, Berger TG, Elston DM: *Andrews' diseases of the skin: Clinical dermatology*, ed 10, Edinburgh, 2006, Saunders.

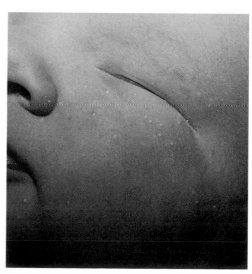

FIGURE **11**   Milia. From White GM, Cox NH: *Diseases of the skin: A color atlas and text*, ed 2, Edinburgh, 2006, Mosby.

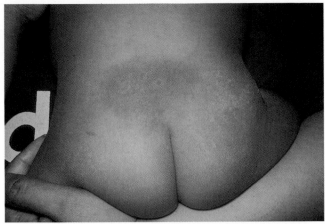

FIGURE **12**    Mongolian spot. From Swartz MH: *Textbook of physical diagnosis: History and examination*, ed 6, Philadelphia, 2009, Saunders.

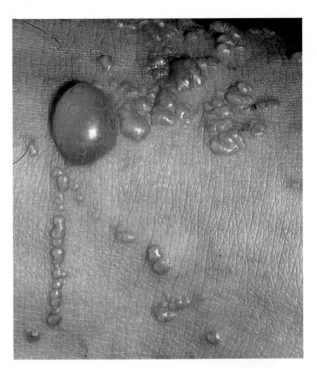

FIGURE **13**    Poison ivy. From Habif T: *Clinical dermatology: A color guide to diagnosis and therapy*, ed 5, Philadelphia, 2010, Mosby.

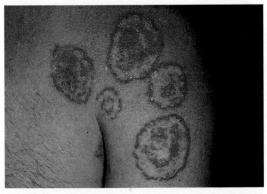

FIGURE **14**    Ringworm. From Callen JP, Greer KE, Paller AS, Swinyer LJ: *Color atlas of dermatology*, ed 2, Philadelphia, 2000, Saunders.

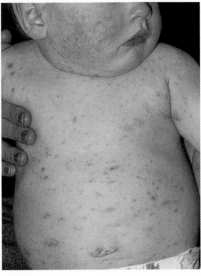

FIGURE **15**    Scabies. From White GM, Cox NH: *Diseases of the skin: A color atlas and text*, ed 2, Edinburgh, 2006, Mosby.

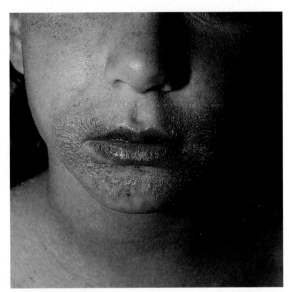

FIGURE **16**    Scalded skin syndrome. From Callen JP, Greer KE, Paller AS, Swinyer LJ: *Color atlas of dermatology*, ed 2, Philadelphia, 2000, Saunders.

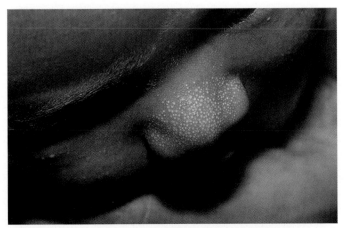

FIGURE **17**    Sebaceous gland hyperplasia. From White GM, Cox NH: *Diseases of the skin: A color atlas and text*, ed 2, Edinburgh, 2006, Mosby.

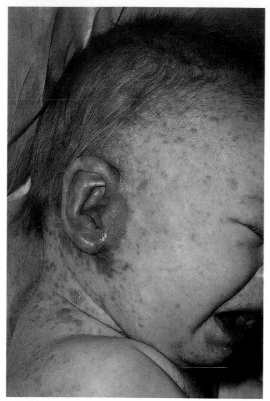

FIGURE **18** Seborrheic dermatitis. From Habif T: *Clinical dermatology: A color guide to diagnosis and therapy*, ed 5, Philadelphia, 2010, Mosby.

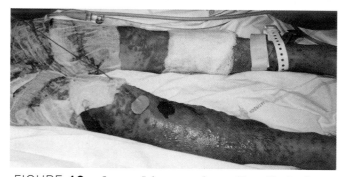

FIGURE **19** Stevens-Johnson syndrome. From Hockenberry MJ, Wilson D: *Wong's nursing care of infants and children*, ed 9, St Louis, 2010, Mosby.

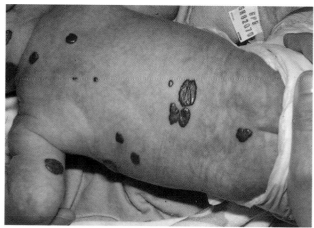

FIGURE **20** Strawberry hemangioma. From Zitelli BJ, Davis HW: *Atlas of pediatric physical diagnosis*, ed 5, St Louis, 2007, Mosby.

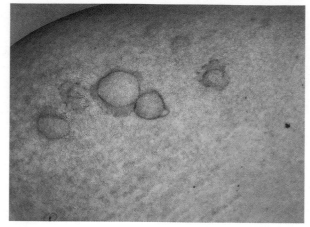

FIGURE **21** Urticaria. From White GM, Cox NH: *Diseases of the skin: A color atlas and text*, ed 2, Edinburgh, 2006, Mosby.

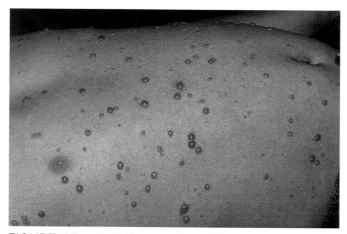

FIGURE **22** Varicella zoster. From White GM, Cox NH: *Diseases of the skin: A color atlas and text*, ed 2, Edinburgh, 2006, Mosby.

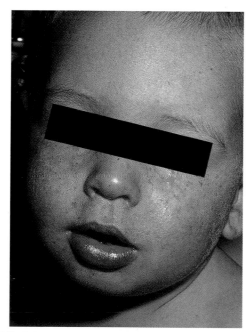

FIGURE **23** Xeroderma pigmentosum. From White GM, Cox NH: *Diseases of the skin: A color atlas and text*, ed 2, Edinburgh, 2006, Mosby.

## GUIDELINES

### Applying a Topical Anesthetic

There are several topical anesthetics available; the time it takes the medication to actually "work" and numb the site varies. LMX4 is a 4% liposomal lidocaine preparation that is applied just like EMLA; the main difference is that LMX4 is reported to numb the skin within 30 minutes. The site should not have any alcohol-based product before application of this anesthetic. See Evolve Evidence-Based Practice: EMLA versus LMX for pain reduction during peripheral IV access in children.

### Equipment

EMLA cream or LMX4 cream
Transparent dressing
Plastic film and tape (if needed)
Ballpoint pen or marker
Tissue or paper towel

### Instructions for EMLA Cream and LMX4 Cream

1. Unscrew the cap, and puncture the metal covering of the tube with the point on the top of the cap.
2. EMLA: Apply ½ of the 5-g tube in a thick layer to about a 2-inch by 2-inch area of skin where the procedure will be done. If the puncture area is very small, such as a finger stick, you can use ⅓ of the tube.

LMX4: Apply a pea-sized amount to the area of skin to be numbed, and rub it in for approximately 30 seconds. Then apply a larger dollop (approximately 2.5 g or ½ of a 5-g tube) over the area and apply the dressing.
3. Remove the center cutout piece of the transparent dressing.
4. Peel the paper liner from the paper-framed dressing.
5. Cover the topical anesthetic cream so that you get a thick layer underneath. Do not spread out the cream. Smooth down the dressing edges carefully, and be sure it is secure to avoid leakage.
6. Remove the paper frame. Mark directly on the occlusive dressing the time you applied the cream.
7. To remove the transparent dressing, grasp opposite sides of the film and pull the sides away from each other to stretch and loosen the film. After the film begins to loosen, grasp the other two sides of the film and pull. This method is easier and more comfortable than pulling the dressing up and off the skin.
8. Wipe off the topical anesthetic cream with a tissue. The numbing effect can last 1 hour or more after removing the dressing.
   EMLA® Cream is a registered trademark of Abraxis BioScience, Inc., and is manufactured by Abraxis BioScience, Inc., for use in the United States only.

This guideline may be photocopied and distributed to families.

## GUIDELINES

### Administering Buffered Lidocaine

**Procedures:** Per Procedural Pain Protocol, may be used prior to PIV insertion, venipuncture, arterial puncture, or AV graft/AV fistula access.

    **Contraindications:** Known hypersensitivity to xylocaine or other amide type local anesthetics such as prilocaine, mepivacaine, bupivacaine, or etidocaine.

    **Dosage:** Inject 0.1 ml intradermally ½ cm below the proposed PIV insertion site.

    **Administration:** Buffered lidocaine 1% prefilled syringes must be refrigerated. Allow medication to warm to room temperature just

prior to administration (rolling syringe between hands to warm the contents is allowable). Insert 30-gauge needle intradermally ½ cm below the proposed insertion site. Aspirate the plunger of the syringe to verify that the vein has not been entered. Instill buffered lidocaine 0.1 ml at a constant rate to form a small wheal. Buffered lidocaine may be used in up to three potential sites (maximum of three 0.1ml injections may be given within 2 hours). Wait at least 1 minute before attempting the insertion/puncture. Perform needlestick with the needle entering the skin within the wheal.

# Sedation for Painful Procedures

Pain associated with invasive procedures and anxiety associated with diagnostic imaging can be managed with sedation and analgesia. Sedation involves a wide range of levels of consciousness (Box 3-1). Commonly used sedation agents are found in Table 3-9.

TABLE 3-9   Sedation Agents

| Agent Table | Moderate Sedation | Deep Sedation | Onset/Duration | Adverse Effects | Comments |
|---|---|---|---|---|---|
| Propofol | Used for general anesthesia | *Children and adults* IV bolus: 1 mg/kg/dose IV infusion: 50-200 mcg/kg/minute; max: 200 mcg/kg/min | Onset: IV: <1 minute Duration: 5-10 minutes | Hypotension, injection site burning, apnea, hypertension, arrhythmia, pruritus, rash | Children and adults >50 kg should be dosed in 20-50 mg increments |
| Fentanyl | *<12 years* IV: 1-2 mcg/kg/dose, may repeat full dose in 5 minutes if needed. Max cumulative dose: 50 mcg *≥12 years or >50 kg* IV: 0.5-1 mcg/kg/dose or 25-50 mcg/dose, may repeat full dose in 5 minutes if needed; Max cumulative dose: 100 mcg | *Neonates, infants, children, and adults* IV: >2 mcg/kg/dose or max cumulative dose 100 mcg | Onset: IV: 1-5 minutes Duration: 20-60 minutes | Respiratory depression, apnea; muscle rigidity and chest wall spasm occur following rapid IV administration; hypotension, bradycardia, seizures, delirium | Provides rapid onset of action with a short duration of action; minimal hemodynamic changes |
| Midazolam | *>6 months to <12 years* IV: 0.05-0.1 mg/kg/dose; Max cumulative dose: 10 mg *≥12 years* IV: 0.5-2 mg/dose; Max cumulative dose: 10 mg | N/A | Onset: IV: 1-2 minutes Duration: 20-30 minutes | Respiratory depression, bitter taste, amnesia, blurred visior, headache, hiccoughs, nausea, vomiting, coughing, sedation; cardiac arrest and hypotension have occurred after premedication with a narcotic | Provides no analgesia; effective anxiolytic, sedative, amnesic; fewer cardiac complications |
| Ketamine | *Children and adults* IV: 0.5-1 mg/kg/dose over 2-3 minutes; May repeat as needed up to max cumulative dose of 100 mg or 2 mg/kg in a 30-minute time period | *Children and adults* IV: >1 mg/kg/dose, or cumulative dose of 100 mg or 2 mg/kg in a 30-minute time period | Onset: IV: 1-2 minutes Duration: 10-15 minutes | Hypertonicity, nystagmus, diplopia; contraindicated in patients in which a rapid rise in blood pressure would be detrimental and in patients with increased ICP | Good sedative, amnesic, analgesic; provides bronchial smooth muscle relaxation; airway protective reflexes remain intact; eyes usually open with blank stare; administer by slow IV push to decrease risk of respiratory depression |

## GUIDELINES

### Pain Management During Neonatal Circumcision*

#### Pharmacologic Interventions

##### Use of Topical Anesthetic Only

1. One hour before the procedure, administer acetaminophen (e.g., Tylenol 15 mg/kg) as ordered by the practitioner.
2. Place a thick layer (1 g) of EMLA† or LMX4‡ cream around the penis where the prepuce (foreskin) attaches to the glans. Avoid placing cream on the tip of the penis where it may come in contact with urethral opening.
3. Cover the penis with a "finger cot" that is cut from a vinyl or latex glove, or a piece of plastic wrap, and secure bottom of covering with tape. Avoid using Tegaderm or large amounts of tape on the skin because removing the adhesive causes pain and can irritate the fragile skin.
4. If the infant urinates during the time EMLA is applied (1 hour) and a significant amount of EMLA is removed, reapply the cream and covering. The total application of EMLA should not exceed a surface area of 10 cm² (1.25 × 1.25 inches).
5. Remove cream with clean cloth or tissue. Blanching of skin is an expected reaction to EMLA's application under an occlusive dressing; erythema and some edema may occur also.
6. Two minutes before starting the procedure, give the infant a sucrose solution; 24% (weight/volume) sucrose solution is available commercially from Children's Medical Ventures (800-345-6443), or it may be easily made by a hospital pharmacy. Use this solution to coat the pacifier (recoat several times before and during the procedure).
7. After the procedure, apply petrolatum or A&D ointment on a 2 × 2 inch dressing before diapering infant to prevent the wound from adhering to the dressing or diaper.
8. Administer acetaminophen as ordered by the practitioner 4 hours after the initial dose; give additional doses as needed but not to exceed five doses in 24 hours or a maximum dose of 75 mg/kg/day.

##### Use of Dorsal Penile Nerve Block (DPNB) or Ring Block

1. One hour before the procedure, administer acetaminophen as ordered by the practitioner.
2. One hour before procedure, apply EMLA. For the DPNB, apply EMLA to the prepuce as described previously and at the penile base. For the ring block, apply EMLA to the prepuce as described previously and to the shaft of the penis. Use a topical anesthetic in conjunction with the DPNB or ring block to avoid the pain of injecting the anesthetic.
3. Use a 30-gauge needle to administer the lidocaine.§ For the DPNB, 0.4 ml of the lidocaine is infiltrated at the 10:30 and 1:30 o'clock positions in Buck fascia at the penile base. For the ring block, 0.4 ml of lidocaine is infiltrated subcutaneously on each side of the shaft of the penis below the prepuce.
4. For maximum anesthesia, wait 5 minutes after injection of lidocaine. An alternative anesthetic agent is chloroprocaine, which is as effective as lidocaine after 3 minutes.
5. Approximately 2 minutes before the circumcision, administer concentrated oral sucrose solution as described previously.
6. After the procedure, apply A&D ointment or petrolatum and administer acetaminophen as described previously.

#### Nonpharmacologic Interventions

In addition to the preceding pharmacologic interventions:

- If using a Circumstraint board, pad with blankets or other thick, soft material such as "lamb's wool." A more comfortable, padded, and physiologic restraint that places the infant semireclining can also decrease distress‖ (Stang, Snellman, Condon, and others, 1997).
- Provide the parents, caregiver, or another staff member with the option to hold the infant during the procedure or to be present during the circumcision.
- Swaddle the upper body and legs to provide warmth and containment and to reduce movement.
- If the patient is not swaddled and is unclothed, use a radiant warmer to prevent hypothermia. Shield infant's eyes from overhead lights.
- Prewarm any topical solutions to be used in sterile preparation of the surgical site by placing in a warm blanket or towel.
- Play infant relaxation music¶ before, during, and after procedure; allow parents or other caregiver the option of choosing the music.
- After the procedure, remove restraints and swaddle. Immediately have the parent, other caregiver, or nursing staff hold the infant. Continue to have the infant suck on pacifier, or offer feeding.

Data from Broadman LM, Hannallah RS, Belman AB, and others: Post-circumcision analgesia—A prospective evaluation of subcutaneous ring block of the penis, *Anesthesiology* 67(3):399-402, 1987; Howard CR, Howard FM, Weitzman ML: Acetaminophen analgesia in neonatal circumcision: The effect on pain, *Pediatrics* 93(4):641-646, 1994; Lander J, Brady-Fryer B, Metcalfe JB, and others: Comparison of ring block, dorsal penile nerve block, and topical anesthesia for neonatal circumcision: A randomized controlled trial, *JAMA* 278(24):2157-2162, 1997; Mintz MR, Grillo R: Dorsal penile nerve block for circumcision, *Clin Pediatr* 28(12):590-591, 1989; Serour F, Mandelberg A, Mori J: Slow injection of local anesthetic will decrease pain during dorsal penile nerve block, *Acta Anesthesiol Scand* 42(8):926-928, 1998; Spencer DM, Miller KA, O'Quinn M, and others: Dorsal penile nerve block in neonatal circumcision: Chloroprocaine versus lidocaine, *Am J Perinatol* 9(3):214-218, 1992; Stang H, Snellman LW, Condon LM, and others: Beyond dorsal penile nerve block: A more humane circumcision, *Pediatrics* 100(2):E3, 1997, available at *www.pediatrics.org/cgi/content/full/100/2/e3* (accessed November 25, 2009); Stevens B, Yamada J, Ohlsson A: Sucrose for analgesia in newborn infants undergoing painful procedures, *Cochrane Database Syst Rev* (3):CD001069, 2004; Taddio A, Stevens B, Craig K, and others: Efficacy and safety of lidocaine-prilocaine cream (EMLA) for pain during circumcision, *N Engl J Med* 336(17):1197-1201, 1997.
*There is sufficient evidence and support for use of a combination of pharmacologic and nonpharmacologic interventions to holistically manage neonatal circumcision pain. Combined analgesia, nonpharmacologic interventions (such as swaddling), and local anesthesia may be used during the procedure to provide holistic pain management (Taddio, Pollock, Gilbert-MacLeod, and others, 2000; Anand and International Evidence-Based Group for Neonatal Pain, 2001; Geyer, Ellsbury, Kleiber, and others, 2002; Razmus, Dalton, and Wilson, 2004).
†On March 11, 1999, the US Food and Drug Administration approved use of EMLA in infants age 37 weeks of gestation, provided practitioners followed recommendations regarding maximal dose and limits for exposure time to the medication. In addition, practitioners are advised not to use EMLA with infants who are receiving methemoglobinemia-inducing medications such as acetaminophen or phenobarbital. Although the package insert warns that patients taking acetaminophen are at greater risk for developing methemoglobinemia, there have been no reported cases of this complication in children taking acetaminophen and using EMLA.
‡LMX4 (previously Ela-Max) is a 4% lidocaine cream reported to be effective within 30 minutes of application for venipuncture. There is no need to apply an occlusive dressing over LMX4 cream as recommended for EMLA (Wong, 2003). Use of LMX4 for pain relief of pediatric meatotomy has been reported previously (Smith and Gjellum, 2004). Despite anecdotal reports of its use in neonatal circumcision, at this time no studies are available regarding the use or effectiveness of LMX4 for neonatal circumcision analgesia.
§In one study, the use of buffered lidocaine, which normally reduces stinging sensation of lidocaine, did not provide effective anesthesia for DPNB (Stang, Snellman, Condon, and others, 1997). The study on slow injection of the anesthetics lidocaine and bupivacaine compared 40 versus 80 seconds in patients ages 15 to 53 years (Serour, Mandelberg, and Mori, 1998).
‖For information on Stang Circ Chair, contact Pedicraft, 4134 Saint Augustine Rd, Jacksonville, FL 32207, 800-223-7649; e-mail: info@pedicraft.com; *www.pedicraft.com*
¶Suggested infant relaxation music: Heartbeat Lullabies by Terry Woodford. Available from Baby-Go-To-Sleep Center, Audio-Therapy Innovations, Inc., PO Box 550, Colorado Springs, CO 80901, 800-537-7748.

**3 - PAIN ASSESSMENT AND MANAGEMENT**

BOX 3-1 | Sedation Categories

**Minimal Sedation (Anxiolysis)**
Patient responds to verbal commands
Cognitive function may be impaired
Respiratory and cardiovascular systems unaffected

**Moderate Sedation (Previously Conscious Sedation)**
Patient responds to verbal commands but may not respond to light tactile stimulation
Cognitive function is impaired
Respiratory function adequate; cardiovascular unaffected

**Deep Sedation**
Patient cannot be easily aroused except with repeated or painful stimuli
Ability to maintain airway may be impaired
Spontaneous ventilation may be impaired; cardiovascular function is maintained

**General Anesthesia**
Loss of consciousness, patient cannot be aroused with painful stimuli
Airway cannot be maintained adequately, and ventilation is impaired
Cardiovascular function may be impaired

3 - PAIN ASSESSMENT AND MANAGEMENT

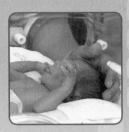

# Evidence-Based Pediatric Nursing Interventions

## ⊜volve WEBSITE

**Evidence-Based Practice**
- Assessing Correct Placement of Nasogastric or Orogastric Tubes in Children
- Intramuscular Injections in Infants, Todders, and Small Children
- Pediatric Pain and Symptom Management at the End of Life
- Reduction of Minor Procedural Pain in Infants

**Nursing Care Plans**
- The Child who is Terminally Ill or Dying
- The Child with Respiratory Failure

**Patient and Family Education— Spanish Translations**
- Giving Aerosolized Medications (Nebulizer Treatments) (Administración de Medicamentos por Aerosol [Tratamiento con Nebulizador])
- Giving Nasogastric Tube Feedings (Administrando Alimentación a Través del Tubo Nasogástrico)
- Giving Nose Drops (Administración de Gotas Nasales)
- Giving Intramuscular (IM) Injections (Administración de Inyecciones Intramusculares [IM])

- Giving Inhaled Medications (Administración de Medicamentos Inhalados)
- Insulin Administration (Administración de Insulina)
- Giving Ear Medications (Administración de Medicinas en el Oído)
- Giving Oral Medications (Administración de Medicamentos por Vía Oral)
- Oral Rehydration Guidelines (Parámetros de Rehidratación Oral)
- Giving Subcutaneous (Sub Q) Injections (Administración de Inyecciones Subcutáneas [Sub Q])

# Preparing Children for Procedures Based on Developmental Characteristics

## Infancy: Developing a Sense of Trust and Sensorimotor Thought
### Attachment to Parent
Involve parent in procedure if desired.*

Keep parent in infant's line of vision.

If parent is unable to be with infant, place familiar object or comfort/security item with infant (e.g., stuffed toy, pacifier, or blanket).*

### Stranger Anxiety
Have usual caregivers perform or assist with procedure.*

Make advances slowly and in nonthreatening manner.

Limit number of strangers entering room during procedure.*

### Sensorimotor Phase of Learning
Use sensory soothing measures during procedure (e.g., stroking skin, talking softly, giving pacifier).

Use analgesics (e.g., topical anesthetic, intravenous opioid) to control discomfort.*

Cuddle and hug infant after stressful procedure; encourage family to comfort infant.

### Increased Muscle Control
Expect older infants to resist.

Restrain adequately.

Keep harmful objects out of reach.

### Memory for Past Experiences
Realize that older infants may associate objects, places, or persons with prior painful experiences and will cry and resist at the sight of them.

Keep frightening objects out of view.*

Perform painful procedures in a separate room (not in crib or bed).*

Use nonintrusive procedures whenever possible (e.g., axillary temperature, oral medication).*

### Imitation of Gestures
Model desired behavior (e.g., opening mouth).

## Toddler: Developing a Sense of Autonomy and Sensorimotor to Preoperational Thought
Use same approaches as for infant in addition to the following.

### Egocentric Thought
Explain procedure in relation to what child will see, hear, taste, smell, and feel.

Emphasize those aspects of procedure that require cooperation (e.g., lying still).

Tell child it is acceptable to cry, yell, or use other means to express discomfort verbally.

Designate one healthcare person to speak during procedure. Hearing more than one can be confusing to child.*

*Applies to any age.

### Negative Behavior

Expect treatments to be resisted; child may try to run away.

Use firm, direct approach.

Ignore temper tantrums.

Use distraction techniques (e.g., singing a song with child).

Restrain adequately.

### Animism

Keep frightening objects out of view. (Young children believe objects have lifelike qualities and can harm them.)

### Limited Language Skills

Communicate using behaviors.

Use a few simple terms familiar to child.

Give one direction at a time (e.g., "Lie down," then "Hold my hand").

Use small replicas of equipment; allow child to handle equipment.

Use play; demonstrate on doll but avoid child's favorite doll, because child may think doll is really feeling the procedure.

Prepare parents separately to avoid child's misinterpreting words.

### Limited Concept of Time

Prepare child shortly or immediately before procedure.

Keep teaching sessions short (about 5 to 10 minutes).

Have preparations completed before involving child in procedure.

Have extra equipment nearby (e.g., alcohol swabs, new needle, adhesive bandages) to avoid delays.*

Tell child when procedure is completed.

### Striving for Independence

Allow choices when they exist but realize that child may still be resistant and negative.

Allow child to participate in care and to help whenever possible (e.g., drink medicine from a cup, hold a dressing).

Provide opportunities/choices for coping/distraction (e.g., bubbles, music, books) <u>before</u> procedure begins.*

## Preschooler: Developing a Sense of Initiative and Preoperational Thought
### Egocentric

Explain procedure in simple terms and in relation to how it affects child (as with toddler, stress sensory aspects).

Demonstrate use of equipment.

Allow child to play with miniature or actual equipment.

Encourage playing out experience on a doll both before and after procedure to clarify misconceptions.

Use neutral words to describe the procedure (Table 4-1).

### Increased Language Skills

Use verbal explanation, but avoid overestimating child's comprehension of words.

Encourage child to verbalize ideas and feelings.

Rephrase questions to make sure of what child is asking.

### Concept of Time and Frustration Tolerance Still Limited

Implement same approaches as for toddler, but may plan longer teaching session (10 to 15 minutes); may divide information into more than one session.

| TABLE 4-1 | Selecting Nonthreatening Words or Phrases |
|---|---|
| **Words and Phrases to Avoid** | **Suggested Substitutions** |
| Shot, bee sting, stick | Medicine under the skin |
| Organ | Special place in body |
| Test | See how [specify body part] is working |
| Incision, cut | Special opening |
| Edema | Puffiness, swelling |
| Stretcher, gurney | Rolling bed |
| Stool | Child's usual term |
| Dye | Special medicine |
| Pain | Hurt, discomfort, "owie," "boo-boo," sore, achy |
| Deaden | Numb, make sleepy |
| Fix | Make better |
| Take (as in "take your temperature or blood pressure") | See how warm you are; check your pressure; hug your arm |
| Put to sleep, anesthesia | Special sleep so you won't feel anything |
| Catheter | Tube |
| Monitor | TV screen |
| Electrodes | Stickers, ticklers |
| Burn | Warm |
| Dressings, dressing change | Bandages |

### *Illness and Hospitalization May Be Viewed as Punishment*

Clarify why each procedure is performed; a child will find it difficult to understand how medicine can taste bad and make him or her feel better at the same time.

Ask for child's thoughts regarding why a procedure is performed.

State directly that procedures are never a form of punishment.

### *Animism*

Keep equipment out of sight, except when shown to or used on child.

### *Fears of Bodily Harm, Intrusion, and Castration*

Point out on drawing, doll, or child where procedure will be performed.

Emphasize that no other body part will be involved.

Use nonintrusive procedures whenever possible (e.g., axillary temperatures, oral medication).

Apply an adhesive bandage over puncture site.

Encourage parental presence.

Realize that procedures involving genitalia produce anxiety.

Allow child to wear underpants with gown.

Explain unfamiliar situations, especially noises or lights.

### *Striving for Initiative*

Involve child in care whenever possible (e.g., to hold equipment, remove dressing).

Give choices when they exist, but avoid excessive delays.

Praise child for helping and for attempting to cooperate; never shame child for lack of cooperation.

## School-Age Child: Developing a Sense of Industry and Concrete Thought
### *Increased Language Skills; Interest in Acquiring Knowledge*

Explain procedures using correct scientific or medical terminology.

Explain reason for procedure using simple diagrams of anatomy and physiology.

Explain function and operation of equipment in concrete terms.

Allow child to manipulate equipment; use doll or another person as model to practice using equipment whenever possible (doll play may be considered childish by older school-age child).

Allow time before and after procedure for questions and discussion.

### *Improved Concept of Time*

Plan for longer teaching sessions (about 20 minutes).

Prepare before procedure.

### *Increased Self-Control*

Gain child's cooperation.

Tell child what is expected.

Suggest ways of maintaining control (e.g., deep breathing, relaxation, counting).

### *Striving for Industry*

Allow responsibility for simple tasks (e.g., collecting specimens).

Include in decision making (e.g., what time of day to perform procedure, the preferred site).

Encourage active participation (e.g., removing dressings, handling equipment, opening packages).

### *Developing Relationships with Peers*

May prepare two or more children for same procedure or encourage one peer to help prepare another.

Provide privacy from peers during procedure to maintain self-esteem.

## Adolescent: Developing a Sense of Identity and Abstract Thought
### *Increasingly Capable of Abstract Thought and Reasoning*

Supplement explanations with reasons why procedure is necessary or beneficial.

Explain long-term consequences of procedures.

Realize that adolescent may fear death, disability, or other potential risks.

Encourage questioning regarding fears, options, and alternatives.

### *Conscious of Appearance*

Provide privacy.

Discuss how procedure may affect appearance (e.g., scar) and what can be done to minimize it.

Emphasize any physical benefits of procedure.

### *Concerned More with Present Than with Future*

Realize that immediate effects of procedure are more significant than future benefits.

### *Striving for Independence*

Involve in decision making and planning (e.g., time and place; individuals present during procedure; clothing; whether they will watch procedure).

Impose as few restrictions as possible.

Suggest methods of maintaining control.

Accept regression to more childish methods of coping.

Realize that adolescent may have difficulty accepting new authority figures and may resist complying with procedures.

### *Developing Peer Relationships and Group Identity*

Same as for school-age child but assumes even greater significance.

Allow adolescents to talk with other adolescents who have had the same procedure.

# Preparing the Family

The process of patient education involves giving the family information about the child's condition, the regimen that must be followed and why, and other health teaching as indicated. The goal of this education is to enable the family to modify behaviors and adhere to the regimen that has been mutually established.

General principles of family education are as follows:

1. Establish a rapport with the family.
2. Avoid using *any* specialized terms or jargon. Clarify all terms with the family.
3. When possible, allow family members to decide how they want to be taught (e.g., all at once or over a day or two). This gives the family a chance to incorporate the information at a rate that is comfortable.
4. Provide accurate information to the family about the illness.
5. Assist family members in identifying obstacles to their ability to comply with the regimen and in identifying the means to overcome those obstacles. Then help family members find ways to incorporate the plan into their daily lives.

If equipment will be needed at home (e.g., suction machines, syringes), begin making the necessary arrangements in advance so that discharge can proceed smoothly. Whenever possible, make arrangements for the family to use the same equipment in the home that they are using in the hospital. This allows them to become familiar with the items. In addition, the staff can help troubleshoot the equipment in a controlled environment. Plan the teaching sessions well in advance of the time the family will be responsible for performing the care. The more complex the procedure, the more time is needed for training.

Review the instructions with family members. Encourage note taking if they desire. Allow ample practice time under supervision. At least one family member, but preferably two members, should demonstrate the procedure before they are expected to care for the child at home. Provide the family with the telephone numbers of resource individuals who are available to assist them in the event of a problem.

## GUIDELINES
### Family Preparation for Procedures

Family education for specific procedures are included throughout this unit. General concepts applicable to most family education sessions include the following:
1. Name of the procedure
2. Purpose of the procedure
3. Length of time anticipated to complete the procedure
4. Anticipated effects
5. Signs of adverse effects
6. Assess the family's level of understanding
7. Demonstrate and have family return demonstration (if appropriate)

# Skin Care and General Hygiene

## Skin Care

### General Guidelines

Keep skin free of excess moisture (e.g., urine or fecal incontinence, wound drainage, excessive perspiration).

Cleanse skin with gentle soap (e.g., Dove) or cleanser (e.g., Cetaphil). Rinse well with plain, warm water.

Provide daily cleansing of eyes, oral area, diaper or perineal area, and any areas of skin breakdown.

Apply non–alcohol-based moisturizing agents after cleansing to retain moisture and rehydrate skin.

Use minimum tape and adhesives. On very sensitive skin, use a protective, pectin-based or hydrocolloid skin barrier between skin and tape and adhesives.

Place pectin-based or hydrocolloid skin barriers directly over excoriated skin. Leave barrier undisturbed until it begins to peel off. With wet, oozing excoriations, place a small amount of stoma powder (as used in ostomy care) on site, remove excess powder, and apply skin barrier. Hold barrier in place for several minutes to allow barrier to soften and mold to skin surface. See Table 4-2 for common wound care products.

Alternate electrode and probe placement sites and thoroughly assess underlying skin, typically every 8 to 24 hours.

Eliminate pressure secondary to medical devices such as tracheostomy tubes, wheelchairs, braces, and gastrostomy tubes.

Be certain fingers or toes are visible whenever extremity is used for IV or arterial line.

Reduce friction by keeping skin dry (may apply absorbent powder such as cornstarch) and using soft, smooth bed linens and clothes.

Use a draw sheet to move a child in bed or onto a stretcher to reduce friction and shearing injuries; do not drag the child from under the arms.

Position in neutral alignment; pillows, cushions, or wedges may be needed to prevent hip abduction and pressure to bony prominences, such as heels, elbows, and sacral and occipital areas. When the child is positioned laterally, pillows/cushions between the knees, under the head, and under the upper arm will help promote neutral body alignment. Avoid donut cushions because they can cause tissue ischemia. Elevate the head of bed 30 degrees or less to reduce pressure, unless contraindicated

Do not massage reddened, bony prominences because this can cause deep tissue damage; provide pressure relief to these areas instead.

Routinely assess the child's nutritional status. A child who is on nothing by mouth (NPO) status for several days and who is receiving only IV fluids is nutritionally at risk. This can also affect the skin's ability to maintain its integrity. Hyperalimentation (TPN, TNA) should be considered for these children at risk.

# EVIDENCE-BASED PRACTICE

## Wound Care

Shannon Stone McCord

### Ask the Question
In children, what dressings are more effective in reducing healing time and pain?

### Search the Evidence
#### Search Strategies
Search selection criteria included English language publications and research-based articles on wound care in the neonatal and pediatric population.

#### Databases Used
National Guideline Clearinghouse (AHRQ), Cochrane Collaboration, PubMed, Medscape

### Critically Analyze the Evidence
**Grade criteria:** Evidence quality low; recommendation strong (Guyatt, Oxman, Vist, and others, 2008)

The studies that were consulted (Winter, 1963; Ovington, 2001; Mertz, Marshall, and Eaglstein, 1985; Berger and others, 2000; Valencia, 2001; Vermeulen, Ubbink, Goossens, and others, 2004; Dickson and Bodnaryk, 2006; Lund, Osborne, Kuller, and others, 2001; Nemeth, Eaglstein, Taylor, and others, 1991; Lawrence, Lilly, and Kidson, 1992) found that moist wound healing is two or three times faster than when wounds are left open to air. Moisture-retentive dressings such as transparent and hydrocolloid dressings accelerate wound healing, protect the wound, decrease bacterial wound contamination and infection, and reduce scarring. Comparatively, wet-to-dry dressings are associated with increases in labor costs, dressing change frequency, wound healing time, infection rates, pain, disruption of newly formed healthy tissue, and dispersal of bacteria on removal.

Dressing type and dressing change frequency should be based on the wound type and location, phase of wound healing, and amount of exudate. Many of the newer dressings allow for reduced dressing changes because they absorb more drainage and promote a moist wound healing environment. In addition, wound gels provide moisture to a wound bed while eliminating dead space. If a wound is infected or bacterial colonization is suspected, antibacterial ointments are indicated to reduce the bacterial bioburden and promote moist wound healing.

Packing wounds with absorptive materials reduces wound exudate and abscess development and prevents skin maceration. There is insufficient evidence to suggest whether one dressing or topical product is more effective at healing a wound than another. There is evidence to suggest that wet-to-dry gauze dressings are more painful to patients on removal (Vermeulen, Ubbink, Goossens, and others, 2004).

Premature and newborn infants are prone to epidermal stripping and skin tears secondary to an immature epidermal-dermal bond. Avoid tape when possible. Secure dressings with a stretchy overwrap, or use Montgomery straps. Frame wounds with a barrier dressing and adhere tape to the barrier. Apply non–alcohol-based skin preparation barriers under tape and dressings (AWHONN, 2007).

### Apply the Evidence: Nursing Implications
- Apply dressings that provide a moist wound environment.
- Pack wounds to eliminate dead space, absorb exudate, and prevent abscess formation.
- Dressing change frequency should be based on wound type and location, amount of pain and exudate, and the need for wound assessment. Most wounds require a daily dressing change.
- Protect the periwound skin with a barrier dressing or protective wipe to prevent epidermal injury.
- Avoid tape and secure dressings with stretchy wraps.

### References
Association of Women's Health, Obstetric and Neonatal Nurses: *Neonatal skin care 2nd edition evidence-based clinical practice guideline*, Washington, DC, 2007, The Association.

Berger RS, Pappert AS, Van Zile PS, and others: A newly formulated topical triple-antibiotic ointment minimizes scarring, *Cutis* 65(6):401-404, 2000.

Dickson D, Bodnaryk K: Neonatal intravenous extravasation injuries: Evaluation of a wound care protocol, *Neonatal Netw* 25(1):13-19, 2006.

Guyatt GH, Oxman AD, Vist GE, and others: GRADE: An emerging consensus on rating quality of evidence and strength of recommendations, *BMJ* 336(7650): 924-926, 2008.

Lawrence J, Lilly H, Kidson A: Wound dressings and airborne dispersal of bacteria, *Lancet* 339:807, 1992.

Lund C, Osborne J, Kuller J, and others: Neonatal skin care: Clinical outcomes of the AWHONN/NANN evidence-based clinical practice guideline, Association of Women's Health, Obstetric and Neonatal Nurses and the National Association of Neonatal Nurses, *J Obstet Gynecol Neonatal Nurs* 30(1):41-51, 2001.

Mertz PM, Marshall DA, Eaglstein WH: Occlusive wound dressings to prevent bacterial invasion and wound infection, *J Am Acad Dermatol* 12(4):662-668, 1985.

Nemeth A, Eaglstein W, Taylor J, and others: Faster healing and less pain in skin biopsy sites treated with an occlusive dressing, *Arch Dermatol* 127(11):1679-1683, 1991.

Ovington L: Hanging wet to dry dressings out to dry, *Home Healthc Nurse* 19(8):477-484, 2001.

Valencia I: New developments in wound care for infants and children, *Pediatr Ann* 30(4):211-218, 2001.

Vermeulen H, Ubbink D, Goossens A, and others: Dressings and topical agents for surgical wounds healing by secondary intention. In *Cochrane Database Syst Rev* 2004, Issue 1. Article No. CD003554. DOI: 10.1002/14651858. CD003554.pub2.

Winter G: Effect of air drying and dressings on the surface area of a wound, *Nature* 197:91-92, 1963.

4 – EVIDENCE-BASED PEDIATRIC NURSING INTERVENTIONS

| TABLE 4-2 | Wound Dressing Category Definitions and Examples of Products | |
|---|---|---|
| **Category** | **Description** | **Examples** |
| Gauze or sponge for external use | Nonresorbable | Pads |
| | Sterile or nonsterile | Island dressings |
| | Strip, piece, or pad | |
| | Woven or nonwoven mesh cotton cellulose | |
| | Simple chemical derivatives of cellulose | |
| | Intended for medical purposes | |
| Hydrophilic wound dressing | Sterile or nonsterile | Alginate dressings |
| | Nonresorbable | Foam dressings |
| | Material with hydrophilic properties | Hydropolymer dressings |
| | No added drugs or biologics | Sheet gel dressings |
| | Intended to cover wound and absorb exudate | Hydrocolloid dressings |
| | | Composite dressings |
| | | Hydrogel dressings |
| Occlusive wound dressing | Sterile or nonsterile | Transparent adhesive dressings |
| | Nonresorbable | Thin film dressings |
| | Synthetic polymeric material with or without adhesive backing | Foam dressings |
| | | Hydrocolloid dressings |
| | Intended to cover wound, provide or support moist wound environment, and allow exchange of gases | Composite dressings |
| | | Hydropolymer dressings |
| Hydrogel wound dressing | Sterile or nonsterile | Alginate dressings |
| | Nonresorbable | Hydropolymer dressings |
| | Matrix of hydrophilic polymers or other material combined with at least 50% water | Hydrogel dressings |
| | | Gauze dressings impregnated with hydrogel (without active ingredients) |
| | Intended to cover wound, absorb wound exudates, control bleeding or fluid loss, and protect against abrasion, friction, desiccation, contamination | |
| Porcine wound dressing | Made from pigskin | |
| | Temporary burn dressing | |

From van Rijswijk L: Recommendations to change the FDA classification of various wound dressings, *Ostomy Wound Manag* 45(3):31, 1999. Used with permission.

Identify children who are at risk for skin breakdown before it occurs. Employ measures such as *pressure-reducing devices* (reduce pressure more than would usually occur on a regular hospital bed or chair) or *pressure-relieving devices* (maintain pressure below that which would cause capillary closing) to prevent breakdown (Table 4-3).

## Adhesives

Decrease use as much as possible.

Use transparent adhesive dressings to secure IV lines, catheters, and central lines.

Consider use of hydrogel electrodes.

Consider pectin barriers (Hollihesive, DuoDerm) beneath adhesives to protect skin.

Secure pulse oximeter probe or electrodes with elasticized dressing material (carefully avoid restricting blood flow).

Do not use adhesive remover, solvents, and bonding agents. Adhesive removal can be facilitated using water, mineral oil, petrolatum, or alcohol-based foam hand cleanser.

Remove adhesives or skin barriers slowly, supporting the skin underneath with one hand and gently peeling away the product from the skin with the other hand. (CAUTION: Do not use scissors for tape or dressing removal because of hazard of cutting skin or amputating tiny digits.)

## Treating Skin Breakdown

Numerous studies have demonstrated that normal saline (NS) is the least damaging cleanser to cells, because it has a neutral pH. Other antiseptics such as povidone-iodine, hydrogen peroxide, Dakin's solution, and alcohol should not be used in open wounds, particularly at full strength, because they are toxic to white cells and fibroblasts and can impair wound healing. Study suggestions (Krasner, Rodeheaver, and Sibbald, 2001; Baranoski and Ayello, 2004; Lineweaver, Howard, Soucy, and others, 1985; Lund, Kuller, Lane, and others, 1999; Bryant, 2002; Bennett, Rosenblum, Perlov, and others, 2001; Fernandez, Griffiths, and Ussia, 2002; Moore and Cowman, 2005) also include the following:

*Text continued on p. 216.*

| TABLE 4-3 | Pressure Reduction and Relief Devices | | |
|---|---|---|---|
| **Description** | **Advantages** | **Disadvantages** | **Examples*** |
| **Overlay†** | | | |
| Foam: Varying density; 3- to 4-inch convoluted and nonconvoluted | Primarily pressure reduction, although in children may have pressure relief advantages; can be cut to fit cribs | Can be soiled by incontinent patient; inability to reduce skin moisture because of lack of airflow | Bio Clinic Brand BioGard (Sunrise Medical), Geo-Matt (Span America), Ultra Form Pediatric (American Health Systems, Inc.) |
| Gel or water filled: Pressure reduction; water or gel conforms to patient's contours | One-time charge; low cost for water; gels are expensive. Relieves pressure and shear; nonpowered, easy cleaning | Mattress is a dense collection of viscous fluid cells; there have been reports that the mattress is cold to the touch; patients may have to spare vital calories to warm the mattress. Heavy | Comfort Zone Gel Overlay (Tele-Made Disposables, Inc.), RIK Fluid Overlay (KCI) |
| Alternating-pressure mattress: An overlay with rows of air cells and pump; pump cycles air to provide inflation and deflation over pressure points | Intent is to relieve pressure points to create pressure gradients that enhance blood flow | Studies show inconsistent results; some have reported very low deflation interface pressures, but only the deflation pressures were used for analysis; tissue interface pressures during inflation are consistently higher and must be incorporated into the statistical analysis; clinical trials indicate higher pressure ulcer incidence rates when compared with other products | Aero Pulse (Medline), AlphaBed (Huntleigh Healthcare), Beta (Volkner Turning Systems), PressureGuard CFT (Span America) |
| Static air: Designed with interlocking air cells that provide dry flotation; inflated with a blower | Mattress overlays that are designed with multiple chambers, allowing air exchange between the compartments | Pressure reduction depends on adequate air volume and periodic reinflation | ROHO (The ROHO Group) Sof-Care (Gaymar) |
| Low–air-loss specialty overlay: Multiple airflow cushions that cover the entire bed; pressures can be set and controlled by a blower | Surface materials are constructed to reduce friction and shear and to eliminate moisture; pressure relief; can be used for prevention and/or treatment of ulcers | Surface mattress and pump are a rental item; not available for cribs | Acucair (Hill-Rom), BioTherapy (BioClinic), First Step Select (KCI), Plexus Aire Select (Gaymar), PressureGuard APM2 (Span America) |
| **Specialty Beds‡** | | | |
| Low–air-loss beds: Bed surface consists of inflated air cushions; each section is adjusted for optimum pressure relief for patient's body size; some models have built-in scales | Provides pressure relief in any position; treatment for stages III and IV pressure ulcers; available in pediatric crib sizes | Bed is more bulky than a hospital bed, and some homes may not be able to accommodate its size; reimbursement is questionable | Clinitron (Hill-Rom), KinAir IV (KCI), TheraPulse ATP (KCI), TotalCare SpO2RT (Hill-Rom) |
| Low–air-loss mattress replacements | Provides pressure relief in any position; fits on hospital frame | Requires mattress storage | First Step Select (KCI), Flexicair Eclipse (Hill-Rom) |
| Air-fluidized beds: Air is blown through beads to "float" patient | Provides pressure relief for oncology patients and for treatment of full-thickness pressure ulcers, postoperative flaps, burns; lighter-weight home care units available | Can be difficult to transfer patient | Clinitron (Hill-Rom), FluidAir Elite (KCI), Skytron (KEISEI Medical) |

*Continued*

| TABLE 4-3 | Pressure Reduction and Relief Devices—cont'd | | |
|---|---|---|---|
| **Description** | **Advantages** | **Disadvantages** | **Examples*** |
| Kinetic therapy: Therapy surfaces that provide continuous gentle side-to-side rotation of 40 degrees or more on each side; table-based or cushion-based | Has been demonstrated to improve mucous transport, redistribute pulmonary blood flow, and mobilize pulmonary interstitial fluid; has been used for trauma victims and unstable spinal cord injuries (should use table-based; once stabilized, may use cushion-based) | Used only in acute care settings | RotoProne (KCI), RotoRest Delta Kinetic (KCI), Synergy Air Elite (Hill-Rom), Triadyne (KCI) |
| Continuous lateral rotation beds (CLRT): Less than 40 degrees side-to-side rotation | Helps reposition unstable spinal cord injury patient; promotes comfort and shifts pressure points | | BariAir (KCI), TotalCare SpO2RT (Hill-Rom), V-Cue Dynamic Air Therapy System (Hill-Rom) |

Material revised by Kathy McLane MSN, RN, CPNP, CWON.

*This list is a representative sampling of products and is not intended to be all-inclusive. No endorsement of any product is intended. Within each category, products must be individually evaluated on their efficacy as comfort, pressure-reducing, or pressure-relieving devices. All products within a category do not necessarily perform equally.

†A device that is made to fit over a regular hospital mattress.

‡High-tech beds used in place of the standard hospital bed. These are normally used on a rental basis and are intended for short-term use. They usually provide pressure relief and eliminate shear, friction, and maceration.

- Cleanse all wounds with NS or a saline-based wound cleanser with surfactant.
- Cleansing with drinkable tap water may be as effective as cleansing with sterile water or sterile saline.
- For intact periwound skin, soap and water may be used.

Irrigate wound every 4 to 8 hours with warm normal saline (NS) using a 30-ml or larger syringe and 20-gauge catheter.

Culture wound and treat if signs of infection are present (excessive redness, swelling, pain on touch, heat, resistance to healing).

Use transparent adhesive dressing for uninfected wounds.

Use hydrocolloid for deep, uninfected wounds (leave in place for 5 to 7 days); warm barrier in hand for several minutes to soften before applying to skin.

Apply hydrogel with or without antibacterial or antifungal ointments (as ordered) for infected wounds (may need to moisten before removal).

Debride wounds of necrotic, devitalized tissue (exception: do not debride stable, dry eschar on feet and heels and on patients at risk for poor wound healing because of diabetes, immunocompromise, ischemia, poor circulation, or poor nutrition).

## Neonatal Guidelines*
### General Skin Care
**Assessment**

Assess skin every day or once per shift for redness, dryness, flaking, scaling, rashes, lesions, excoriation, or breakdown. Standardized scales, such as the Neonatal Skin Condition Score (NSCS) measure skin condition objectively, but may not be clinically relevant as they typically remain the same from day to day.

Evaluate and report abnormal skin findings, and analyze for possible causation.

Intervene according to interpretation of findings or as ordered.

### Bathing
**Initial Bath**

- Assess for stable temperature and vital signs; may take 2 to 4 hours.
- Use cleansing agents with neutral pH and minimal dyes or perfume, in water.
- Do not remove vernix; allow to wear off with normal care and handling.
- Bathe preterm infant <32 weeks in warm water alone.
- Wear gloves.

**Routine**

- Decrease frequency of baths to every second or third day by daily cleansing of eye, oral, and diaper areas and pressure points.
- Use cleanser or soaps no more than two or three times a week.
- Avoid rubbing skin during bathing or drying.
- Immerse stable infants fully except the head and neck to decrease evaporative heat loss.

*Modified from Association of Women's Health, Obstetric and Neonatal Nurses: *Neonatal skin care 2nd edition evidence-based clinical practice guideline,* Washington, DC, 2007, The Association.

## GUIDELINES

### Incontinence-Associated Diaper Dermatitis (IDD)

Imma Arbilo BSN, RN; Erika Guidry BSN, RN, WOCN; Robbie Norville MSN, RN, CPON; Barbara Richardson BSN, RN, CPN, WOCN; Jasmin Westcott BSN, RN, WOCN

**Definition:** Inflammation of the skin within the diaper area

### Etiology
- Contact irritants (enzyme activity of urine/stool, increased pH, medications)
- Friction
- Infection (bacterial, viral, fungal; primarily *Candida*)
- Underlying medical conditions (e.g., incontinence, gastroenteritis, neurogenic bladder/bowel, ileostomy/colostomy closure, short gut syndrome)

### Clinical Features
#### Signs and Symptoms
- Erythema in diaper area
- Pruritis
- Irritability

### Complications
- *Candida* infection (well-demarcated lesions; papule or pustule satellite lesions)
- Denuded skin

### IDD Grading
- Mild: slight erythema in diaper area; intact skin
- Moderate: shiny erythema in diaper area; patchy denuded areas
- Severe: severe erythema in diaper area; large denuded areas; macerated skin; bleeding; ulcerations

### Prevention
#### A—Air
- Schedule time for diaper area to air-dry (20 minutes 2 to 3 times a day).

#### B—Barrier
- Apply layer of skin barrier with every diaper change.
- Use petroleum jelly–based product or zinc oxide–based product or nonalcohol barrier film (e.g., Aloe Vesta Skin Protectant, Sensicare, Desitin, 3M No Sting Barrier).
- 3M No Sting Barrier must be allowed to dry before applying other barrier product; can be applied to skin only 1 to 2 times per day; not approved for infants younger than 30 days of age.

#### C—Cleanser
- Use pH balanced, no-rinse product (e.g., Aloe Vesta Cleansing Foam) or mild soap (unscented Dove, Cetaphil).
- Infants/young children: Use mild soap and water with disposable nonwoven washcloths or unscented, alcohol-free baby wipes or Aloe Vesta Cleansing Foam with disposable nonwoven washcloths.
- Older children: Use perineal wipes with dimethicone moisture barrier* (Shield Barrier Cloths) or Aloe Vesta cleansing foam with disposable nonwoven washcloths or mild soap and water with disposable nonwoven washcloths.

#### D—Diapers
- Use super absorptive diapers
- Change at least every 3 to 4 hours

#### E—Education
- Provide verbal and written family education.

### Management
#### A—Air
- Schedule time for diaper area to air-dry (20 minutes 2 to 3 times a day).

#### B—Barrier
- Mild:
  - Apply thick layer of skin barrier with every diaper change.
  - Use petroleum jelly–based product or zinc oxide–based product or nonalcohol barrier film (Aloe Vesta Skin Protectant, Sensicare, Desitin, 3M No Sting Barrier).
  - 3M No Sting Barrier must be allowed to dry before applying other barrier product; can be applied to skin only 1 to 2 times per day; not approved for infants younger than 30 days of age
  - If *Candida* present, apply nystatin ointment or Aloe Vesta with miconazole 2% directly to skin before applying barrier; medical order required.
- Moderate:
  - Apply thick layer of zinc oxide–based product (Sensicare) with every diaper change.
  - May seal ulcers with nonalcohol barrier film (3M No Sting Barrier); must be allowed to dry before applying other barrier product; can be applied to skin only 1 to 2 times per day; not approved for infants younger than 30 days of age.
  - If *Candida* present, apply nystatin ointment or Aloe Vesta with miconazole 2% directly to skin before applying barrier; medical order required.
- Severe:
  - Apply thick layer of zinc oxide–based product (e.g., Sensicare, Criticaid Paste, Ilex Skin Protectant Paste) with every diaper change; apply like "icing" and only remove soiled product to minimize mechanical trauma.
    Sensicare—Apply if not used in previous IDD grade.
    Criticaid—Apply ostomy powder, followed by Criticaid, followed by ostomy powder (ostomy powder holds paste to moist skin and prevents removal by diaper).
    Ilex—Apply directly to skin, followed by layer of petroleum jelly to prevent buttocks from sticking together.
  - May seal ulcers with nonalcohol barrier film (3M No Sting Barrier); must be allowed to dry before applying other barrier product; can be applied to skin only 1 to 2 times per day; not approved for infants younger than 30 days of age.
  - If *Candida* present, apply nystatin powder directly to skin before applying barrier; medical order required.

#### C—Cleanser
- Use pH balanced, no-rinse product (e.g., Aloe Vesta Cleansing Foam) or mild soap (e.g., unscented Dove, Cetaphil).
- Infants/Young Children: Use mild soap and water with disposable nonwoven washcloths or unscented, alcohol-free baby wipes or Aloe Vesta Cleansing Foam with disposable nonwoven washcloths.

*Continued*

4 - EVIDENCE-BASED PEDIATRIC NURSING INTERVENTIONS

## GUIDELINES

### Incontinence-Associated Diaper Dermatitis (IDD)—cont'd

- Older Children: Perineal wipes with dimethicone moisture barrier* (Shield Barrier Cloths) or Aloe Vesta cleansing foam with disposable nonwoven washcloths or mild soap and water with disposable nonwoven washcloths
- Once a day bathe child to soak off all product; may use mineral oil to help remove product.

#### D—Diapers
- Use super absorptive diapers.
- Change every 2 hours at a minimum.

#### E—Education
- Provide verbal and written family education.

### Bibliography

Adam R: Skin care of the diaper area, *Pediatr Dermatol* 25(4):427-433, 2008.

Atherton DJ: A review of the pathophysiology, prevention and treatment of irritant diaper dermatitis, *Curr Med Res Opin* 20(5): 645-649, 2004.

Atherton D, Mills K: What can be done to keep babies' skin healthy? *RCM Midwives* 7(7):288-290, 2004.

Boiko S: Treatment of diaper dermatitis, *Dermatol Clin* 17(1):235-240, 1999.

Campbell RL, Seymour JL, Stone LC, and others: Clinical studies with disposable diapers containing absorbent gelling materials: Evaluation of effects on infant skin condition, *J Amer Acad Dermatol* 17(6):978-987, 1987.

Davis JA, Leyden JJ, Grove GL, and others: Comparison of disposable diapers with fluff absorbent and fluff plus absorbent polymers: Effects of skin hydration, skin pH, and diaper dermatitis, *Pediatr Dermatol* 6(2): 102-108, 1989.

Gray M, Bliss DZ, Doughty DB, and others: Incontinence-associated dermatitis: A consensus. *J Wound Ostomy Continence Nurs* 34(1):45-54, 2007.

Gupta AK, Skinner AR: Management of diaper dermatitis, *Int J Dermatol* 43(11): 830-834, 2004.

Humphrey S, Bergman JN, Au S: Practical management strategies for diaper dermatitis. *Skin Therapy* Letter.com 11(7), September 2006, available at *http://www.skintherapyletter.com/download/stl_11_7.pdf* (accessed November 17, 2008).

Junkin J, Selekof JL: Prevalence of incontinence and associated skin injury in the acute care inpatient, *J Wound Ostomy Continence Nurs* 334(3):260-267, 2007.

Lund C, Kuller J, Lane A, and others: Neonatal skin care: The scientific basis for practice, *Neonatal Netw* 18(4):15-27, 1999.

McLane KM, Bookout K, McCord S, and others: The 2003 national pediatric pressure ulcer and skin breakdown prevalence survey, a multisite study, *J Wound Ostomy Continence Nurs* 31(4):168-178, 2004.

Nield LS, Kamat D: Prevention, diagnosis, and management of diaper dermatitis, *Clin Pediatr* 46(6):480-486, 2007.

Noonan C, Quigley S, Curley MAQ: Skin integrity in hospitalized infants and children, a prevalence survey. *J Pediatric Nurs* 21(6), 445-453. (2006).

Odio M, Streicher-Scott J, Hanson RC: Disposable baby wipes: Efficacy and skin mildness, *Dermatol Nurs* 13(2):107-121, 2001.

Ratliff C, Dixon M: Treatment of incontinence-associated dermatitis (diaper rash) in a neonatal unit, *J Wound Ostomy Continence Nurs* 34(2):158-162, 2007.

Scheinfeld N: Diaper dermatitis: A review and brief summary of eruptions of the diaper area, *American Journal of Clinical Dermatology* 6(5):273-281, 2005.

Wilson PA, Dallas MJ: Diaper performance: Maintenance of healthy skin, *Pediatr Dermatol* 7(3):179-184, 1990.

*Dimethicone moisture barrier (Shield Barrier Cloths) can be used for any age child; however, the product is five times more expensive than alcohol-free baby wipes.

---

- Immediately after bathing, dry the newborn and place in a diaper and cap and wrap in two warm blankets; after 10 minutes, dress the infant and apply dry cap and blankets.

### Emollients

- Apply petroleum-based ointment without preservative, perfume, or dye sparingly to body (avoid face, head) for dry, flaking or fissured areas every 12 hours or as needed.
- Emollients may be used for infants on warmers or receiving phototherapy.

### Disinfectants

All disinfectants have the potential to cause irritation or burns in newborns and should be *removed with water or saline after an invasive procedure is performed.*

- For infants less than 34 weeks gestation, use 2% aqueous chlorhexidine gluconate (CHG) or povidone-iodine. CHG with alcohol is approved for use in infants older than age 2 months, and use in neonates is considered off-label use. Avoid use of alcohol as the primary disinfectant or to remove other disinfectants.
- Apply CHG for 30 seconds or with two applications. Aqueous CHG will not dry and can be removed with sterile gauze. Apply povidone-iodine with two applications and allow to dry.

### Transepidermal Water Loss

Minimize transepidermal water loss (TEWL) and heat loss in small premature infants younger than 30 weeks by:
- Using humidified incubators (70% to 90% first 7 days, then 50% until 28 days of life).
- Applying transparent dressings to chest, abdomen, and back.
- Using heated water pads or mattresses.

### Skin Breakdown Prevention

Decrease pressure from externally applied forces using water, air, or gel mattresses, sheepskin, or cotton bedding.

Provide adequate nutrition, including protein, fat, and trace minerals such as zinc.

Apply transparent adhesive dressings to protect elbows and knees from friction injury.

Use tracheostomy and gastrostomy dressings for drainage and relief of pressure from tracheostomy or gastrostomy tube (Hydrasorb or Lyofoam).

Use emollient in the diaper area (groin, thighs) of very low–birth-weight infants to reduce urine irritation.

### *Other Skin Care Concerns*
#### Use of Substances on Skin

Evaluate all substances that come in contact with infant's skin.

Before using any topical agent, analyze components of preparation and:

- Use sparingly and only when necessary.
- Confine use to smallest possible area.
- Whenever possible and appropriate, wash off with water.
- Monitor infant carefully for signs of toxicity and systemic effects.

### Use of Thermal Devices

Avoid heat lamps because of increased potential for burns. If needed, measure actual temperature of exposed skin every 15 minutes.

When using heating pads:

- Change infant's position every 15 minutes initially, then every 1 to 2 hours.

- Preset temperature of heating pads to <40° C (<104° F).

When using preheated transcutaneous electrodes:

- Avoid use on infants <1000 g.
- Set at lowest possible temperature (<44° C [<111.2° F]), and secure with plastic wrap.
- Use pulse oximetry rather than transcutaneous monitoring whenever possible.

When prewarming heels before phlebotomy, avoid temperatures >40° C (>104° F).

Warm ambient humidity, direct away from infant; use aerosolized sterile water, and maintain ambient temperature so as not to exceed 40° C.

## Bathing

Never leave infant or small child unattended in a bathtub.

Hold infant who is unable to sit alone.

Support infant's head securely with one hand or grasp the infant's farther arm firmly and rest the head comfortably on your wrist.

Closely supervise the infant or child who is able to sit without assistance.

Place a pad in the bottom of the tub to prevent slipping and loss of balance.

Offer older children the option of a shower, if available.

Use judgment regarding the amount of supervision older children require.

Children with mental and/or physical limitations such as severe anemia or leg deformities and suicidal or psychotic children (who may commit bodily harm) require close supervision.

Clean the ears, between skinfolds, the neck, the back, and the genital area carefully.

Retract the foreskin of uncircumcised boys gently once it is mobile (usually older than age 3 years), clean the exposed surfaces, and replace the foreskin. Never forcefully retract the foreskin.

Provide more extensive assistance with bathing and other aspects of hygienic care to children who are debilitated: Encourage them to perform as much as they are capable of without overtaxing their energies.

Expect increasing involvement with improved strength and endurance.

## Hair Care

Brush and comb hair, or help children with hair care at least once daily.

For African-American children with curly hair, use a comb with widely spaced teeth. Comb, braid, plait, or weave loosely after shampooing when hair is wet. Use special hair dressing or pomade by rubbing on the hands and transferring to hair; consult parents regarding the usual preparation. Petroleum jelly should not be used.

Style hair for comfort and in a manner pleasing to the child and parents.

Do not cut hair without parental permission, although clipping hair to provide access to scalp vein for needle insertion is permissible.

Shampoo hair in the tub or shower, or transport the child by stretcher to an accessible sink or washbasin. If the child is unable to be transported, shampoo in the bed with adequate protection and/or with specially adapted equipment or positioning.

Wash hair of the newborn every 2 to 3 days as part of the bath.

Wash hair and scalp as needed in later infancy and childhood.

Teenagers may need more frequent hair care and shampoos.

Use commercial dry shampoo products on a short-term basis.

## Skin Closure (Suture or Staple) Removal Procedure

Determine that sutures have been in place an adequate length of time. This length of time varies depending on area of the body sutured. Some guidelines are 3 days for the eyelids; 3 to 4 days for the neck; 5 days for the face and scalp; 7 days for the trunk and upper extremities; and 8 to 10 days for the lower extremities.

Position patient to allow access to stitches without putting undue tension on incision.

Assess wound for any signs of infection (redness, swelling, heat, drainage) or of wound not healing (dehiscence).

Clean wound with NS or antiseptic. Hydrogen peroxide may be used to remove any scabs over stitches.

Remove stitches (technique varies based on type of stitch).

## Simple Interrupted Sutures

Simple interrupted sutures are the most widely used type of stitch; each stitch is placed and tied individually.

Use forceps to firmly grasp knot and pull taught to expose underside of knot. Insert scissors underneath stitch to side of knot. Clip stitch with scissors while continuing to pull on knot with forceps. Gently pull knot with forceps to remove stitch completely. To minimize infection, cut stitch as close to skin as possible so that external parts of stitch do not pass through wound. Repeat process for additional sutures.

## Simple Continuous Sutures

Simple continuous sutures consist of a series of stitches; only the first and last stitches are tied.

Use forceps to firmly grasp knot and pull taught to expose underside of knot. Insert scissors underneath stitch to side of knot. Clip stitch with scissors. To minimize infection, stitch should be cut as close to skin as possible so that external parts of stitch do not pass through wound. Move down to the next suture in line, keeping on the same side of wound. Clip this stitch with scissors. Gently pull stitch with forceps to remove. Continue this process of cutting and removing stitches, working down the same side of wound.

## Staples

Insert lower jaw of staple extractor underneath first staple. Push jaws of staple remover together. Once jaws are firmly closed, pull extractor toward you to remove staple. Continue this process, removing every other staple, and then remove the remainder.

Assess for possible complications. If incision begins to separate, leave remainder of stitches in place and use skin closure strips (Steri-Strips) to secure opening area of wound. Notify physician.

Use dressing as needed if wound is draining.

# Procedures Related to Maintaining Safety

Ensure that environmental safety measures are in operation, such as the following:

- Good illumination
- Floors clear of fluid or objects that might contribute to falls
- Nonskid surfaces in showers and tubs
- Furniture that is scaled to the child's proportions and sturdy and well balanced to prevent tipping over
- Beds of ambulatory patients locked in place and at a height that allows easy access to the floor
- Electrical equipment maintained in good working order, used only by personnel familiar with its use, and not in contact with moisture or near tubs
- Electrical outlets covered to prevent burns
- A well-organized fire plan known to all staff members
- All windows secure
- Blind and curtain cords out of reach with split cords to prevent strangulation
- Proper care and disposal of small objects, such as syringes, caps, needle covers, and temperature probes

Be sure child is wearing a proper identification band.

Check bath water carefully before placing child in the bath.

Securely strap infants and small children into infant seats, feeding chairs, and strollers.

Do not leave infants, young children, and children who are agitated or cognitively impaired unattended on treatment tables, on scales, or in treatment areas.

Keep portholes in incubators securely fastened when not attending the infant.

Do not use baby walkers; they provide access to hazards or may tip over, causing injury.

Keep crib sides up and fastened securely. Use cribs that meet federal safety standards (*www.cpsc.gov/info/cribs/index.html.*)

- Leave crib sides up regardless of child's ability to get out, and even when the crib is unoccupied, to remove the temptation for the child to climb in.
- Never turn away from an infant or small child in a crib that has the sides down without maintaining contact with the child's back or abdomen to prevent rolling, crawling, or jumping from the open crib.

Place the child who may climb over the side of the crib in a specially constructed crib with a cover or one that has a safety net placed over the top.

- Tie net to the frame in such a manner that there is ready access to the child in case of emergency.
- Never tie nets to the movable crib sides or use knots that do not permit quick release.

Do not tie balloons or other objects with long ties or strings to cribs because they can pose an entanglement hazard.

Do not tie pacifiers around the infant's neck or attach them to the infant with a string.

Do not place cribs within reach of heating units, appliances, dangling cords, outlets, or other objects that can be reached by curious hands.

Pillows should not be placed in cribs with children chronologically or developmentally less than age

12 months except to therapeutically position a patient per medical orders.

Assess the safety of toys brought to the hospital for children, and determine whether they are appropriate to the child's age and condition. Electrical or friction toys should not be allowed for children receiving oxygen therapy since sparks can cause oxygen to ignite.

Inspect toys to make certain they are allergy-free, washable, and unbreakable and that they have no small removable parts that can be aspirated or swallowed.

All objects within reach of children younger than age 3 years should pass the choke tube test. A toilet paper roll is a handy guide. If a toy or object fits into the cylinder (items less than $1\frac{1}{4}$ inches across or balls smaller than $1\frac{3}{4}$ inches), it is a potential choking danger to the child.

Latex balloons pose a choking hazard to children of all ages; if a balloon breaks, latex can be aspirated or swallowed, resulting in choking.

Set limits for the child's safety.

Make sure children understand where they are permitted to go and what they are permitted to do in the hospital.

Prevent child's access to tubs, laundry bags or chutes, elevators, medication rooms, and medication and cleaning carts.

Enforce the limitations consistently, and repeat them as frequently as necessary to make certain that they are understood.

## Transporting

Carry infants and small children for short distances within the unit:

- In the horizontal position, hold or carry small infants with the back supported and the thighs grasped firmly by the carrying arm (Figure 4-1, A).
- In the football hold, support the infant on the nurse's arm with the head supported by the hand and the body held securely between the body and elbow (Figure 4-1, B).
- In the upright position, hold the infant with the buttocks on the nurse's forearm and the front of the body resting against the chest. Support the infant's head and shoulders with the other arm to allow for any sudden movement by the infant (Figure 4-1, C).

For more extended trips, use a suitable conveyance:

- Determine the method of transporting children by considering their age, condition, and destination.
- Use appropriate safety belts and/or raised sides to secure the child.
- Transport infants in their incubators, cribs, strollers, or in wagons with raised sides.

Use wheelchairs or stretchers with side rails for older children.

Ambulation may be appropriate for children who are not on cardiac or pulse oximetry monitors.

Critically ill children should always be transported on a stretcher or bed by at least two staff members with monitoring continuing during transport. A blood pressure monitor (or standard blood pressure cuff), pulse oximeter, cardiac monitor/defibrillator, airway equipment, and emergency medications should accompany the patient.

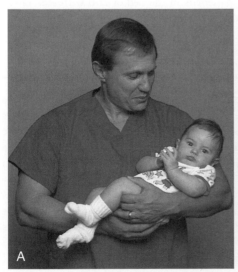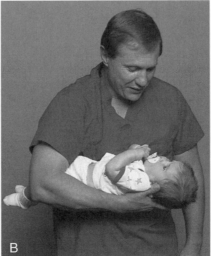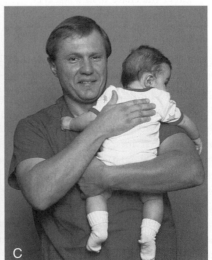

FIGURE **4-1**    Transporting infants. A, Infant's thigh firmly grasped in nurse's hand. B, Football hold. C, Back supported.

4 - EVIDENCE-BASED PEDIATRIC NURSING INTERVENTIONS

## Preventing Falls

Multiple interventions are needed to minimize pediatric patients' risk of falling. Once individual children are identified as at risk for falling, visual identification and communication of the risk among all health care providers is essential. Reduce the risk of falling through patient, family, and staff education.

Identify children at risk for falling. Perform a fall risk assessment on patients on admission and throughout hospitalization to identify patients at high risk for falls. Risk factors for hospitalized children include the following:

- Medication effects: postanesthesia or sedation; analgesics or narcotics, especially in those who have never had narcotics in the past and in whom effects are unknown
- Altered mental status: secondary to seizures, brain tumors, or medications
- Altered or limited mobility: reduced skill at ambulation secondary to developmental abilities, disease process, tubes, drains, casts, splints, or other appliances; new to ambulating with assistive devices such as walkers or crutches
- Postoperative children: risk of hypotension or syncope secondary to large blood loss, a heart condition, or extended bed rest
- History of falls
- Infants or toddlers in cribs with side rails down or on the daybed with family members

Visually identify patients at risk with one or more of the following:

- Post signs on the door and at the bedside.
- Apply a special armband labeled "Fall Precautions."
- Label the chart with a sticker.
- Document information on the chart.

Alter the environment:

- Keep bed in lowest position, breaks locked, and side rails up.
- Place call bell within reach.
- Ensure that all necessary and desired items are within reach (e.g., water, glasses, tissues, snacks).
- Offer toileting on a regular basis, especially if patient is on diuretics or laxatives.
- Keep lights on at all times, including dim lights while sleeping.
- Lock wheelchairs before transferring patients.
- Ensure that patient has appropriate size gown and nonskid footwear. Do not allow gowns or ties to drag on the floor when ambulating.
- Keep floor clean and free of clutter. Post "wet floor" sign if floor was recently mopped or is wet.
- Ensure that patient has glasses on if he or she normally wears them.

Educate patients and family members:

- Patients (as age appropriate):
  - Assist with ambulation even though the child may have ambulated well before hospitalization.
  - Patients who have been lying in bed will need to get up slowly, sitting on the side of the bed before standing.
- Family members:
  - Call the nursing staff for assistance, and do not allow patients to get up independently.
  - Keep the side rails of the crib or bed up whenever patient is in the crib or bed.
  - Do not to leave infants on the daybed; put them in the crib with the side rails up.
  - When all family members need to leave the bedside, notify the nursing staff before leaving and ensure that the patient is in the bed or crib with side rails up and call bell within reach (if appropriate).

## Restraining Methods and Therapeutic Holding

The Joint Commission (2001) defines restraint as "any method, physical or mechanical, which restricts a person's movement, physical activity, or normal access to his or her body." Before initiating restraints, the nurse completes a comprehensive assessment of the patient to determine whether the need for a restraint outweighs the risk of not using one. Restraints can result in loss of dignity, violation of patient rights, psychological harm, physical harm, and even death.

Alternative methods should first be considered and documented in the patient's record. Some examples of alternative measures include bringing a child to the nurses' station for continuous observation, providing diversional activities such as music, encouraging the participation of the parents, or therapeutic holding. Therapeutic holding is the use of a secure, comfortable, temporary holding position that provides close physical contact with the parent or caregiver for 30 minutes or less. The use of restraints can often be avoided with adequate preparation of the child; parental or staff supervision of the child; or adequate protection of a vulnerable site, such as an infusion device. The nurse needs to assess the child's development, mental status, potential to hurt others or self, and safety. The nurse is responsible for selecting the least restrictive type of restraint (Figure 4-2). Using less restrictive restraints is often possible by gaining the cooperation of the child and parents. Examples of less restrictive restraints are in Table 4-4.

The two types of restraints used with children are classified as medical-surgical and behavioral restraints. When a standard or protocol states that immobilization is required 100% of the time as a part of the procedure or postprocedural care process, the restraint device is considered a part of routine care. For example, the postoperative use of elbow restraints after a cleft lip repair, if written in the protocol or standard of care and used in 100% of patients, would not fall under the Joint Commission or Centers for Medicare and Medicaid Services mandates for restraints.

Medical-surgical restraints are used for children with an artificial airway or airway adjunct for delivery of oxygen, indwelling catheters, tubes, drains, lines, pacemaker wires, or suture sites. The medical-surgical restraint is used to ensure that safe care is given to the patient. The potential risks of the restraint are offset by the potential benefit of providing safer care. Criteria have been developed that outline when medical-surgical restraints may be instituted. These situations include the following:

- Risk for interruption of therapy used to maintain oxygenation or airway patency
- Risk of harm if indwelling catheter, tube, drain, line, pacemaker wire, or sutures are removed, dislodged, or ruptured
- Patient confusion, agitation, unconsciousness, or developmental inability to understand direct requests or instructions

Medical-surgical restraints can be initiated by an individual order or by protocol; the use of the protocol must be authorized by an individual order. Continued use of restraints must be renewed each day. Patients are monitored at least every 2 hours.

Behavioral restraints are limited to situations with a significant risk of patients physically harming themselves or others because of behavioral reasons and when nonphysical interventions are not effective. Before initiating a behavioral restraint, the nurse should assess the patient's mental, behavioral, and physical status to determine the cause for the child's behavior that may be harmful to the patient or others. If behavioral restraints are indicated, a collaborative approach involving the patient, if appropriate, the family, and the health care team should be used. An order must be obtained as soon as possible, but no longer than 1 hour after the initiation of behavioral restraints. Behavioral restraints for children must be reordered every 1 to 2 hours, based on age. A Licensed Independent Practitioner (LIP) must conduct an in-person evaluation within 1 hour and again every 4 hours until restraints are discontinued. Children in behavioral restraints must be *continuously* observed and assessed every 15 minutes. Assessment components include signs of injury associated with applying restraint, nutrition/hydration, circulation and

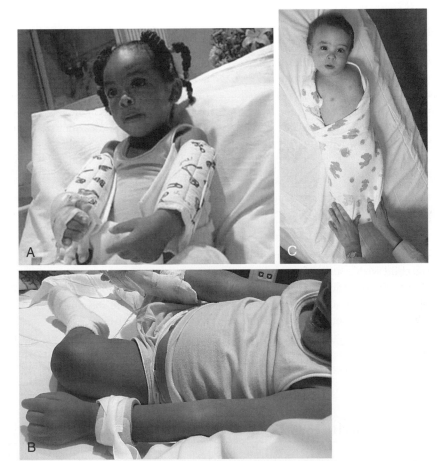

FIGURE **4-2** Restraint examples from least restrictive to most restrictive. A, Elbow restraints. B, Wrist restraints. C, Mummy restraint.

**TABLE 4-4 Restraining Children: Less Restrictive to More Restrictive Techniques**

| Technique or Device | Less Restrictive to More Restrictive | | | | | | |
|---|---|---|---|---|---|---|---|
| **Extremities** | | | | | | | |
| Sleeves | | X | | | | | |
| Hand mitts/mittens | | X | | | | | |
| Stockinette | | | X | | | | |
| Elbows (no-no's) | | | | X | | | |
| Arm board | | | | | X | | |
| 1-2 Limbs | | | | | | X | |
| 3-4 Limbs | | | | | | | X |
| **Chest/Body** | | | | | | | |
| Belts/safety belts | X | | | | | | |
| Posey vest/safety jacket | | | | X | | | |
| Mummy restraint | | | | | | | X |
| Papoose board | | | | | | | X |
| **Environment** | | | | | | | |
| Side rails | | | X | | | | |
| Crib tops | | | X | | | | |
| Seclusion | | | | | | | X |
| **Other** | | | | | | | |
| Chemical | | | | | | X | |

Adapted from Selekman J, Snyder B: Uses of and alternatives to restraints in pediatric settings, *AACN Clin Issues* 7(4):603-610, 1996.



range-of-motion of extremities, vital signs, hygiene and elimination, physical and psychological status and comfort, and readiness for discontinuation of restraint. Use clinical judgment in setting a schedule of when each of these parameters needs to be evaluated because every parameter must be assessed during each 15-minute physical assessment.

Restraints with ties must be secured to the bed or crib frame, not the siderails. Suggestions for increasing safety and comfort while the child is in a restraint include leaving one finger breadth between skin and the device; tying knots that allow for quick release; ensuring the restraint does not tighten as the child moves; decreasing wrinkles or bulges in the restraint; placing jacket restraints over an article of clothing; placing limb restraints below waist level, below knee level, or distal to the IV; and tucking in dangling straps (Selekman and Snyder, 1997).

# Positioning for Procedures

Placing a child in a comfort or nonthreatening position (with a trusted adult) provides the child with a sense of control and minimizes anxiety. Comfort positioning encourages opportunities for the child to cope more effectively and promotes cooperation and success with procedures. Concepts of positioning include the following:

- Ensure patient and staff safety.
- Provide a secure, comforting, hugging hold with firm control of limb or access area.
- Facilitate close physical contact with parent or caregiver.
- Allow the child to have a sense of control, as appropriate to the situation; sitting upright enhances sense of control.
- Offer the child choices, such as type of distraction to use (e.g., book, counting, or singing).
- Family members should provide positive support, not negative restraint.

## Extremity Venipuncture or Injection

Place child on parent's (or assistant's) lap, with the child facing toward the parent and in the straddle position (Figure 4-3, A).

For venipuncture, place child's arm on a firm surface such as the treatment table (for support) and on top of a soft cloth or towel.

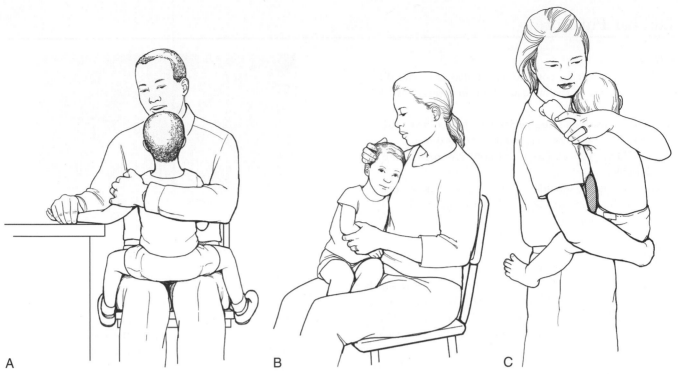

FIGURE **4-3**    Procedural positioning. A, Chest-to-chest straddle position. B, Side-sitting position with head and legs secured. C, Chest-to-chest straddle standing position.

Have assistant or parent immobilize child's arm for venipuncture.

Have parent hug the child around the back to hold the child's free arm.

Place child on parent's (or assistant's) lap, with the child facing away from the parent.

To hold the child's legs still, place them between the parent's legs. This position is appropriate for an injection into the thigh; or, for an injection into the arm, place child in parent's (or assistant's) lap, with the child facing sideward (Figure 4-3, B).

Place the child's arm closest to the parent under the parent's arm, and wrap toward the back.

Have the parent hold the arm receiving the injection against the child's body.

### ATRAUMATIC CARE
#### Analgesia and Sedation

For painful procedures, the child should receive adequate analgesia or sedation to minimize pain and the need for excessive restraint. For local anesthesia, use buffered lidocaine to reduce stinging sensation, or apply LMX or EMLA. (See Evidence-Based Practice boxes.)

Some painful procedures, such as bone marrow tests, can be performed without restraint using general anesthesia with proper anesthesia monitoring availability (e.g., propofol [Diprivan]).

## Femoral Venipuncture

Place infant supine with legs in frog position to provide extensive exposure of the groin.

Restrain legs in frog position with hands while controlling the child's arm and body movements with downward and inward pressure of forearms.

Cover genitalia to protect the operator and the venipuncture site from contamination if the child urinates during the procedure.

Site is not advisable for long-term venous access in mobile child because of risk of infection and trauma to flexion area.

## Subdural Puncture (Through Fontanel or Bur Holes)

Place active infant in mummy restraint.
Position supine with head accessible to examiner.

Control head movement with firm hold on each side of the head.

# Lumbar Puncture

## Infant

Place infant in sitting position with buttocks extended over the edge of the table and head in neutral position (Figure 4-4).

In neonates, use side-lying position with modified head extension to decrease respiratory distress during procedure. Pulse oximetry and heart rate monitoring are advisable.

Hold infant at the shoulders (not the head or neck), and immobilize arms and legs with nurse's hands.

Observe infant for difficulty in breathing.

## Child

A flexed sitting or side-lying position may be used, depending on the child's ability to cooperate and whether sedation will be used. In the sitting position with the hips flexed, the interspinous space is maximized (Abo, Chen, Johnston, and others, 2010). Neck flexion is not necessary.

For sedated children and those who are unable to safely sit throughout the procedure, place child on side with back close to or extended over the edge of examining table, head flexed, and knees drawn up toward the chest.

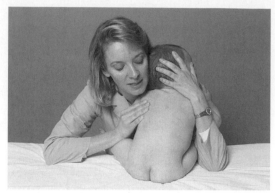

FIGURE **4-4**    Infant sitting position allows flexion of lumbar spine.

Reach over the top of the child, and place one arm behind child's neck and the other behind the knees.

Stabilize this position by clasping own hands in front of the child's abdomen.

Take care that excessive pressure does not compromise circulation or breathing and that the nose and mouth are not covered by the restrainer's body.

# Bone Marrow Aspiration or Biopsy

The position for a bone marrow aspiration or biopsy depends on the chosen site. In children, the posterior or anterior iliac crest is most frequently used, although in infants the tibia may be selected because of easy access to the site and holding of the child.

If the posterior iliac crest is used, position the child prone. Sometimes a small pillow or folded blanket is placed under the hips to facilitate obtaining the bone marrow specimen. Children should receive adequate analgesia or anesthesia to relieve pain. If the child may awaken, holding may be needed and is best done with two people—one person to immobilize the upper body and a second person to immobilize the lower extremities.

# Nose and/or Throat Access

Position child supine with face accessible to examiner.

Control head and arms by holding child's extended arms over and close to the head, thus immobilizing both head and arms.

# Ear Access

Place child in parent's (or assistant's) lap with the child's body sideways and the ear to be examined away from the parent (see Figure 4-3, B). Place the child's arm closest to the parent under the parent's arm, and wrap it toward the back.

Have the parent hold the other arm against the child's body and use the free arm to hold the head against the parent's chest.

To hold the child's legs still, place them between the parent's legs.

This can also be performed with the parent standing (Figure 4-3, C).

# Collection of Specimens

## Fundamental Procedure Steps Common to all Procedures

The following steps are very important for every procedure and should be considered fundamental aspects of care. These steps, while important, are not listed in each of the specimen collection procedures.

1. Assemble necessary equipment.
2. Identify the child using two patient identifiers (e.g., patient name and medical record or birth date; neither can be a room number). Compare the same two identifiers to the specimen container and order.
3. Perform hand hygiene, maintain aseptic technique, and follow Standard Precautions.
4. Explain procedure to parents and child according to the developmental level of the child; reassure child that the procedure is not punishment.
5. Provide atraumatic care, and position the child securely.
6. Prepare area with antiseptic agent.
7. Place specimens in appropriate containers, and apply a patient identification label to the specimen container in the presence of the child and family.
8. Discard puncture device in puncture-resistant container near site of use.
9. Wash procedural preparation agent off if povidone-iodine is used, if skin is sensitive, and for infants.
10. Remove gloves, and perform hand hygiene after the procedure. Have children wash their hands if they have helped.
11. Praise the child for helping.
12. Document pertinent aspects of the procedure, such as number of attempts, site and amount of blood/urine withdrawn, as well as type of test performed.

## Urine

See Safety Alert.

### Non–Toilet-Trained Child
#### *Materials Needed to Use a Urine Collection Bag*
Urine specimen cup
Urine collection bag
Soap and water
Washcloths or diaper/perineal wipes
Clean diaper

#### *Instructions*
If the child is very active, you will need help to put on the urine bag.

1. Place the child supine.
2. Remove the child's diaper.
3. Clean the child's genital area with soap and water or a diaper/perineal wipe. For girls, spread the child's labia with your fingers and wash from front to back (Figure 4-5). For boys, wash the tip of the penis; if uncircumcised, pull back the foreskin only as far as it will easily go, cleanse, and push foreskin back toward the tip after cleansing.
4. Have your helper hold the child's legs apart while you apply the bag.
5. Hold the urine collector with the bag portion downward.
6. Remove the bottom half of the adhesive protector.
7. For girls, spread the labia and buttocks, keeping the skin tight (Figure 4-6). For boys, place the boy's penis and scrotum into the bag if possible (Figure

!  **SAFETY ALERT**
The American Academy of Pediatrics recommends that urine collected by the bag can be used to determine whether it is necessary to obtain a catheterized urine specimen for culture. For best results, the perineal area should be washed thoroughly before applying the urine collection bag, with prompt removal of the bag as soon as voiding occurs. Leaving the device in situ for more than 1 hour is more likely to yield a contaminated urine specimen.

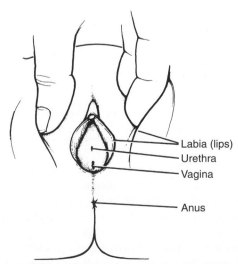

FIGURE **4-5**   Finger position to spread labia for cleaning before obtaining a urine sample.

4 - EVIDENCE-BASED PEDIATRIC NURSING INTERVENTIONS

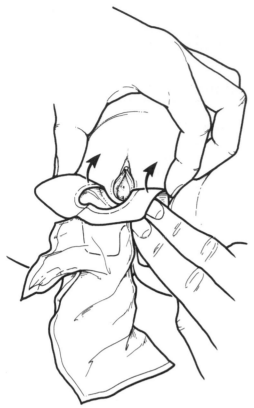

FIGURE **4-6**   Putting the urine bag on a girl, starting from back and proceeding to front.

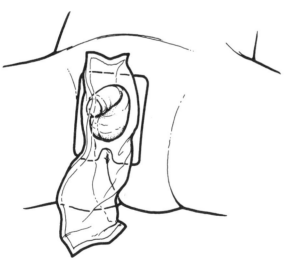

FIGURE **4-7**   Putting the urine bag on a boy, with the penis and scrotum inside the bag.

4-7). If only the penis fits in the bag, put the sticky part of the bag on the scrotum.

8. Begin with the bottom of the adhesive. Place the sticky portion of the bag as flat as possible against the skin.

9. Smooth the plastic to avoid any wrinkles.

10. Remove the top half of the adhesive protector, and smooth it also on the skin, taking care to avoid making any wrinkles.

11. Cut a small slit in the diaper, and pull the bag through to allow room for urine to collect and to facilitate checking the contents. Check the bag often, and remove it as soon as the child urinates.

12. To remove the bag, hold it against the child's skin at the bottom and carefully peel it off by pulling the sticky part parallel to the skin.

13. Pour the urine into the specimen cup after opening the specimen drain or cutting the bag.

Small amounts of urine can be obtained using a syringe without a needle to aspirate urine directly from the diaper; if diapers with absorbent gelling material that traps urine are used, place a small gauze dressing, pad, or some cotton balls inside the diaper to collect urine, and then aspirate the urine with a syringe.

Urine should be tested within 30 minutes, refrigerated, or placed in a sterile container with a preservative.

## Toilet-Trained Child

Children who are 8 years of age and older may be able to obtain the sample by themselves. Children under 8 years of age will need help. Young children may not be able to urinate on request. To help the child urinate, have her blow through a straw or listen to running water while the specimen cup is held for her. Do not give the child more than one glass of liquid to drink. Large amounts of liquid can affect the result of the urine test.

### *Materials Needed*

Urine specimen cup
Potty chair, potty hat, or toilet
Soap and water
Washcloth or diaper/perineal wipes

### *Routine Urine Sample (Boys and Girls)*

1. Put on nonsterile gloves. If the child is able to obtain the sample of urine, have the child wash her hands.

2. Open the urine container, taking care not to touch the inside of the cup or lid.

3. If a clean-catch specimen is needed:
   - For boys, wash the tip of the penis with a wipe or soap and water. If uncircumcised, pull back the foreskin only as far as it will easily go, then wash the tip of the penis. Rinse well if soap is used. Make sure the foreskin is pushed back toward the tip after cleaning.
   - For girls, spread the child's labia with your fingers. Wash the area from front to back with a wipe or soap and water. Rinse well if soap is used.
   - Have the child begin to urinate in the potty chair or toilet.
   - Tell the child to stop the stream. If he cannot stop the flow of urine, place the urine cup so that you can catch some of the urine.

4. Have the child urinate directly into the cup (or potty hat if more convenient for female and clean-catch not needed).

5. Replace the lid on the cup.

# Bladder Catheterization

Bladder catheterization is employed for the following reasons:

- Collection of a urine specimen
- Diagnostic testing
- Continuous urinary drainage
- Intravesical instillation of medications or chemotherapeutic agents

## Materials Needed

Sterile gloves (Safety Alert)
Catheter (see Safety Alert)

> **! SAFETY ALERT**
> Nonlatex catheters and sterile gloves should be used for all infants and children with known latex allergy, with latex sensitivity, or on latex precautions (e.g., children with conditions associated with frequent exposure to latex-containing products).

- Select a catheter based on the purpose of the procedure, the age and gender of the child, and any history of prior urologic surgery.
- When collecting a urine specimen or completing a diagnostic test requiring catheterization for a brief period, use:
  - A 4-5 French catheter for the infant
  - A 5-8 French catheter for the toddler or school-age child
  - An 8-12 French in-and-out catheter for the adolescent girl
  - An 8-12 French, straight-tipped or coudé-tipped in-and-out catheter for the adolescent boy
- When placing an indwelling catheter, use:
  - A 6-8 French Foley catheter with a 3-ml retention balloon for the infant
  - A 6-8 French Foley catheter with a 3-5-ml retention balloon for the toddler or school-aged child
  - An 8-12 French Foley catheter with a 5-ml retention balloon for the adolescent girl
  - An 8-16 French Foley catheter with a 5-ml retention balloon for the adolescent boy
  - Larger French sizes (14 to 16) are reserved for older adolescents with more fully developed prostates. A coudé-tipped catheter is selected for the adolescent boy with a history of urologic surgery.

Catheter tray

- Catheter insertion trays are available that provide a cost-effective alternative to gathering individual supplies for catheterization. These kits may come with or without a catheter, and both should be available for use with children. When a tray is not accessible, the following materials are needed in addition to the catheter: Betadine cleanser with cotton balls, sterile draping, a syringe with 5 ml of sterile water, and sterile, water-soluble lubricating jelly.

Container for urine collection

- When collecting a specimen or completing a diagnostic test, an appropriate urine specimen container and 500-ml basin are used; when inserting an indwelling catheter, a bedside drainage bag is obtained before the procedure. When inserting a Foley catheter, it is preferable to use a preconnected (closed) system containing catheter and bedside drainage bag.

## Procedure

1. Special procedural explanation considerations
   - Explain before preparation of the perineum.
   - Reassure parents that catheterization will not harm their child or damage the urethra or hymen.
   - Reassure child that insertion of the catheter will not feel like having a sharp object inserted but will produce a feeling of pressure and desire to urinate.
   - Give instruction on pelvic muscle relaxation whenever possible.
   - Young child is taught to blow (using a pinwheel is helpful) and to press the hips against the bed or procedure table during catheterization in order to relax the pelvic and periurethral muscles.
   - Older child or adolescent is taught to contract and relax the pelvic muscles, and the relaxation procedure is repeated during catheter insertion. If the child vigorously contracts the pelvic muscles when the catheter reaches the striated sphincter (proximal urethra in boys and mid-urethra in girls), catheter insertion is temporarily stopped. The catheter is neither removed nor advanced; instead the child is assisted to press the hips against the bed or examining table and relax the pelvic muscles. The catheter is then gently advanced into the bladder.
2. Place the infant or child in a supine position with the perineum adequately exposed. Girls may bend the knees and abduct the legs in a froglike position; boys should lie with the penis lying above the upper thighs. Use rolled towels or blankets to support the legs. As an alternative, for a young child, have the parent sit on the bed or examining table with a back support. Place the child leaning back in the parent's lap with the parent's arms hugging the child's upper body. When the child's legs are in the frog position, the parent's legs can be placed over the child's to stabilize them. In this comfortable position, the perineum is exposed for the procedure and the child is helped to lie still.
3. Put on a pair of sterile gloves. (See Safety Alert.)
4. Place a sterile drape over the perineum of girls, ensuring that the vagina, labia, and urethral meatus remain exposed. Most catheter insertion kits provide a sterile drape with a diamond-shaped hole in the middle to assist with this. For boys, the sterile drape is placed over the upper aspect of the thighs.
5. Place 5 ml of sterile lubricating jelly on the sterile drape. During catheterization of an adolescent or child accustomed to the procedure, the catheter may be

placed on the sterile drape laid over the perineum. When an anxious child is being catheterized, the catheter should remain on a sterile field that will not be upset should the child move during the procedure.

6. Cleanse the perineum of girls, including the labia, vaginal introitus, and urethral meatus. Use a new cotton ball for each wipe, moving in a front-to-back motion along each side of the labia minora, along the sides of the urinary meatus, and finally straight down over the urethral opening. For boys, cleanse the entire glans penis in an outward circular fashion, using one cotton ball for each wipe. The foreskin is retracted in the uncircumcised boy just far enough to visualize the urethral opening. If the foreskin cannot be easily retracted, particular care is taken to ensure that the glans penis is adequately cleaned before catheter insertion.

7. Wipe the cleanser from the skin using sterile cotton balls.

8. *Girls:* Spread the labia (if necessary) using one hand in order to clearly visualize the urethral meatus. With the other hand, grasp the catheter and apply a small amount of sterile lubricant from the sterile field onto the tip of the catheter. (It is rarely necessary to spread the labia in infants; instead, locate the urethra, which often appears as a dimple above the hymen.) Gently insert the catheter until urine return is seen. If inserting an indwelling catheter, advance the catheter an additional 1 to 2 inches before attempting to fill the retention balloon.

9. *Boys:* Hold the penile shaft just under the glans to prevent the foreskin from contaminating the area. Grasp the catheter with the other hand, and apply a small amount of sterile lubricant from the sterile field onto the tip of the catheter. Insert the catheter while gently stretching the penis and lifting it to a 90-degree angle to the body. Resistance may occur when the catheter meets the urethral sphincter. Ask the patient to inhale deeply and advance the catheter at that time. Insert the catheter until urine return occurs; this may take several seconds longer because of the additional lubricant present in the urethra. If inserting an indwelling catheter, advance until urine return is noted and then advance to the bifurcation of the filling port before filling the retention balloon.

10. When catheterizing for specimen collection, allow 15 to 30 ml for urinalysis and urine culture. Drain bladder, and record postvoid urinary volume if collected soon after urination. Cap the specimen, label it, and send it to the laboratory.

11. When inserting an indwelling catheter, gently pull catheter back until resistance is met; this ensures that the retention balloon lies just above the bladder neck. Tape tubing to the leg to avoid pulling, or use a commercially available catheter securement device. Hang drainage apparatus to bed frame (avoid bed rails to prevent pulling on catheter).

> **! SAFETY ALERT**
>
> Do not advance the catheter too far into the bladder. Knotting of catheters and tubes within the bladder has been reported in several case studies. Feeding tubes should not be used for urinary catheterization as they are more flexible, longer, and prone to knotting compared to commercially designed urinary catheters (Kilbane, 2009; Lodha, Ly, Brindle, Daneman, & McNamara, 2005; Levison & Wojtulewicz, 2004; Turner, 2004; Gonzalez & Palmer, 1997; Foster, Ritchey, & Bloom, 1992).

## 24-Hour Urine Collection

Begin and end collection with an empty bladder:
- At time collection begins, instruct child to void, and discard specimen.
- Twenty-four hours after that specimen was discarded, instruct child to void for last specimen.

Save all voided urine during the 24 hours in a refrigerated container marked with date, total time, and child's name.

### Non–Toilet-Trained Child

Prepare skin with thin coating of skin sealant (unless contraindicated, such as in premature infant or on irritated and/or nonintact skin), and apply a urine collection bag with a collection tube that allows urine to drain into a large receptacle.

If a collection tube is not available, insert a small feeding tube through a puncture hole at the top of the bag; use a syringe without a needle to aspirate urine through the feeding tube.

# Stool

Collect stool without urine contamination, if possible.

## Non–Toilet-Trained Child

Put on nonsterile gloves.

Apply a urine collection bag, and apply diaper over bag. Stool specimens may also be collected directly from the diaper.

After bowel movement, use a gloved hand and tongue blade or specimen stick to collect stool. If the stool is liquid, collect as many small pieces of fecal matter as possible, using a disposable spoon. If liquid stool soaks into diaper, line the inside of a clean diaper with plastic wrap. Place the clean diaper on the child and collect the next stool sample from the plastic liner.

Place specimen in specimen container. Replace the lid on the cup.

Wash child's diaper area with warm water and soap after each stool to prevent skin irritation.

### Toilet-Trained Child

Children who are age 8 years and older may be able to obtain the sample by themselves. Tell the child how to clean herself and how to obtain the sample. Young children may not be able to defecate on request. Use the child's words and usual place for defecating to obtain the sample, if possible. Have the child tell the parent when they think they are going to have a bowel movement. To help the child defecate, have the child bear down or hold his or her breath to facilitate evacuation of the stool.

Have child urinate, and then flush the toilet.

Perform hand hygiene, and put on nonsterile gloves.

Have child defecate into bedpan or potty hat in reverse position in the toilet.

After bowel movement, use tongue depressor or specimen stick to collect stool.

Place specimen in specimen container. Replace the lid on the cup.

Apply a patient identification label to the cup.

Remove gloves, and perform hand hygiene. Have the child wash his or her hands.

Praise the child for helping.

## Respiratory (Nasal) Secretions

To obtain nasal secretions using a nasal washing:

- Place child supine if maximal restraint needed; upright or semireclining allows the child more control and causes less anxiety.
- Instill 1 to 3 ml sterile NS with a sterile syringe (without needle or with 2 inches of 18- or 20-gauge tubing) into one nostril.
- Aspirate contents with a small, sterile bulb syringe.
- Place in sterile container.

## Sputum

Older children and adolescents are able to cough as directed and supply specimens when given proper direction.

Specimens can sometimes be collected from infants and young children who have an endotracheal (ET) tube or tracheostomy by means of tracheal aspiration with a mucous trap or suction apparatus.

## Blood

### Heel or Finger

Heel lancing has been shown to be more painful than venipuncture; consider venipuncture when the amount of blood from the heel would require much squeezing (e.g., genetic tests).

Puncture should be no deeper than 2 mm.

To increase blood flow, warm heel by using a commercial heel warmer for 3 minutes before puncture. May hold finger under warm water for a few seconds before puncture.

Prepare area for puncture with antiseptic agent.

Perform puncture on heel or finger in proper location with an automatic lancet device:

- Usual site for heel puncture is outer aspects of heel (Figure 4-8, A). Boundaries can be marked by an imaginary line extending posteriorly from a point between the fourth and fifth toes and running parallel to the lateral aspect of the heel and another line extending posteriorly from the middle of the great toe and running parallel to the medial aspect of the heel.
- Usual site for finger puncture is just to the side of the finger pad (see Figure 4-8, B), which has more blood vessels and fewer nerve endings. Avoid steadying the finger against a hard surface.

Collect blood sample in appropriate specimen container.

Apply pressure to puncture site with a dry, sterile gauze pad until bleeding stops.

### Vein

Apply tourniquet; alternative tourniquet for neonate is a rubber band.

Visualize or palpate vein.

Insert needle with bevel up; a slight pop may be felt when entering a child's vein; in small and preterm infants this may not occur.

Withdraw required amount of blood, and place in appropriate container.

Release tourniquet.

Withdraw needle from site, and apply dry, sterile gauze or cotton ball to site with firm pressure until bleeding stops. If antecubital site is used, keep arm extended to reduce bruising.

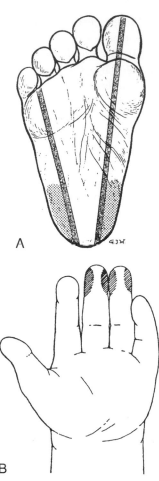

FIGURE **4-8**   A, Puncture sites (shaded areas) on infant's heel. B, Puncture sites on fingers. B from Smith DP, Wong DL: *Comprehensive child and family nursing skills,* St Louis, 1991, Mosby.

### Artery

Arterial blood samples from punctures are painful and often cause crying and breath holding, which affect the accuracy of blood gas values (decreased $PaO_2$). Provide pain intervention with buffered lidocaine, and for infants use sucrose before stick.

Arterial punctures may be performed using the radial, brachial, or femoral arteries.

Palpate artery for puncture.

Perform *Allen test* to determine adequacy of collateral circulation prior to radial puncture:

- Elevate extremity distal to puncture site, and blanch by squeezing gently (e.g., making a fist); two arteries supplying blood flow to the extremity (radial and ulnar arteries of the wrist) are then occluded.
- Lower extremity, and remove pressure from one artery (ulnar); color return to the blanched extremity in less than 5 seconds indicates adequate collateral circulation.

Prepare area for puncture with antiseptic agent.

Insert needle at a 60- to 90-degree angle.

Withdraw required amount of blood into syringe (or specimen container, as appropriate).

Withdraw needle, and apply pressure to site with a dry, sterile gauze pad for 5 to 10 minutes until bleeding stops. NOTE: Pressure must be applied at the site to prevent a hematoma.

Place specimen in heparinized syringe after removing bubbles from the syringe.

Place specimen on ice if it will not be processed immediately.

# Procedures Related to Administration of Medications

## General Guidelines

### Approaches to Pediatric Patients

Children's reactions to treatments are affected by the following:

- Developmental characteristics, such as physical abilities and cognitive capabilities
- Environmental influences
- Past experiences
- Current relationship with the nurse
- Perception of the present situation

Expect success: use a positive approach.

Provide an explanation appropriate to the child's developmental level.

Allow the child choices whenever they exist.

Be honest with the child.

Involve the child in the treatment in order to gain cooperation.

Allow the child the opportunity to express his or her feelings.

Hold and comfort the child after medication administration.

Praise the child for doing his or her best.

Provide distraction for a frightened or uncooperative child.

Spend some time with the child after administering the medication.

Let the child know that he or she is accepted as a person of value. (See also section on preparing children for procedures, pp. 209-211.)

## Safety Precautions

Take a drug allergy history.

Check the following five *R*'s for correctness:

- Right drug
- Right dosage
- Right time
- Right route
- Right child (Always check identification band and use 2 patient identifiers.)

Double-check drug and dosage with another nurse.

Always double-check the following:

- Antiarrhythmics (e.g., Digoxin)
- Insulin
- Anticoagulants (e.g., Heparin)
- Blood
- Chemotherapy
- Cardiotoxic drugs

Some institutions also double-check the following:

- Vasopressors
- Opioids (narcotics)
- Sedatives

Identify the child using two patient identifiers (e.g., patient name and medical record or birth date; neither can be a room number). Compare the same two identifiers to the medication label and order.

Be aware of drug-drug or drug-food interactions.

Document all drugs administered.

Monitor child for side effects.

Be prepared for serious side effects (e.g., respiratory depression, anaphylaxis).

Dispose of any plastic covers that may be on the ends of syringes. These covers are small enough to be aspirated by young children.

Measure liquid medications with a syringe or other specific medication dropper or calibrated spoon; instruct families to not use household teaspoons or tablespoons.

## Family Education: Medication Administration

In addition to the General Principles of Family Education on page 212, families need to know the following:

- Amount of the drug to be given
- Length of time to be administered
- Time(s) to give the drug; assist family in scheduling the time for administration around the family routine.
- Positioning
- Administration procedure
- Postadministration care
- Safe storage of drug (Safety Alert)
- What to do and whom to contact if any side effects occur

> **! SAFETY ALERT FOR HOME CARE**
>
> Do not tell children that medications are candy; if the bottle is ever left in a place where it can be reached, a child may take an overdose. Tell the child to take drugs *only* from parents or other special people, such as grandparents, babysitters, or nurses. Store *all* drugs in a safe place such as a locked cabinet. The storage area should be cool and dry. Bathrooms are usually too warm and moist for storing tablets or capsules. *Always* keep drugs in the original container, with the childproof cap tightly closed. Place drugs that need to be refrigerated on a high shelf toward the back of the refrigerator, not in the door.

## Oral Administration

1. Follow safety precautions for administration.
2. Select appropriate vehicle, for example, calibrated cup, oral medication syringe, dropper, measuring spoon, or nipple (Safety Alert).
3. Prepare medication:
   - Measure into appropriate vehicle. (Figure 4-9)
   - Crush tablets (except when contraindicated, e.g., time-released or enteric-coated preparations) for children who will have difficulty swallowing if a liquid medication is unavailable; mix with syrup, juice, and so on (Atraumatic Care box) At home, crushing can be done using two spoons or one spoon and wax paper
   - Capsules should not be opened and sprinkled into food prior to checking with a pharmacist.
   - Avoid mixing medications with essential food items, such as milk and formula.
4. Employ safety precautions in identification and administration (Safety Alert).

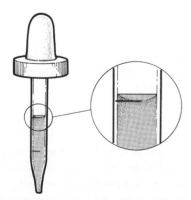

FIGURE **4-9**    Checking correct amount in a dropper.

**ATRAUMATIC CARE**

### Encouraging a Child's Acceptance of Oral Medications

Give the child a flavored ice pop or a small ice cube to suck to numb the tongue before giving the drug.

Mix the drug with a small amount (about 1 teaspoon) of sweet-tasting substance such as honey (except in infants because of the risk of botulism), flavored syrup, jam, fruit puree, sherbet, or ice cream; avoid essential food items, such as formula or milk, because the child may later refuse to eat or drink them.

Give a chaser of water, juice, soft drink, flavored ice pop, or frozen juice bar after the drug.

If nausea is a problem, give a carbonated beverage poured over finely crushed ice before or immediately after the medication.

When medication has an unpleasant taste, have the child pinch the nose and drink the medicine through a straw. (Much of what we taste is associated with smell.)

Flavorings such as apple, banana, and bubble gum can be added at many pharmacies (e.g., FLAVORx) at nominal additional cost. Another alternative is to have the pharmacist prepare the drug in a flavored, chewable troche or lozenge.*

Infants will suck medicine from a needleless syringe or dropper in small increments (0.25 to 0.5 ml) at a time. Use a nipple or special pacifier with a reservoir for the drug.

*For information about compounding drugs, contact Technical Staff, Professional Compounding Centers of America (PCCA), 9901 S. Wilcrest Dr., Houston, TX 77099; 800-331-2498; *www.pccarx.com.*

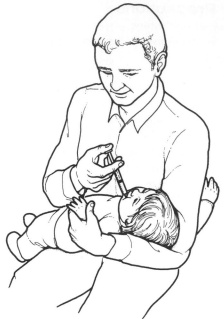

FIGURE **4-10**  Giving oral medication using a syringe. Note how the child's arms are placed.

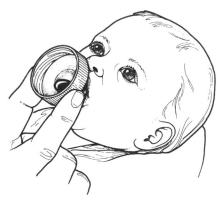

FIGURE **4-11**  Giving oral medication using a bottle nipple.

5. Give the medicine to the child in a quiet place so that you will not be disturbed.

6. Tell the child what you are going to do.

7. If needed, hold the infant or young child in your lap. Place whichever of her arms is closer to you behind your back. Firmly hug her other arm and hand with your arm and hand; snuggle her head between your body and your arm (Figure 4-10). Sometimes you may also want to grasp her legs between yours. Your other hand remains free to give the child the drug.

8. Gently place the dropper or syringe in the child's mouth along the inside of the cheek. Allow the child to suck the liquid from the dropper or syringe. If the child does not suck, squeeze a small amount of the drug at a time. This takes longer, but the child will swallow the medicine and be less likely to spit it out or choke on it.

OR

Place an empty bottle nipple in the child's mouth, add the drug to the nipple, and allow the child to suck the nipple (Figure 4-11).

OR

Allow the child to sip the drug from the spoon. Make sure that the child takes all of the drug.

9. Rinse the child's mouth with plain water to remove any of the sweetened drug from the gums and teeth. This can be done by wrapping a paper towel around your finger, soaking it in plain water, then swabbing the gums, cheeks, palate, and tongue.

## Infants

Hold in semireclining position.

Place oral syringe, measuring spoon, or dropper in mouth well back on the tongue or to the side of the tongue.

Administer slowly to reduce likelihood of choking or aspiration.

Allow infant to suck medication placed in a nipple.

## Older Infant or Toddler

Administer with oral syringe, measuring spoon, or dropper (as with infants).

Use mild or partial restraint with reluctant children.

Do not force actively resistive children because of danger of aspiration; postpone 20 to 30 minutes, and offer medication again.

## Preschool Children

Use straightforward approach.

For reluctant children, use the following:

- Simple persuasion
- Innovative containers
- Reinforcement, such as stars, stickers, or other tangible rewards for compliance

*Rudy C: A drop or a dropper: The risk of overdose, *J Pediatr Health Care* 6(1):40, 51-52, 1992.
†Shonna YH, Mendelsohn AL, Wolf MS, and others: Parents' medication administration errors: Role of dosing instruments and health literacy. *Arch Pediatr Adolesc Med* 164(2):181-186, 2010.
**Yin HS, Wolf MS, Dreyer BP, and others: Evaluation of consistency in dosing directions and measuring devices for pediatric nonprescription liquid medications, *JAMA* 304(23): E1-E8, 2010.

**4 - EVIDENCE-BASED PEDIATRIC NURSING INTERVENTIONS**

## Family Education: Administering Digoxin at Home

Give digoxin at regular intervals (usually every 12 hours, such as at 8 AM and 8 PM; in some children it may be given every 24 hours).

Plan the times so that the drug is given *1 hour before* or *2 hours after* feedings.

Use a calendar to mark off each dose that is given; or post a reminder, such as a sign on the refrigerator.

Have the prescription refilled *before* the medication is completely used.

Do not mix it with other foods, formula or other fluids, because refusal to consume these results in inaccurate intake of the drug.

If the child has teeth, give water after administering the drug; whenever possible, brush the teeth to prevent tooth decay from the sweetened liquid.

If a dose is missed and more than 4 hours have elapsed, withhold the dose and give the next dose at the regular time; if less than 4 hours have elapsed, give the missed dose.

If the child vomits within 1 hour of receiving the dose, do not give a second dose.

If more than two consecutive doses have been missed, notify the physician or other designated health professional.

Do not increase or double the dose for missed doses.

Avoid administration with herbal preparations such as St. John's wort or Siberian ginseng because these may change the medication's intended effect on the heart.

Notify your child's health practitioner if you need to give the child any over-the-counter medications.

If the child becomes ill with any of the following, notify the physician or other designated health professional immediately:

- Diarrhea
- Nausea
- Vision changes
- Lack of appetite
- Vomiting

Keep digoxin in a safe place, preferably a locked cabinet.

In case of accidental overdose of digoxin, call the nearest Poison Control Center immediately or the national number: 800-222-1222; the number is usually listed in the front of the telephone directory.

# ⊜ Nasogastric, Orogastric, or Gastrostomy Tube Administration

Use elixir or suspension preparations of medication (rather than tablets) whenever possible (Safety Alert).

Dilute viscous medication or syrup with a small amount of water if possible.

Avoid oily medications because they tend to cling to the sides of the tube.

If administering tablets, crush them to a very fine powder and dissolve drug in a small amount of warm water.

Never crush enteric-coated or sustained-release tablets or capsules.

Do not mix medication with enteral formula unless fluid is restricted. If adding a drug:

- Check with pharmacist for compatibility.
- Shake formula well, and observe for any physical reaction (e.g., separation, precipitation).
- Label formula container with name of medication, dosage, date, and time infusion started.

Check for correct placement of nasogastric (NG) or orogastric tube.

Attach syringe (with adaptable tip but without plunger) to tube.

Pour medication into syringe.

Unclamp tube, and allow medication to flow by gravity.

Adjust height of container to achieve desired flow rate (e.g., increase height for faster flow).

> **⚠ SAFETY ALERT**
>
> Sprinkle-type medications should be avoided. However, if there is no other option and the tube is large gauge (18 French or greater), but usually not a Foley catheter, the medication may be given by mixing the sprinkles with a small amount of pureed fruit and thinning with water. The fruit keeps the sprinkles suspended so they do not float to the top. Flush well. This procedure is not recommended for skin-level gastrostomy devices.

As soon as syringe is empty, pour 10 ml of water to flush tubing.

- Amount of water depends on length and gauge of tubing.
- Determine amount before administering any medication by using a syringe to completely fill an unused NG or orogastric tube with water. The amount of flush solution is usually $1\frac{1}{2}$ times this volume.
- With certain drug preparations (e.g., suspensions), more fluid may be needed.

If administering more than one drug at the same time, flush the tube between each medication with clear water.

Clamp tube after flushing, unless tube is left open.

# Rectal Administration

## Suppository

Medications may need to be administered rectally if the oral route is not available. If half a suppository is to be used, cut it in half *lengthwise*.

### Insertion Procedure

1. Position the child on his or her left side, with the right leg slightly bent.
2. Remove the wrapper from the suppository.
3. Use a gloved index or pinky (fifth) finger to insert the suppository; families may use gloves, finger cots, or plastic wrap at home.
4. Wet the glove or plastic covering and the suppository with warm (not hot) water. Do not use lubricant as it may affect medication absorption.
5. Insert with the apex (pointed end) first; 1 inch into a child's rectum and slightly less for an infant.
6. If the child is too young to help, hold the buttocks together for at least five minutes to prevent expulsion of the suppository.

## Enemas and Constipation

Simple constipation in children should not be treated with enemas but with changes in the child's diet. Increasing the amount of liquids to at least 1 quart each day and the amount of fiber in foods (especially whole grains, bran cereals, fresh vegetables, and fruit with the skin on) should increase the size and number of the child's bowel movements. Fruit juices such as apple, pear, and prune juices contain sorbitol and can prevent or relieve constipation. Oral medications such as mineral oil and polyethylene glycol electrolyte solutions are also effective in relieving constipation. No controlled trials have demonstrated the effectiveness of magnesium hydroxide, magnesium citrate, lactulose, sorbitol, senna, or bisacodyl, but these laxatives are widely thought to be effective. Infants should not be given stimulant laxatives or mineral oil. Glycerin suppositories are effective in infants, and bisacodyl suppositories are used in children. Phosphate soda enemas, saline enemas, or mineral oil enemas are effective. Soap suds, tap water, and magnesium enemas are not recommended because of potential toxicity (North American Society for Pediatric Gastroenterology, Hepatology, and Nutrition, 2006).

### Enema Procedure

1. Dilute drug in smallest amount of solution possible.
2. Place the child in one of the following positions:
   - Lying face-down on belly with the knees and hips bent toward the chest (Figure 14-12, A)
   - Lying on the left side with the left leg straight and the right leg bent at the hip and knee and

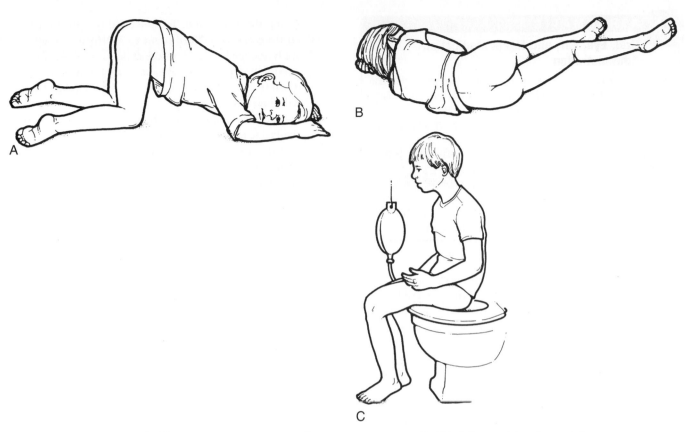

FIGURE **4-12**    A, Knee-chest position for receiving an enema. B, Side-lying position for receiving an enema. C, Position for receiving an enema on toilet.

placed comfortably on top of the left leg (Figure 14-12, B)

- Sitting on the potty chair or toilet (Figure 14-12, C)

1. Place a small amount of lubricant on your finger or on a tissue, and spread the lubricant around the tip of the tube, being careful not to plug the holes with lubricant; prepackaged enema tips are already lubricated.
2. Insert into rectum (Guidelines box). Depending on volume, may use syringe with rubber tubing, enema bottle, or enema bag.
3. If using an enema bag, hold the bottom of the container no more than 4 inches above the child; open the clamp and allow the liquid to flow, holding the tube in place.
4. When the container is empty, remove it.
5. Have the child keep the liquid inside for 3 to 5 minutes. If the child is too young to follow instructions, then hold

### GUIDELINES
#### Administration of Enemas to Children

| Age | Amount (ml) | Insertion Distance in Centimeters (inches) |
|---|---|---|
| Infant | 120-240 | 2.5 (1) |
| 2-4 years | 240-360 | 5.0 (2) |
| 4-10 years | 360-480 | 7.5 (3) |
| 11 years | 480-720 | 10.0 (4) |

the buttocks together to keep the liquid inside. For an older child, encourage slow deep breathing, or read a book to take the child's mind off the time.

6. Help the child to the toilet or potty chair, or allow the child to release the liquid into a diaper.

## Eye, Ear, and Nose Administration

See Atraumatic Care box.

### Eye Medication

Eye drops are administered in the same manner as to adults. Children, however, require additional preparation (Nursing Alert). When both drops and ointment are needed, give the drops first, wait 3 minutes, and then apply the ointment. This allows each drug time to work. When possible, administer eye ointments before bedtime or naptime, because the child's vision will be blurred for a while.

#### Eye Drop Instillation Procedure

1. Remove any discharge from the eye with a clean tissue. Wipe from nose to ear. If the eye has crusted material

### ATRAUMATIC CARE

#### Oral, Eye, Ear, and Nasal Medication Administration

To administer oral, nasal, ear, or optic medication when only one person is available to restrain the child, use the following procedure:
- Place child supine on flat surface (bed, couch, floor).
- Sit facing child so that child's head is between operator's thighs and child's arms are under operator's legs.
- Place lower legs over child's legs to restrain lower body if necessary.
- To administer oral medication, place small pillow under child's head to reduce risk of aspiration.
- To administer nasal medication, place small pillow under child's shoulders to aid flow of liquid through nasal passages.

around it, wet a washcloth with warm water and place over the eye. After 1 minute, gently wipe the eye from the nose side outward with the washcloth, place it on the eye, and wait again. If you cannot remove the crusting, rewet the washcloth. Continue using the warm, moist washcloth and gently wiping until all the crusting is removed. If both eyes need cleaning, use separate cloths for each eye.

2. Position supine with a pillow under the child's shoulders, or a rolled-up towel under his neck so that the head is tilted back and to the same side as the eye to be treated (i.e., right eye, turn head to right; left eye, turn head to left). Eye drops should flow *away* from the child's nose.
3. Open the medication container.
4. Steady your hand on the child's forehead.
   - Position a bottle so that the drops will fall into the lower eyelid, *not* directly onto the eyeball.
   - Position an ointment tube at the inner part of the eye near the nose
5. Gently pull down the child's lower eyelid with the other hand by placing gentle downward pressure below the eyelashes (Figure 4-13).
   - For drops: Tell the child to look up and to the other side (away from the eye into which you are putting the drops). Choose something specific for the child to look at. If the child is young, you can make a game of

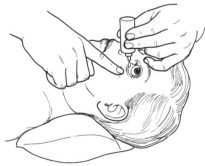

FIGURE **4-13**  Medication container and hand position for administering eye drops or ointment.

giving the medication. Tell the child to open his eyes on the count of 3. Then count to 3. When you say 3, apply the medication into the child's eye. Even if the child will not open the eyes on 3, keep him lying down until he decides to open the eyes. The medicine will flow in the eye.
   - For ointment: Squeeze a ribbon of the ointment onto the inside of lower eyelid. Begin at the side of the eye near the nose, and go toward the outer edge of the eye. Avoid touching the eye with the ointment container. Give the tube a half-turn. This helps "cut" the ribbon of medicine.
6. Tell the child to close the eye, then to blink. This helps spread the drug around the eye.
7. Remove any extra drug with a clean tissue, wiping from the nose outward. Putting gentle pressure on the inner corner of the eye for 1 minute prevents any medicine from dripping into the back of the throat and causing an unpleasant taste.
8. If both eyes are to be given the drug, repeat with the other eye.

### ⊖ Ear Medication

Depending on the child's age, the pinna is pulled differently.

#### Ear Medication Instillation Procedure

1. Ear medication may be warmed by placing medication bottle in a container of warm water. Feel a drop to ensure the medication is not uncomfortably cold or hot.
2. Have the child lie on the side opposite the ear into which the medication will be placed (e.g., right ear, on left side).
3. If any drainage is present, remove it with a clean tissue or cotton-tipped applicator. *Do not* clean any more than the outer ear.
4. Open the bottle of ear drops. Do not let the dropper portion touch anything.
5. Steady your hand by placing your wrist on the child's cheek or head.
6. Straighten the child's ear canal.
   - For children 3 years old and younger, pull the outer ear *down* and toward the *back* of the head (Figure 4-14, A).
   - For older children, pull the outer ear *up* and toward the *back* (Figure 4-14, B).
7. Position the bottle so that the drops will fall against the side of the ear canal.
8. Squeeze the bottle for the right number of drops.
9. Keep the child lying on that side with the medicated ear up for 1 minute. Gently rub the skin in front of the ear (Figure 4-14, C). This helps the drug flow to the inside of the ear.
10. If any drug has spilled on the skin, wipe the outer ear. A cotton ball can be loosely placed in the ear, but it must be changed each time drops are administered.
11. If both ears need the medication, repeat with the other ear after a one-minute wait.

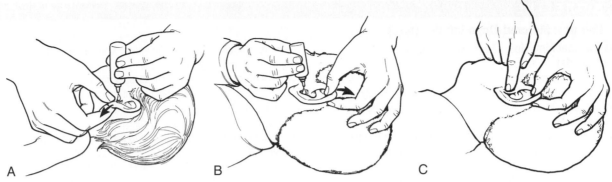

FIGURE **4-14**    Instilling ear medication. A, Hand and dropper position for children 3 years old and younger, with earlobe pulled down and back. B, Hand and dropper position for older children, with earlobe pulled up and back. C, Rubbing ear to help drug flow to inside of ear.

## ⊖ Nose Drops

Nose drops are administered in the same manner as to adults. Different positions may be used, depending on the child's age.

1. Remove any mucus from the nose with a clean tissue. If the nose has crusted material around it, wet a washcloth with warm water and place this around the nose. Wait about one minute. Gently wipe the nose with the washcloth. If you cannot remove the crusting, rewet the washcloth and again place it around the nose. Continue using the warm, moist washcloth and gently wiping until all of the crusting is removed.
2. Place the child on his back. Tilt the child's head backward by placing a pillow or rolled-up towel under the child's shoulders or letting the head hang over the side of a bed or your lap (Figure 4-15).
3. Place the right number of drops in each side of the nose.
4. Keep the child's head tilted back for at least one minute to prevent gagging or tasting the medication.

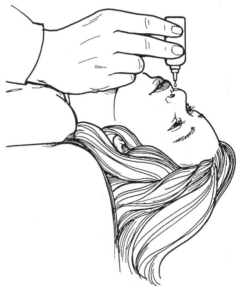

FIGURE **4-15**    Correct position of child's head and neck for giving nose drops.

## ⊖ Aerosol Therapy

The purpose is the inhalation of a solution in droplet (particle) form for direct deposition in the tracheobronchial tree.

Aerosols consist of liquid medications (e.g., bronchodilators, steroids, mucolytics, decongestants, antibiotics, antiviral agents) suspended in a particulate form in air.

Aerosol generators propelled by air or air-oxygen mixtures generally fall into three categories:

- Small-volume jet nebulizers or handheld nebulizers
- Ultrasonic nebulizers for sterile water or saline aerosol only
- Metered-dose inhalers (MDIs) (sometimes with a "spacer" device that acts as a reservoir and simplifies use of the inhaler; devices such as the Rotohaler or Turbuhaler eliminate the need for a spacer device and are easier for young children to use)

Deposition of aerosol is maximized by instructing the child to breathe through the mouth with slow, deep inhalations, followed by holding the breath for 5 to 10 seconds, then slow exhalations while in an upright position.

Using an incentive spirometer can help a cooperative child learn this ventilatory pattern.

For infants and young children, activities to produce deep breathing and coughing include feet tapping, tactile stimulation, and crying. The infant must be held upright.

Assessment of breath sounds and work of breathing is performed before and after treatments.

## GUIDELINES

### Use of a Metered-Dose Inhaler (MDI)

**Steps for Checking How Much Medicine Is in the Canister**

1. If the canister is new, it is full.
2. If the canister has been used repeatedly, it might be empty. (Check product label to see how many inhalations should be in each canister.)
3. The most accurate way to determine how many doses remain in an MDI is to count and record each actuation as it is used.
4. Many dry powder inhalers have a dose-counting device or dose indicator on the canister to let you know when the canister is empty.
5. Placing dry powder inhalers or MDIs with hydrofluoroalkanes in water will destroy these inhalers.

**Steps for Using the Inhaler\***

1. Remove the cap, and hold inhaler upright.
2. Shake the inhaler.
3. Tilt the head back slightly, take a deep breath, and breathe out slowly.
4. With the inhaler in an upright position, insert the mouthpiece:
   - About 3 to 4 cm from the mouth (Figure 4-16, A) or
   - Into an aerochamber (Figure 4-16, B) or

- Into the mouth, forming an airtight seal between the lips and the mouthpiece (Figure 4-16, C)
5. At the end of a normal expiration, depress the top of the inhaler canister firmly to release the medication (into either the aerochamber or the mouth), and breathe in slowly (about 3 to 5 seconds). Relax the pressure on the top of the canister.
6. Hold the breath for 10 seconds to allow the aerosol medication to reach deeply into the lungs.
7. Remove the inhaler, and breathe out slowly through the nose.
8. Wait 1 minute between puffs (if additional one is needed).
   Tips to avoid common inhaler mistakes:
   - Breathe out before pressing your inhaler.
   - Inhale slowly, evenly, and deeply.
   - Breathe in through your mouth, not your nose.
   - Press down on your inhaler at the start of inhalation (or within the first second of inhalation).
   - Keep inhaling as you press down on inhaler.
   - Press your inhaler only once while you are inhaling (one breath for each puff).
   - Make sure you breathe in evenly and deeply.

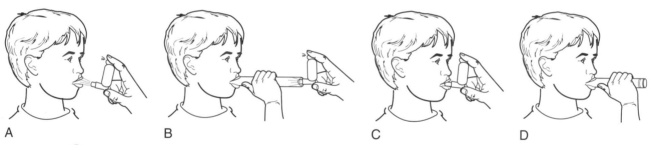

⊖ FIGURE **4-16** A, Open mouth with inhaler 3 to 4 cm away. B, Spacer or aerochamber (recommended especially for young children and for people using corticosteroids). C, Into the mouth. Do not use for corticosteroids. D, Inhaled dry powder capsule. Figures redrawn from the National Asthma Education and Prevention Program.

Modified from *Nurses' Asthma Education Working Group: Nurses: partners in asthma care,* NIH Publication No. 95-3308, Bethesda, Md, 1995, National Heart Lung and Blood Institute, National Institutes of Health.
\*NOTE: Inhaled dry powder such as Pulmicort requires a different inhalation technique. To use a dry powder inhaler, the base of the device is turned until a click is heard. It is important to close the mouth tightly around the mouthpiece of the inhaler and inhale rapidly (Figure 4-16, D).

## Intramuscular Administration

Explain procedure to child as developmentally appropriate, and provide atraumatic care (Atraumatic Care box).

Use safety precautions in administering medications. (See p. 233.)

Determine the site of injection (Table 4-5); make certain muscle is large enough to accommodate volume and type of medication.
- Older children—Select site as with the adult patient; allow child some choice of site, if feasible.
- Following are acceptable sites for infants and small or debilitated children (See Safety Alert):

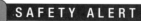

### SAFETY ALERT
Do not use the dorsal gluteal site even in children who are walking.

  ○ Vastus lateralis muscle
  ○ Ventrogluteal muscle

Select needle and syringe appropriate to the following (Table 4-6):
- Amount of fluid to be administered (syringe size)
- Viscosity of fluid to be administered (needle gauge)

**Evidence-Based Practice—Reduction of Minor Procedural Pain in Infants**

## ATRAUMATIC CARE

### Injections

Select a method to anesthetize the puncture site:
- Apply EMLA on site 2½ hours before intramuscular (IM) injection, or apply LMX on site for at least 30 minutes before injection.
- Use a vapocoolant spray* (e.g., Fluori-Methane or ethyl chloride) just before injection.
- For young infants, use sucrose before injection.
- Breastfeeding prior to and during the injection.

Prepare site with antiseptic and allow to dry completely before skin is penetrated.

Have medication at room temperature.

Use a new, sharp needle with smallest gauge that permits free flow of the medication and safe penetration of muscle.

Decrease perception of pain:
- Distract child with conversation; excessive parental reassurance, criticism, or apology increases distress, whereas humor and distraction decrease distress (Schechter, Zempsky, Cohen, and others, 2007).
- Give child something on which to concentrate (e.g., squeezing a hand or bed rail, pinching own nose, humming, counting, yelling "ouch!").
- Apply pressure at the site with a finger or device.

- Say to child, "If you feel this, tell me to take it out."
- Have child hold a small bandage and place it on puncture site after IM injection is given.

Enlist parents' assistance if they wish to participate and/or assist.

Restrain child *only as needed* to perform procedure safely. (See restraining methods and therapeutic hugging, p. 222.)

Insert needle quickly using a dartlike motion.

Avoid tracking any medication through superficial tissues:
- Replace needle after withdrawing medication, or wipe medication from needle with sterile gauze.
- If withdrawing medication from an ampule, use a needle equipped with a filter that removes glass particles; then use a new, nonfilter needle for injection.
- Use the Z track and/or air-bubble technique as indicated.
- Avoid any depression of the plunger during insertion of the needle.

Place a small bandage on puncture site (unless skin is compromised, e.g., in low-birth-weight infant); with young children decorate bandage by drawing a smiling face or other symbol of acceptance.

Hold and cuddle young child, and encourage parents to comfort child; praise older child.

*Abbott K, Fowler-Kerry S: The use of a topical refrigerant anesthetic to reduce injection pain in children, *J Pain Symptom Manage* 10(8):584-590, 1995; Cohen Reis E, Holubkov R: Vapocoolant spray is equally effective as EMLA cream in reducing immunization pain in school-aged children, *Pediatrics* 100(6):E5, 1997.

- Amount of tissue to be penetrated (needle length)
- If withdrawing medication from an ampule, use a needle equipped with a filter that removes glass particles; then use a new nonfilter needle for injection. Replace needle after withdrawing medication from a vial.

Maintain aseptic technique, and follow Standard Precautions.

Provide for sufficient help in restraining the child; children are often uncooperative, and their behavior is usually unpredictable.

Prepare area for puncture with antiseptic agent and allow to dry completely.

Administer the medication:
- Expose injection area for unobstructed view of landmarks.
- Select a site where the skin is free of irritation and danger of infection; palpate for and avoid sensitive or hardened areas. With multiple injections, rotate sites.
- Place the child in a lying or sitting position; the child is not allowed to stand for the following reasons:
  o Landmarks are more difficult to assess.
  o Restraint is more difficult.
  o The child may faint and fall.
- Grasp the muscle firmly between the thumb and fingers to isolate and stabilize the muscle for deposition of the drug in its deepest part; in obese

children spread the skin with the thumb and index finger to displace subcutaneous tissue and grasp the muscle deeply on each side.
- Insert needle quickly using a dartlike motion.
- Avoid tracking any medication through superficial tissues:
  o Use the Z track and/or air-bubble technique as indicated.
  o Avoid any depression of the plunger during insertion of the needle.
- Aspirate for blood.
  o If blood is found, remove syringe from site, change needle, and reinsert into new location.
  o If no blood is found, inject into a relaxed muscle.
- Inject medication slowly over several seconds.

Remove needle quickly; hold gauze firmly against skin near needle when removing it to avoid pulling on tissue.

Apply firm pressure with dry gauze to the site after injection; massage the site to hasten absorption unless contraindicated (e.g., with iron, dextran).

Clean area of prepping agent with water to decrease absorption of agent in neonate.

Praise child for cooperation.

Discard syringe and needle in puncture-resistant container near site of use.

Record date, time, dose, drug, and site of injection.

## TABLE 4-5  ⊖ Intramuscular Injection Sites in Children

| Site | Discussion |
|---|---|

### *Vastus Lateralis*

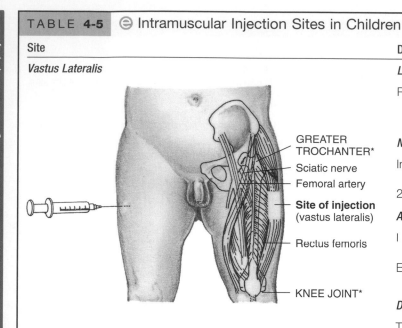

GREATER TROCHANTER*
Sciatic nerve
Femoral artery
**Site of injection** (vastus lateralis)
Rectus femoris
KNEE JOINT*

#### Location*

Palpate to find greater trochanter and knee joints; divide vertical distance between these two landmarks into thirds; inject into middle one third.

#### Needle Insertion and Size

Insert needle at 90-degree angle between syringe and upper thigh in infants and in young children.
22-25 gauge, ⅝-1 inch

#### Advantages

Large, well-developed muscle that can tolerate larger quantities of fluid (0.5 ml [infant] to 2 ml [child])
Easily accessible if child is supine, side lying, or sitting

#### Disadvantages

Thrombosis of femoral artery from injection in midthigh area (rectus femoris muscle)
Sciatic nerve damage from long needle injected posteriorly and medially into small extremity
More painful than deltoid or gluteal sites

### *Ventrogluteal*

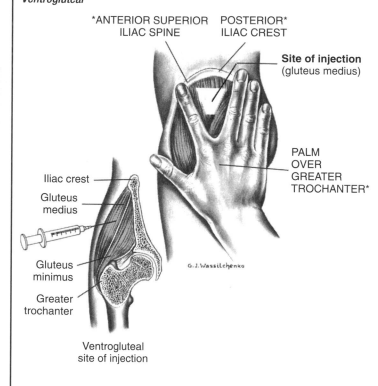

*ANTERIOR SUPERIOR ILIAC SPINE    POSTERIOR* ILIAC CREST
**Site of injection** (gluteus medius)
PALM OVER GREATER TROCHANTER*

Iliac crest
Gluteus medius
Gluteus minimus
Greater trochanter

G.J.Wassilchenko

Ventrogluteal site of injection

#### Location*

Palpate to locate greater trochanter, anterior superior iliac tubercle (found by flexing thigh at hip and measuring up to 1 to 2 cm above crease formed in groin), and posterior iliac crest; place palm of hand over greater trochanter, index finger over anterior superior iliac tubercle, and middle finger along crest of ilium posteriorly as far as possible; inject into center of *V* formed by fingers.

#### Needle Insertion and Size

Insert needle perpendicular to site but angled slightly toward greater trochanter.
22-25 gauge, ½ to 1 inch

#### Advantages

Free of important nerves and vascular structures
Easily identified by prominent bony landmarks
Thinner layer of subcutaneous tissue than in dorsogluteal site, thus less chance of depositing drug subcutaneously rather than intramuscularly
Can accommodate larger quantities of fluid (0.5 ml [infant] to 2 ml [child])
Easily accessible if child is supine, prone, or side lying
Less painful than vastus lateralis

#### Disadvantages

Health professionals' unfamiliarity with site

*Locations of landmarks are indicated by asterisks on illustrations.

## TABLE 4-5   ⊖ Intramuscular Injection Sites in Children—cont'd

| Site | Discussion |
|---|---|
| **Deltoid** 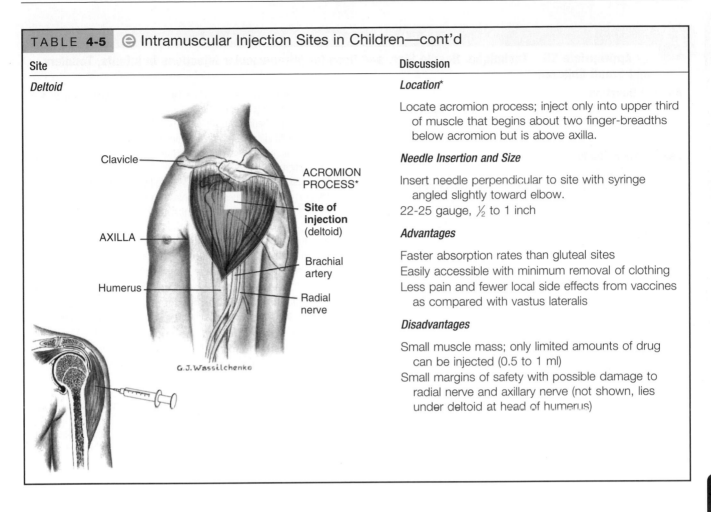 G.J.Wassilchenko | **Location*** <br><br> Locate acromion process; inject only into upper third of muscle that begins about two finger-breadths below acromion but is above axilla. <br><br> **Needle Insertion and Size** <br><br> Insert needle perpendicular to site with syringe angled slightly toward elbow. <br> 22-25 gauge, ½ to 1 inch <br><br> **Advantages** <br><br> Faster absorption rates than gluteal sites <br> Easily accessible with minimum removal of clothing <br> Less pain and fewer local side effects from vaccines as compared with vastus lateralis <br><br> **Disadvantages** <br><br> Small muscle mass; only limited amounts of drug can be injected (0.5 to 1 ml) <br> Small margins of safety with possible damage to radial nerve and axillary nerve (not shown, lies under deltoid at head of humerus) |

## TABLE 4-6   Intramuscular Administration: Location, Needle Length, Gauge, and Fluid Administration Amount

| | Location of Injection | Needle Length (inches) | Needle Gauge (G) | Suggested Maximum Amount (ml) |
|---|---|---|---|---|
| Preterm newborn | Anterolateral thigh | ⅝ | 23-25 | 0.25-0.5* |
| Term newborn | Anterolateral thigh | ⅝ | 23-25 | 0.5-1* |
| Infant (1 month to 12 months) | Anterolateral thigh | ⅝-1 | 22-25 | 1* |
| Toddler (13 to 36 months ) | Deltoid | ⅝-1 | 22-25 | 0.5-1* |
| | Anterolateral thigh or ventrogluteal | ⅝-1† <br> 1-1¼‡ | 22-25 | 1-2* |
| Preschool and older children | Deltoid | ⅝-1 | 22-25 | 0.5-1* |
| | Anterolateral thigh or ventrogluteal | 1-1¼‡ | 22-25 | 2-3* |
| Adolescent | Deltoid | ⅝-1 <br> 1-1½† <br> 1-1¼§ | 22-25 | 1-1.5* <br> 2§ |
| | Anterolateral thigh or ventrogluteal | 1-1¼‡ <br> 1-1½† | 22-25 | 2-3* <br> 2-5§ |

Modified from Becton-Dickinson Media Center: *A guide for managing the pediatric patient: Reducing the anxiety and pain of injections,* Franklin Lakes, NJ, 1998, Becton-Dickinson; Centers for Disease Control and Prevention: General recommendations on immunization: Recommendations of the Advisory Committee on Immunization Practices (ACIP), *MMWR* 55(RR-15):16-18, 2006; American Academy of Pediatrics; *Red book, 2006 Report of the Committee on Infectious Diseases,* ed 27, Elk Grove Village, IL, 2006, American Academy of Pediatrics, pp 19-21; and Nicoll LH, Hesby A: Intramuscular injection: An integrative research review and guideline for evidence-based practice, *Appl Nurs Res* 16(2):149-162, 2002.
*Evaluate size of muscle mass before administration.
†Centers for Disease Control and Prevention, 2006.
‡American Academy of Pediatrics, 2006.
§Nicoll and Hesby, 2002.

## Appropriate Site, Technique, Needle Size, and Dose for Intramuscular Injections in Infants, Toddlers, and Small Children

### Ask the Question

In infants, toddlers, and small children what is the best site, technique, needle size and gauge, and dosage for intramuscular (IM) injections?

### Search the Evidence
#### Search Strategies

Literature from 1990 to 2009 was reviewed to obtain clinical research studies related to this issue.

#### Databases Used

CINAHL, PubMed

### Critically Analyze the Evidence

**Grade criteria:** Evidence quality low; recommendation strong (Guyatt, Oxman, Vist, and others, 2008)

The searches reviewed were mostly small studies. There were no randomized trials, double-blinded trials, or large clinical studies addressing the subject of IM injections in children.

- Studies in adults indicate that injection pain can be minimized by deep IM administration, since muscle tissue has fewer nerve endings and medications are absorbed faster than those administered subcutaneously (Zuckerman, 2000). Immunizations such as diphtheria-tetanus–acellular pertussis (DTaP) and hepatitis A and B contain an aluminum adjuvant that, if injected into subcutaneous tissue, increases the incidence of local reactions. Inadvertent injection into subcutaneous tissue may be caused by use of a needle too short to reach IM tissue (Zuckerman, 2000).
- One study found that 4-month-old infants experienced fewer local side effects (redness, tenderness, and swelling) when immunizations were administered into the anterior aspect of the thigh with a 25-mm (1-inch) needle as opposed to the shorter 16-mm (⅝-inch) needle (Diggle and Deeks, 2000).
- Another study comparing needle length and injection method found that a longer needle (25 mm) was preferred for injection when bunching the skin and injecting, whereas a shorter needle (16 mm) was perceived as causing fewer localized reactions when the injection was administered with the skin being held taut (Groswasser, Kahn, Bouche, and others, 1997). However, the study's conclusions fail to address whether needle lengths were applicable to both the deltoid and vastus lateralis muscles.
- Cook and Murtagh (2002) made ultrasound measurements of the subcutaneous and muscle layer thickness in 57 children ages 2, 4, 6, and 18 months. These researchers concluded that a 16-mm needle was sufficient to penetrate the anterolateral thigh muscle if the needle is inserted at a 90-degree angle without pinching the muscle, whereas thigh measurements demonstrated that a 25-mm needle was necessary to penetrate the muscle when a 45-degree injection technique was employed. This study supports the concept of longer needle length to fully deposit the medication into the muscle.
- In a study by Davenport (2004), needle length proved to be the most significant variable for local reactions in children after injection with 16-mm and 25-mm needles; the 25-mm needle was associated with fewer localized reactions.
- Diggle, Deeks, and Pollard (2006) likewise found that when long needles (25 mm) were used for infant immunizations, localized

vaccine reactions were significantly reduced in comparison to the shorter needles (16 mm).
- Beecroft and Redick (1990) cited numerous differences of opinion regarding IM injection technique among pediatric nurses, highlighting how little agreement there is among nursing texts evaluated in regards to injection site and technique.
- In a nursing journal column, a nurse noted discrepancies in IM administration technique when injections were given to her child, further highlighting the differences in opinion regarding IM injection technique among pediatric nurses (Winslow and Jacobson, 1997).
- In a study of diphtheria-tetanus-pertussis (DTP) immunizations administered to infants 7 months and younger, only 84.6% of injections were administered at the correct site (anterior thigh); an alarming number were given in the dorsogluteal (5.1%) and deltoid (2.6%) muscles (Daly, Johnston, and Chung, 1992).
- Beecroft and Kongelbeck (1994) evaluated pediatric IM injections and concluded that the ventrogluteal site is the site of choice in children of all ages; they found no reports of complications at this site in the literature. The ventrogluteal site is relatively free of important nerves and vascular structures, the site is easily identified by landmarks, and the subcutaneous tissue is thinner in that area. To date, no reports can be found in the literature to refute the claims made by these researchers.
- The American Academy of Pediatrics (2009) and the Centers for Disease Control and Prevention (2002) recommend that vaccines containing adjuvants such as aluminum (e.g., DTaP, hepatitis A and B, diphtheria-tetanus [DT or Td]) be given deep into the muscle to prevent local reactions. In addition, a 16-mm needle may be adequate for injections in small infants, and a 22- to 25-mm (⅞ to 1 inch) needle can be used in infants 2 months and older. The Centers for Disease Control and Prevention (2002) recommends that toddlers receive injections with a 22- to 32-mm (⅞- to 11/4-inch) needle in the deltoid if muscle size is adequate; a minimum of a 25-mm long needle is recommended for anterolateral thigh injection in toddlers. Both the American Academy of Pediatrics (2009) and the Centers for Disease Control and Prevention (2002) recommend a 22- to 25- guage needle for all IM childhood immunizations. The deltoid muscle may be used for immunizations in toddlers, older children, and adolescents.
- Diggle (2003) recommends the deltoid muscle for IM injections in children older than age 1 year. When multiple vaccines are given, two may be given in the thigh (anterior and lateral) because of its larger size. The American Academy of Pediatrics (2009) recommends that injections in the anterolateral thigh be given at least 2.5 cm (1 inch) apart so local reactions are less likely to overlap. The dorsogluteal muscle should be avoided in infants and toddlers, and perhaps even in smaller preschoolers with smaller muscle mass, because of the possibility of damaging the sciatic nerve.

No research or supportive data were found regarding the amount of medication to be given at the different sites in infants and toddlers. In general, 1 ml of medication is recommended for infants less than 12 months; however, no data can be found to refute or support such a recommendation. Furthermore, small and preterm infants may only tolerate up to 0.5 ml in each muscle to prevent local complications.

In summary, some discrepancy remains in actual clinical practice regarding IM injection sites, amount of drug injected, and needle size in infants and toddlers. Further research is needed to address the following issues:

## EVIDENCE-BASED PRACTICE

### Appropriate Site, Technique, Needle Size, and Dose for Intramuscular Injections in Infants, Toddlers, and Small Children—cont'd

- What is the appropriate muscle in which an IM injection can be administered with fewest adverse effects in infants and toddlers?
- What is the appropriate needle size based on the infant or toddler's age and weight?
- What is the largest safe amount of medication that can be given to infants and toddlers based on weight and muscle size?

### Apply the Evidence: Nursing Implications

Based on the evidence in the literature, the recommendation is to continue administering IM injections to children in the anterolateral thigh (up to 12 months old), deltoid (12 months and older), and ventrogluteal site.

Needle length is an important factor in decreasing local reactions; the length should be adequate to deposit the medication into the muscle for IM injections. Recommendations are for a 25-mm (1-inch) needle in infants, a 25- to 32-mm (1- to 1¼-inch) needle for toddlers, and a 38- to 51-mm (1½- to 2-inch) needle for older children; preterm and small emaciated infants may require a shorter needle (16 to 25 mm [⅝ to 1 inch]) based on weight and muscle mass size.

### References

American Academy of Pediatrics, Committee on Infectious Diseases, Pickering L, editor: *2009 Red book: Report of the Committee on Infectious Diseases*, ed 28, Elk Grove Village, Ill, 2009, The Academy.

Beecroft PC, Kongelbeck SR: How safe are intramuscular injections? *AACN Clin Issues* 5(2):207-215, 1994.

Beecroft PC, Redick SA: Intramuscular injection practices of pediatric nurses: Site selection, *Nurs Educ* 15(4):23-28, 1990.

Centers for Disease Control and Prevention: General recommendations on immunization, *MMWR* 51(RR-2):12-14, 2002.

Cook IF, Murtagh J: Needle length required for intramuscular vaccination of infants and toddlers: An ultrasonographic study, *Austral Fam Phys* 31(3):295-297, 2002.

Daly JM, Johnston W, Chung Y: Injection sites utilized for DPT immunizations in infants, *J Comm Health Nurs* 9(2):87-94, 1992.

Davenport JM: A systematic review to ascertain whether the standard needle is more effective than a longer or wider needle in reducing the incidence of local reaction in children receiving primary immunization, *J Adv Nurs* 46(1):66-77, 2004.

Diggle L: The administration of child vaccines, part 11, Childhood vaccinations, *Practice Nurse* 25(12):63-69, 2003.

Diggle L, Deeks J: Effect of needle length on incidence of local reactions to routine immunisation in infants aged 4 months: Randomised controlled trial, *BMJ* 321(7266):931-933, 2000.

Diggle L, Deeks JJ, Pollard AJ: Effect of needle size on immunogenicity and reactogenicity of vaccines in infants: Randomized controlled trial, *BMJ* 333(7568): 571, 2006.

Groswasser J, Kahn A, Bouche B, and others: Needle length and injection technique for efficient intramuscular vaccine delivery in infants and children evaluated through an ultrasonographic determination of subcutaneous and muscle layer thickness, *Pediatrics* 100(3 Pt 1):400-403, 1997.

Guyatt GH, Oxman AD, Vist GE, and others: GRADE: An emerging consensus on rating quality of evidence and strength of recommendations, *BMJ* 336(7650): 924-926, 2008.

Winslow EH, Jacobson AF: Research for practice: Pediatric IM injections: One size does not fit all, *Am J Nurs* 97(11):20, 1997.

Zuckerman J: The importance of injecting vaccines into muscle, *BMJ* 321(7271): 1237-1238, 2000.

## Subcutaneous and Intradermal Administration

Obtain necessary equipment.

Explain procedure to child as developmentally appropriate, and provide atraumatic care. (See Atraumatic Care box on p. 241.)

Maintain aseptic technique, and follow Standard Precautions.

Any site may be used where there are relatively few sensory nerve endings and large blood vessels and bones are relatively deep.

Suggested sites:

- Center third of lateral aspect of upper arm
- Abdomen
- Center third of anterior thigh
- (Avoid the medial side of arm or leg, where skin is more sensitive.)

After injection:

- Clean area of prepping agent with water to decrease absorption of agent in neonate.
- Praise child for cooperation.
- Discard syringe and needle in puncture-resistant container near site of use.
- Record date, time, dose, drug, and site of injection.

### Needle Size and Insertion

Use 26- to 30-gauge needle; change needle before skin puncture if it pierced a rubber stopper on a vial.

Prepare area for puncture with antiseptic agent. Inject small volumes (up to 0.5 ml).

### Subcutaneous Administration

Pinch tissue fold with thumb and index finger.

Using a dartlike motion, insert needle at a 90-degree angle (Figure 4-17). (Some practitioners use a 45-degree angle on children with little subcutaneous tissue or those who are dehydrated. However, the benefit of using the 45-degree angle rather than the 90-degree angle remains controversial.)

Aspirate for blood. (Some practitioners believe it is not necessary to aspirate before injecting subcutaneously; however, this is not universally accepted. Automatic injector devices do not aspirate before injecting.)

Inject medication slowly without tracking through tissues.

### Intradermal Administration

Spread skin site with thumb and index finger if needed for easier penetration.

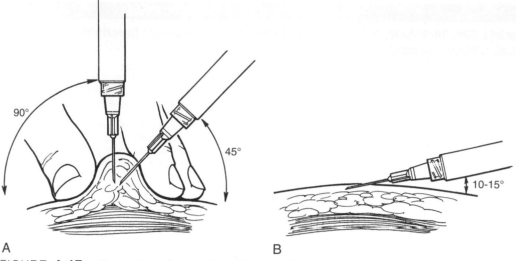

FIGURE **4-17** Comparison of the angles of insertion for injections. A, Subcutaneous (90 degrees or 45 degrees). B, Intradermal (10 to 15 degrees).

Insert needle with bevel up and parallel to skin.

Aspirate for blood.

Inject medication slowly.

### Use of Indwelling Catheter (Insuflon) for Subcutaneous Administration of Insulin

Small indwelling catheter is placed in the subcutaneous tissues.

The average indwelling time is 3 to 5 days.

The catheter is most often inserted in the abdomen, but the buttocks and other areas can also be used. Topical anesthetic cream is recommended before insertion.

Needles 10 mm or shorter should be used for injecting to avoid penetration of the tubing of the catheter.

Using indwelling catheters for up to 4 to 5 days does not affect the absorption of insulin.

The long-term (measured by HbA1c) and short-term glucose control (measured by blood glucose profiles and insulin levels) is not altered.

The dead space of the catheter is about 0.5 unit of U100, so it may be necessary to give 0.5 units extra with the first dose after insertion if the child uses small doses.

### Family Education: Safe Disposal of Needles and Lancets

The growing number of persons being cared for in home settings has increased the amount of medical waste that communities must properly dispose of to prevent accidental needlesticks and the spread of diseases such as hepatitis and human immunodeficiency virus. Many states have programs to assist with the disposal of sharps such as needles and lancets to prevent environmental contamination and accidental mishaps involving needle exposures. Contact one of the resources listed below to obtain further information about needle disposal in your state, or discuss the proper disposal of sharp medical equipment with your local home care agency.

If your state or community does not have programs for safe needle disposal, an option is to place sharps such as needles or lancets in a rigid container such as a bleach bottle or aluminum coffee can. Place the lid on the container to prevent accidental needle exposure. Once the container is about three-quarters full and ready to be discarded, you may add to it a liquid mixture such as cement or plaster to harden the contents and prevent needle exposure. Special devices that break off the needle into a rigid container are also available in some communities.

Additional information is available at Coalition for Safe Community Needle Disposal, 800-643-1643, *www.safeneedledisposal.org;* and Environmental Protection Agency, *www.epa.gov/osw/nonhaz/industrial/medical/disposal.htm.*

## Intravenous Administration

SASH is one way to remember several key steps in IV medication administration: Saline-Administer medication-saline-Heparin, if indicated.

Inspect insertion site to make certain the catheter is secure.

Assess the status of IV infusion to determine that it is functioning properly; this may be done by flushing the line with Saline or flushing and then aspirating a blood return.

Dilute the drug in an amount of solution according to the following:

- Compatibility with infusion fluids or other IV medications child is receiving
- Size of the child
- Size of the vein being used for infusion
- Length of time over which the drug is to be administered (e.g., 30 minutes, 1 hour, 2 hours)
- Rate at which the drug is to be infused
- Strength of the drug or the degree to which it is toxic to subcutaneous tissues
- Need for fluid restriction

Administer the medication

Medication is not completely administered until solution in tubing has infused also (amount of solution depends on tubing length and diameter). Flush the tubing with saline to clear the tubing of the medication.

If the line is a dormant or intermittent line that does not have fluids continuously infusing, heparin may be indicated to ensure patency; see Evidence-Based Practice box and Table 4-7.

## COMMUNITY FOCUS

### Preventing Intravenous Site Infection

With the increasing use of intravenous (IV) therapy in the community, preventing infection is essential. The most effective ways to prevent infection of an IV site are to cleanse hands and wear gloves when inserting an IV catheter. Proper education of the patient and family regarding signs and symptoms of an infected IV site can help prevent infections from going unnoticed.

| TABLE 4-7 | IV Catheter Flushes for Lines without Continuous Fluid Infusions |
|---|---|
| Peripheral lines (Heplock/Saline locks) | Normal saline* after medications or every 8 hours for dormant lines; Instill 2½ times tubing volume |
| | 24 g catheters: Normal saline* or heparin 2 units/ml 2 ml |
| Midline | Heparin 10 units/ml; 3 ml in a 10-ml syringe† after medications or every 8 hours if dormant |
| | Newborns: Heparin 1-2 units/ml to run continuously at ordered rate |
| External central line (nonimplanted, nontunneled, tunneled, or peripherally inserted central catheter [PICC]) | Heparin 10 units/ml; 3 ml in a 10-ml syringe† after medications or once daily if dormant |
| | Newborns: Heparin 2 units/ml; 2-3 ml after medications or to check line patency OR heparin 1-2 units/ml to run continuously at ordered rate |
| Totally implanted central line (TIVAS, implanted port) | Heparin 10 units/ml; 5 ml after medications or once daily if dormant and accessed. If not accessed, Heparin 100 units/ml; 5 ml every month |
| Arterial and central venous pressure continuous monitored lines | Heparin 2 units/ml in 55-ml syringe to run continuously at 1 ml/hr |

*Use $D_5W$ when medication is incompatible with saline.
†Smaller syringes may be used when flush is delivered by a pump.

## EVIDENCE-BASED PRACTICE

### Normal Saline or Heparinized Saline Flush Solution in Pediatric Intravenous Lines

**Ask the Question**

Is there a significant difference in the longevity of intravenous (IV) intermittent infusion locks in children when normal saline (NS) is used as a flush instead a heparinized saline (HS) solution?

**Search for the Evidence**

*Search Strategies*

Selection criteria included evidence during the years 1992 to 2008 with the following terms: *saline versus heparin intermittent flush, children's heparin lock flush, heparin lock patency, peripheral venous catheter in children.*

*Databases Used*

CINAHL, PubMed

**Critically Analyze the Evidence**

**Grade criteria:** Evidence quality moderate; recommendation strong (Guyatt, Oxman, Vist, and others, 2008)

- A systematic Cochrane Review by Shah, Ng, and Sinha (2005) revealed 10 studies that were randomized or quasi-randomized trials of HS administration versus NS, placebo, or no treatment in neonates. The authors of the review concluded that the heterogeneity among the studies, variability in methodologic quality and clinical details, and variability in reporting outcomes resulted in no strong evidence regarding the effectiveness and safety of heparin in prolonging catheter life in neonates.
- No significant statistical difference was found between HS and NS flushes for maintaining catheter patency in children (Hanrahan, Kleiber, and Fagan, 1994; Kotter, 1996; Schultz, Drew, and Hewitt, 2002; Hanrahan, Kleiber, and Berends, 2000; Heilskov, Kleiber, Johnson, and others, 1998; Mok, Kwong, and Chan, 2007).
- Several studies reported increased incidence of pain or erythema with HS flushing of infusion devices (Hanrahan, Kleiber, and Fagan, 1994; Robertson, 1994; Nelson and Graves, 1998; McMullen, Fioravanti, Pollack, and others, 1993).
- Several studies found increased patency and/or longer dwell times with HS solutions versus NS in 24-gauge catheters (Mudge, Forcier,

*Continued*

4 - EVIDENCE-BASED PEDIATRIC NURSING INTERVENTIONS

# EVIDENCE-BASED PRACTICE

## Normal Saline or Heparinized Saline Flush Solution in Pediatric Intravenous Lines—cont'd

and Slattery, 1998; Danek and Noris, 1992; Beecroft, Bossert, Chung, and others, 1997; Gyr, Burroughs, Smith, and others, 1995; Hanrahan, Kleiber, and Berends, 2000; Tripathi, Kaushik, and Singh, 2008).

- Younger children and preterm neonates with lower gestational ages were associated with shorter patency of IV catheters (Paisley, Stamper, Brown, and others, 1997; Robertson, 1994; McMullen, Fioravanti, Pollack, and others, 1993; Tripathi, Kaushik, and Singh, 2008).
- Infusion devices flushed with NS lasted longer than those flushed with HS (Nelson and Graves, 1998; Le Duc, 1997; Goldberg, Sankaran, Givelichian, and others, 1999).
- When measured and reported, length of time between flushing peripheral devices affected dwell time (Crews, Gnann, Rice, and others, 1997; Gyr, Burroughs, Smith, and others, 1995).
- None of the studies cited anticoagulation-associated complications with HS, which is a concern in preterm neonates, who are at higher risk for development of clotting problems as a result of heparin (Klenner, Fusch, Rakow, and others, 2003).
- The American Society of Hospital Pharmacists (ASHP) 2006 Position Statement asserts that 0.9% sodium chloride injection is safe for maintaining patency of peripheral locks in adults and children over age 12 years.
- The 2006 Infusion Nurses Society policy manual indicates that either preservative-free heparin or preservative-free 0.9% sodium chloride may be used to flush a peripheral IV; however, the appendix includes a notation that catheter patency may be maintained by flushing with saline when converting from continuous to intermittent use.

## Apply the Evidence: Nursing Implications

- Further research is still needed with larger samples of children, especially preterm neonates, using small-gauge catheters (24 gauge) and other gauge catheters, flushed with NS and HS as intermittent infusion devices only (no continuous infusions); variables to be considered include catheter dwell time; medications administered; period between regular flushing and flushing associated with medication administration; pain, erythema, or other localized complications; concentration and amount of heparin solutions used; flush method (positive pressure technique versus no specific technique); reason for IV device removal; and complications associated with either solution.
- NS is a safe alternative to HS flush in infants and children with intermittent IV locks larger than 24 gauge; smaller neonates may benefit from HS flush (longer dwell time), but the evidence is inconclusive for all weight ranges and gestational ages.

## References

ASHP Commission on Therapeutics: ASHP therapeutic position statement on the institutional use of 0.9% sodium chloride injection to maintain patency of peripheral indwelling intermittent infusion devices, *Am J Health Syst Pharm* 63(13):1273-1275, 2006.

Beecroft PC, Bossert E, Chung K, and others: Intravenous lock patency in children: Dilute heparin versus saline, *J Pediatr Pharm Practice* 2(4):211-223, 1997.

Crews BE, Gnann KK, Rice MH, and others: Effects of varying intervals between heparin flushes on pediatric catheter longevity, *Pediatr Nurs* 23(1):87-91, 1997.

Danek GD, Noris EM: Pediatric IV catheters: efficacy of saline flush, *Pediatr Nurs* 18(2):111-113, 1992.

Goldberg M, Sankaran R, Givelichian L, and others: Maintaining patency of peripheral intermittent infusion devices with heparinized saline and saline: A randomized double blind controlled trial in neonatal intensive care and a review of literature, *Neonatal Intensive Care* 12(1):18-22, 1999.

Guyatt GH, Oxman AD, Vist GE, and others: GRADE: An emerging consensus on rating quality of evidence and strength of recommendations, *BMJ* 336(7650): 924-926, 2008.

Gyr P, Burroughs T, Smith K, and others: Double blind comparison of heparin and saline flush solutions in maintenance of peripheral infusion devices, *Pediatr Nurs* 21(4):383-389, 1995.

Hanrahan KS, Kleiber C, Berends S: Saline for peripheral intravenous locks in neonates: Evaluating a change in practice, *Neonat Netw* 19(2):19-24, 2000.

Hanrahan KS, Kleiber C, Fagan C: Evaluation of saline for IV locks in children, *Pediatr Nurs* 20(6):549-552, 1994.

Heilskov J, Kleiber C, Johnson K, and others: A randomized trial of heparin and saline for maintaining intravenous locks in neonates, *J Soc Pediatr Nurs* 3(3):111-116, 1998.

Infusion Nurses Society: *Policies and procedures for infusion nursing*, ed 3, Norwood, Mass, 2006, The Society.

Klenner AF, Fusch C, Rakow A, and others: Benefit and risk of heparin for maintaining peripheral venous catheters in neonates: A placebo-controlled trial, *J Pediatr* 143(6):741-745, 2003.

Kotter RW: Heparin vs. saline for intermittent intravenous device maintenance in neonates, *Neonat Netw* 15(6):43-47, 1996.

Le Duc K: Efficacy of normal saline solution versus heparin solution for maintaining patency of peripheral intravenous catheters in children, *J Emerg Nurs* 23(4): 306-309, 1997.

McMullen A, Fioravanti ID, Pollack D, and others: Heparinized saline or normal saline as a flush solution in intermittent intravenous lines in infants and children, *MCN* 18(2):78-85, 1993.

Mok E, Kwong TK, Chan ME: A randomized controlled trial for maintaining peripheral intravenous lock in children, *Int J Nurs Pract* 13(1):33-45, 2007.

Mudge B, Forcier D, Slattery MJ: Patency of 24-gauge peripheral intermittent infusion devices: A comparison of heparin and saline flush solutions, *Pediatr Nurs* 24(2):142-149, 1998.

Nelson TJ, Graves SM: 0.9% Sodium chloride injection with and without heparin for maintaining peripheral indwelling intermittent infusion devices in infants, *Am J Heath Syst Pharm* 55:570-573, 1998.

Paisley MK, Stamper M, Brown T, and others: The use of heparin and normal saline flushes in neonatal intravenous catheters, *J Pediatr Nurs* 23(5):521-527, 1997.

Robertson J: Intermittent intravenous therapy: A comparison of two flushing solutions, *Contemp Nurs* 3(4):174-179, 1994.

Schultz AA, Drew D, Hewitt H: Comparison of normal saline and heparinized saline for patency of IV locks in neonates, *Appl Nurs Res* 15(1):28-34, 2002.

Shah PS, Ng E, Sinha AK: Heparin for prolonging peripheral intravenous catheter use in neonates, *Cochrane Database Syst Rev* (4):CD002774, 2005.

Tripathi S, Kaushik V, Singh V: Peripheral IVs: factors affecting complications and patency—A randomized controlled trial, *J Infus Nurs* 31(3):182-188, 2008.

# Procedures Related to Fluid Balance, Blood Administration, or Nutrition Support

## Intravenous Fluid Administration

Characteristics of pediatric administration sets may be as follows:

- Small-gauge catheters (22 to 24 gauge)
- For longer-term administration, consider a midline catheter, peripherally inserted central catheter (PICC), central venous catheter, or implanted port

Sites are as follows:

- Superficial veins of the upper extremities are preferred, then the foot
- Scalp veins (infants)
- A site is chosen that restricts the child's movements as little as possible (e.g., avoid a site over a joint)
- For extremity veins, start with most distal site, especially if irritating or sclerosing agents are to be used

Maintain integrity of IV site.

Maintain strict asepsis, and follow Standard Precautions.

Use small, padded armboard if IV is inserted at a joint or movement restricts flow.

Provide adequate protection of site.

Observe for signs of infiltration, which may include erythema, pain, edema, blanching, streaking on the skin along the vein, and darkened area at the insertion site.

Change IV tubing and solution at regular intervals (no less than 72 hours) according to institution's policy.

Electronic infusion pumps are routinely used with infants and children.

### Precautions

Assess drip rate by assessing amount infused in a given length of time.

Excess buildup of pressure can occur when the:

- Drip rate is faster than vein can accommodate
- Catheter is out of vein lumen

## Procedure for Inserting and Taping a Peripheral Intravenous Catheter

Choose catheter insertion site and an alternative site in case the initial attempt is unsuccessful. A transilluminator can be useful in identifying suitable veins.

Prepare insertion site by applying with friction an antiseptic solution.

Allow solution to dry completely, but do not blow, blot dry, or fan the area.

Put on gloves.

Apply tourniquet when site is ready for catheter insertion.

Stretch the skin taut downward below the point of insertion, upward above the site of insertion, or from underneath level with the point of insertion. This technique helps stabilize veins that roll or move away from the catheter as attempts are made to enter the vein.

Inspect catheter, looking for damage (e.g., bent stylet, shavings on the catheter, frayed catheter tip [follow employer's policy for reporting defective devices]). Look closely at the IV catheter before inserting it, and note that the stylet tip is slightly longer than the catheter. It is necessary to have both pieces inside the vein before the catheter is advanced.

Insert catheter through the skin, bevel up, at a 30-degree angle, and enter the vein. This direct approach is best for large veins and allows the skin and vein to be entered in one step. The indirect approach for smaller veins enables the catheter to enter the vein from the side perpendicularly. It is sometimes helpful with short veins

to start the catheter below the intended site and advance through the superficial layers of skin so that the advancement of the catheter in the vein is a shorter distance. In infants or children with very small veins, insert the catheter bevel down, which prevents the needle from puncturing the back wall of the vein and provides an earlier flashback of blood as the vein is entered.

Watch for blood return in the flashback chamber; brands and sizes of safety catheters vary in the way flashback is seen.

Once the flashback is seen, lower the angle between the skin and catheter to 15 degrees. Advance the catheter another $\frac{1}{16}$ to $\frac{1}{8}$ inch to ensure that both the metal stylet and the catheter are inside the vein. Holding the stylet steady, push the catheter off the stylet and into the vein until the catheter hub is situated against the skin at the insertion site. Activate safety mechanism if necessary (some safety catheters are passive and activate automatically), remove the stylet, and discard into sharps container. Apply pressure to catheter within the vein to prevent backflow of blood before attachment of tubing.

Collect blood if ordered. Remove the tourniquet. Flush the IV line with NS to check for patency (ease of flushing fluid, lack of resistance while flushing), complaints of pain, or swelling at the site. If line flushes easily, proceed to secure the catheter to the skin.

Connect the T-connector, J-connector, injection cap, or tubing, and reinforce connection with a junction securement device (Luer-Lok, clasping device, threaded device) to prevent accidental disconnection and subsequent air embolism or blood loss.

Place transparent dressing across catheter hub, up to but not including the junction securement device, and surrounding skin.

Further secure the catheter to the skin using tape or adhesive securement devices (e.g., StatLock). Follow manufacturer's directions for adhesive anchors.

Place a $\frac{1}{4}$- to $\frac{1}{2}$-inch strip of clear tape across the width of the transparent dressing and the catheter hub, but avoid the insertion site. This will serve as an anchor tape strip, and all other tape will be affixed to this strip (tape-on-tape method). This strip will not compromise the transparent dressing properties or interfere with visual inspection of the catheter-skin insertion site.

To stabilize the catheter and junction securement device, attach 1 to $1\frac{1}{2}$ inches of clear tape that is $\frac{1}{4}$ to $\frac{1}{2}$ inch wide, adhesive side up, to the underneath side of the catheter hub and junction securement device at their connection. Wrap the ends of the tape around the connections, and meet on top to form a **V** shape (sometimes referred to as a *chevron*); secure the overlapping ends onto the anchor tape strip.

Loop the IV tubing away from the catheter hub and toward the IV fluid source. Secure the looped tubing with a piece of tape on the anchor tape strip. Be certain fingers or toes are visible whenever extremity is used.

Consider use of a commercial protective device (e.g., I.V. House) over the catheter hub and looped tubing. Bending one corner of the tape over and onto itself provides a free tab to lift the tape easily for site visualization.

---

# EVIDENCE-BASED PRACTICE

## Use of Transillumination Devices in Obtaining Vascular Access

Jennifer L. Sanders

### Ask the Question
In children, do transillumination devices decrease the number of attempts needed to obtain vascular access?

### Search the Evidence
**Search Strategies**
Search selection criteria included English language publications, research-based articles on children undergoing venipuncture.

**Databases Used**
PubMed, Cochrane Collaboration, MD Consult, BestBETs

### Critically Analyze the Evidence
**Grade criteria:** Evidence quality low; recommendation strong (Guyatt, Oxman, Vist, and others, 2008)

Five articles were found regarding the efficacy of transillumination. All concluded that transillumination aids in decreasing the number of access attempts.

- Forty cases were described in which transillumination was used to decrease the number of peripheral intravenous (PIV) attempts. In these patients, small superficial veins that were not previously visualized or palpated were visualized using the transillumination device. Far fewer attempts were needed, and PIV access of infants and obese children was easier for staff (Kuhns, Martin, Gildersleeve, and others, 1975).
- One article reviewed the safety (related to heat and burns) of transillumination devices. No burns were reported in a sample of 10 neonates, even when the transillumination device was used for up to 20 minutes (Curran, 1980).
- A letter to the editor focused on the method of using two fiberoptic lights as a venous transilluminator. PIV access was usually successful on the first attempt because of the increased visualization of the superficial venous anatomy (Dinner, 1992).
- A sample of 100 infants ages 2 to 36 months was evaluated for PIV access using a simple otoscope for transillumination. In 40 of the 100 infants, a vein was visible using the otoscope for transillumination. In 23 of these children, transillumination was used after a vein could not be visualized or palpated. In 17 others, one previous attempt to gain

PIV access had failed. With transillumination, 39 of 40 PIV attempts were successful on the first attempt. One patient required a second attempt (Goren, Laufer, Yativ, and others, 2001).
- A sample of 240 patients was randomized to receive PIV access either with or without transillumination with the Veinlite. Patients were either younger than age 3 years and required elective insertion of an IV, or were ages 3 to 21 years with a chronic illness who were previously identified as having difficult access. Those patients in the Veinlite group were significantly more likely to have a successful IV insertion on the first or second attempt (Katsogridakis, Seshadri, Sullivan, and others, 2005).

### Apply the Evidence: Nursing Implications
- Transillumination should be used before PIV access to decrease the number of attempts needed to successfully obtain access.
- Education and practice in this technique are needed for success. Since the veins stand out so clearly with transillumination, they appear more superficial than they are.
- An assistant may be needed to hold the device when using the transilluminator to obtain PIV access.
- The heat and temperature of the transilluminator should be monitored to prevent injury to the patient's skin.
- Appropriate equipment should be used to increase the likelihood of visualization of the vasculature.

### References
Curran JS: A restraint and transillumination device for neonatal-arterial/venipuncture: Efficacy and thermal safety, *Pediatrics* 66(1):128-130, 1980.

Dinner M: Transillumination to facilitate venipuncture in children (letter to editor), *Anesthesiol Analg* 74(3):467-477, 1992.

Goren A, Laufer J, Yativ N, and others: Transillumination of the palm for venipuncture in infants, *Pediatr Emerg Care* 17(2):130-131, 2001.

Guyatt GH, Oxman AD, Vist GE, and others: GRADE: An emerging consensus on rating quality of evidence and strength of recommendations, *BMJ* 336(7650):924-926, 2008.

Katsogridakis Y, Seshadri R, Sullivan C, and others: Veinlite transillumination in the pediatric emergency department: A therapeutic interventional trial, available at *www.veinlite.com/public.html* (accessed August 2005).

Kuhns LR, Martin AJ, Gildersleeve S, and others: Intense transillumination for infant venipuncture, *Radiology* 116(3):734-735, 1975.

## EVIDENCE-BASED PRACTICE

### Peripheral Intravenous Care

Joy Hesselgrave

### Ask the Question
In children, what site preparation and stabilization measures for peripheral intravenous catheters (PIVs) are optimum for preventing complications and extending dwell time?

### Search for Evidence
#### Search Strategies
Search selection criteria included English language and research-based publications within the past 20 years on PIV site care.

#### Databases Used
National Guidelines Clearinghouse (AHQR), Cochrane Collaboration, Joanna Briggs Institute, PubMed, TRIP Database Plus, MD Consult, PedsCCM, BestBETs

### Critically Analyze the Evidence
Grade criteria: Evidence quality low; recommendation strong (Guyatt, Oxman, Vist, and others, 2008)

#### Site Preparation
Multiple studies cited as the basis of the Centers for Disease Control and Prevention recommendations by O'Grady, Alexander, Dellinger, and others (2002) indicate that the skin should be disinfected with an appropriate antiseptic before PIV catheter insertion. A 2% chlorhexidine-based preparation is preferred, but tincture of iodine, an iodophor, or 70% alcohol can be used. Allow the antiseptic to air dry before catheter insertion. There is no recommendation at this time for the use of chlorhexidine in infants younger than 2 months old.

The Infusion Nurses Society (2006) recommends cleansing the skin with a preparation that combines alcohol with either chlorhexidine gluconate or povidone-iodine before PIV insertion. For neonates, all disinfectants have risks. Chlorhexidine gluconate with alcohol should not be used in neonates; aqueous chlorhexidine or povidone-iodine should be used in premature infants. Remove cleansers from infants using sterile water or NS to prevent absorption of the disinfectant (Association of Women's Health, Obstetric and Neonatal Nurses, 2007).

#### Stabilization or Securement Devices
A prospective study of 105 PIV placements compared a control group using traditional transparent dressing (Tegaderm) and tape with a study group that used transparent dressings and a catheter securement device (StatLock) (Wood, 1997). The control group had a 65% complication rate (dislodgments, infiltration, and phlebitis) versus a 20% complication rate in the study group, indicating a 45% reduction in overall PIV therapy complications in the study group.

When comparing tape, StatLock, and Hub-Guard for a 96-hour PIV protocol change, researchers found that PIVs with StatLock produced a statistically significant improved survival rate (52%) compared with tape (8%) or HubGuard (9%) (Smith, 2006). Securement devices may extend the life of a PIV.

#### Dwell Time
In pediatric patients, PIV catheters may remain in place until a complication occurs or the therapy is complete (O'Grady, -Alexander, Dellinger, and others, 2002).

Results of a prospective study of 525 pediatric patients with PIVs determined that the overall risk of PIV catheter complication was extremely low and would not be reduced substantially by routine catheter replacement (Shimandle, Johnson, Baker, and others, 1999).

### Apply the Evidence: Nursing Implications
- For children older than 2 months, chlorhexidine is the preferred skin cleanser. For younger infants, nonalcohol-based cleansers are preferred and should be removed with sterile water or sterile NS to prevent absorption.
- Select a vein that is most distal on the extremity and allows the child optimum movement (avoid over the joint). Veins on the scalp may be used in infants. Subsequent PIVs should be proximal to the previous IV site.
- If the child is mobile, consider using a securement or protection device (e.g., StatLock, HubGuard, Ray-Marshall Shield, IV House, IV Shield, IV Pro).
- Discontinue PIV if complications occur or when it is no -longer needed.

### References
Association of Women's Health, Obstetric and Neonatal Nurses: *Neonatal skin care 2nd edition evidence-based clinical practice guideline*, Washington, DC, 2007, The Association.

Guyatt GH, Oxman AD, Vist GE, and others: GRADE: An emerging consensus on rating quality of evidence and strength of recommendations, *BMJ* 336(7650):924-926, 2008.

Infusion Nurses Society: *Policies and procedures for infusion nursing*, ed 3, South Norwood, Mass, 2006, The Society.

O'Grady N, Alexander M, Dellinger E, and others: Guidelines for the prevention of intravascular catheter–related infections, *MMWR Morb Mortal Wkly Rep* 51(32), 2002.

Shimandle R, Johnson D, Baker M, and others: Safety of peripheral intravenous catheters in children, *Infect Control Hosp Epidemiol* 20:736-740, 1999.

Smith B: Peripheral intravenous catheter dwell times: a comparison of three securement methods for implementation of a 96-hour scheduled change protocol, *J Infus Nurs* 29(1):14-17, 2006.

Wood D: A comparative study of two securement techniques for short peripheral intravenous catheters, *J Intraven Nurs* 20(6):280-285, 1997.

4 - EVIDENCE-BASED PEDIATRIC NURSING INTERVENTIONS

## EVIDENCE-BASED PRACTICE

### Frequency of Changing Intravenous Administration Sets

Brandi Horvath

### Ask the Question

In children, should intravenous (IV) administration sets be changed at 24, 48, 72, or 96 hours to safely prevent patient infection while containing costs?

### Search the Evidence

#### Search Strategies

Search selection criteria included English language publications within past 10 years, and research-based articles on frequency of changing IV administration sets.

#### Databases Used

National Guideline Clearinghouse (AHRQ), Cochrane Collaboration, Joanna Briggs Institute, PubMed, Infusion Nurses Society, Oncology Nurses Society, MD Consult, BestBETs, TRIP Database Plus, PedsCCM

### Critically Analyze the Evidence

**Grade criteria:** Evidence quality moderate; recommendation strong (Guyatt, Oxman, Vist, and others, 2008)

A systematic Cochrane review by Gillies, O'Riordan, Wallen, and others (2005) identified the optimum interval for the routine replacement of IV administration sets when infusate or parenteral nutrition solutions are administered. Data results from 13 randomized or quasi-randomized controlled trials were pooled to compare different time intervals of administration set changes: every 24 hours versus 48 hours or greater, 48 hours versus at least 72 hours, and 72 hours versus 96 hours. Findings revealed no evidence that changing IV administration sets more often than every 96 hours reduces the incidence of bloodstream infection. There were no differences in results between patients with central and peripheral catheters and those who did or did not receive parenteral nutrition. For IV administration sets including blood or blood products and lipids, the researchers recommend changing the sets every 24 hours.

The Centers for Disease Control and Prevention (O'Grady, Alexander, Dellinger, and others, 2002) recommends changing IV administration sets for crystalloids at no more than 72-hour intervals. Rates of phlebitis were not substantially different for administration sets left in place 96 hours compared with 72 hours. For tubing used to administer blood and blood products or lipid emulsions, replace tubing within 24 hours of starting the infusion.

The Infusion Nurses Society (2006) and Alexander (2006) recommend replacing continuously infusing IV administration sets no more frequently than every 72 hours. Administration sets used intermittently should be changed every 24 hours. Secondary piggyback sets may be changed no more frequently than every 72 hours when attached to a continuously infusing line; once detached from the primary set, they should be changed at 24 hours. Exceptions include sets used with lipids (change at 24 hours if continuous or after each unit if intermittently infused) and blood or blood components (change at the end of 4 hours if continuous or after each intermittent component). All sets should be changed immediately if contamination is suspected.

The Oncology Nursing Society (Camp-Sorreli, 2004) recommends replacing IV administration sets every 96 hours or with catheter change, except for fluids that enhance microbial growth. Tubing used to administer blood, blood products, lipids, or total parenteral nutrition should be replaced 24 hours after initiation of therapy.

### Apply the Evidence: Nursing Implications

- Replace IV administration sets every 96 hours.
- Replace tubing used for lipid emulsions, blood, and blood products every 24 hours.
- Replace blood tubing with in-line filters after 2 units or 4 hours, whichever comes first.

### References

Alexander M, editor: Infusion nursing standards of practice, *J Infus Nurs* 29(1S):S48-S50, 2006.

Camp-Sorreli D, editor: *Access device guidelines: Recommendations for nursing practice and education*, ed 2, Pittsburgh, 2004, Oncology Nursing Society.

Gillies D, O'Riordan L, Wallen M, and others: Optimal timing for intravenous administration set replacement. In *The Cochrane Database of Systematic Reviews* 2005, Issue 4, Article No. CD003588.pub2. DOI: 10.1002/14651858. CD003588.pub2.

Guyatt GH, Oxman AD, Vist GE, and others: GRADE: An emerging consensus on rating quality of evidence and strength of recommendations, *BMJ* 336(7650): 924-926, 2008.

Infusion Nurses Society: *Policies and procedures for infusion nursing*, ed 3, South Norwood, Mass, 2006, The Society.

O'Grady N, Alexander M, Dellinger E, and others: Guidelines for the prevention of intravascular catheter-related infections, *MMWR Morb Mortal Wkly Rep* 51(RR-10):1-29, 2002.

# Hydration

Diarrheal illnesses are a common cause of dehydration in infants and children. Vomiting may precede diarrhea in acute gastroenteritis. Prevention of dehydration may be possible with increased fluid intake early after onset of illness. Dehydration signs and treatments are presented in Chapter 1, pages 80-81.

Preventing dehydration during diarrheal illnesses

1. Provide more fluids than usual to prevent dehydration: Pedialyte, Gastrolyte, Infalyte, other commercial oral rehydration solution (ORS), or World Health Organization oral rehydration salt packet mixed in 1 liter of water.
   - Avoid fluids high in sugar or caffeine: carbonated drinks (non-diet sodas), sports drinks, fruit juices or flavored juice drinks, tea, and coffee.
   - After every loose stool, provide
     - Children younger than 2 years: 50 to 100 ml
     - Children 2 to 10 years: 100 to 200 ml
     - Children older than10 years: as much as child wants
2. Give the child plenty of food to prevent undernutrition.
   - Breast-feeding should be continued without interruption.
   - Infants taking a cow milk–based formula should continue the full-strength formula.
   - For children old enough to eat, give soft or semisolid foods and offer small, frequent feedings every 3 to 4 hours.

3. Change the plan if the child's diarrhea stops (return to normal diet) or if the child develops signs of dehydration.

## Correcting Mild to Moderate Dehydration during Diarrheal Illnesses

1. Provide more fluids than usual; give only rehydration fluids for first 3 to 4 hours (see above for types to give and to avoid).
2. If the child is vomiting, give the following
   - Children younger than 2 years: 5 ml every 3 to 5 minutes by medication spoon or syringe (without needle)
   - Children over 2 years: 5 to 10 ml every 5 to 10 minutes; increase amount as tolerated.
   - If the child is breast-fed, continue breast-feeding in addition to administering oral rehydration fluids.
3. If the child will drink more than the estimated amount of fluid and is not vomiting, give more.
4. If the child vomits again, wait 10 minutes and then continue giving oral fluid.
5. Reassess at 4 hours. If sufficient rehydration has been achieved, progress to the refeeding diet (Table 4-8). If ORS therapy has failed or if severe dehydration occurs, then boluses of isotonic IV fluid will likely be required. Subsequent IV fluid therapy will typically be administered at 1.5 to 2 times maintenance in order to accomplish sufficient rehydration (Box 4-1).

---

| TABLE 4-8 | Foods to Consider for a Child with Gastroenteritis |
|---|---|
| **Foods to Consider** | **Foods to Keep Away From** |
| 1% to 2% milk or skim milk; low-fat yogurt; Lactaid milk if suspected lactose intolerance | Whole milk and whole milk products; if lactose intolerance is suspected, avoid all regular milk and milk products |
| Breast milk, all infant formulas if tolerated (Isomil DF, Lactofree, or Similac Lactose Free if symptoms of lactose intolerance are present); Pediasure or other appropriate supplements | |
| Gatorade, oral rehydration solutions such as Pedialyte, Enfalyte, Rehydralyte; diet sodas in limited quantities | Regular soft drinks, caffeine-containing drinks, fruit juices, high sugar–containing drinks . |
| Low-fat grilled or baked meat, fish, or poultry; boiled or poached eggs | High-fat or fried meats, fish, or poultry; fried eggs |
| Low-fat cheeses | High-fat or fried cheeses |
| Any boiled or baked legumes without added fat; peanut butter in small amounts (<2 Tbsp) | Peanut butter in large amounts |
| Low-fat soups and broth with other allowed foods | High-fat creamed soups or chowders |
| Canned (packed in own juice) peaches, pears, applesauce, bananas | Canned fruit packed in heavy syrup; fruit juices |
| Most breads or cereals | Donuts, muffins, bran muffins, wheat germ |
| Rice, baked or mashed potatoes, pasta | Cereal with nuts, coconut, or granola; bran cereals, high-sugar cereals |
| | Fried foods |
| Angel food cake, vanilla wafers, graham crackers, and other low-fat cookies, cakes, and desserts; diet Jello and sugar-free popsicles in limited quantities | Ice cream, sherbet, pies, popsicles, puddings, chocolate, and other high-fat/high-sugar desserts |
| Spices, salt, mustard, ketchup, pickles in limited amounts | Highly seasoned foods, sugar, honey, jelly, syrup |

## ⊝ Family Education: Dehydration and Diarrhea*

- Limit exposure to other children (e.g., day care).
- Encourage continued breastfeeding with infants.
- Use ORS for mild and moderate dehydration.
- Begin refeeding diet once oral fluids are tolerated and sufficient rehydration is achieved.
- Encourage the use of the refeeding diet until symptoms have resolved 1 to 3 days.
- Advance to regular diet once symptoms have resolved.

| BOX 4-1 | Holliday-Segar Method |
|---|---|

4 mL/kg/h for first 10 kg of body weight
2 mL/kg/h for second 10 kg of body weight
1 mL/kg/h for each kg over 20 kg

From Johns Hopkins Hospital: *The Harriet Lane handbook,* ed 19, St Louis, 2011, Elsevier.

# Blood Product Administration

Nursing administration of blood components and nursing care of the child receiving blood components are discussed in Tables 4-9 and 4-10.

## EVIDENCE-BASED PRACTICE

### Catheter Gauge for Blood Transfusions in Children

Marilyn J. Hockenberry

#### Ask the Question
In children, what is the smallest gauge catheter that can be used to administer blood products?

#### Search the Evidence
**Search Strategies**
Search selection criteria included English language research-based studies.

**Databases Used**
PubMed, American Association of Blood Banks, Intravenous Nurses Society, MD Consult

#### Critically Analyze the Evidence
**Grade criteria:** Evidence quality low; recommendation strong (Guyatt, Oxman, Vist, and others, 2008)

Six research-based articles were reviewed (1981 to 2004). All studies used an in vitro experimental design to evaluate hemolysis during simulated transfusion of red blood cells (RBCs). Two studies (Levin, Jesurun, Darden, and others, 1986; Herrera and Corless, 1981) used catheters as small as 27 gauge and found no significant hemolysis. Wong, Schreiber, Criss, and others (2004) evaluated the feasibility of RBC transfusion through a small-bore central venous catheter (1.9F = 23-gauge catheter) and found no significant hemolysis. Three additional studies used catheters larger than 23 gauge and also found no hemolysis (Frelich and Ellis, 2001; De la Roche and Gauther, 1993; Wilcox, Barnes, and Mondanlou, 1981).

A search for national published guidelines found that the American Association of Blood Banks (2004, 1999) states that RBCs can be administered safely through 23- to 25-gauge needles.

#### Apply the Evidence: Nursing Implications
Small-gauge intravenous catheters can be used to safely to administer PRBCs. Considerations should be made for pediatric patients requiring massive transfusions.

#### References
American Association of Blood Banks: *Primer of blood administration,* Bethesda, Md, 2004, The Association.
American Association of Blood Banks: *Blood transfusion therapy,* Bethesda, Md, 1999, The Association.
De la Roche MR, Gauther L: Rapid transfusion of packed red blood cells: Effects of dilution, pressure and catheter size, *Ann Emerg Med* 22(10):1551-1555, 1993.
Frelich R, Ellis MH: The effect of external pressure, catheter gauge, and storage time on hemolysis in RBC transfusion, *Transfusion* 41(6):799-802, 2001.
Guyatt GH, Oxman AD, Vist GE, and others: GRADE: An emerging consensus on rating quality of evidence and strength of recommendations, *BMJ* 336(7650):924-926, 2008.
Herrera AJ, Corless J: Blood transfusions: Effect of speed of infusion and of needle gauge on hemolysis, *J Pediatr* 99(5):757-758, 1981.
Levin GS, Jesurun CA, Darden J, and others: Hemolysis of transfused packed red blood cells, *Perinatol Neonatol* 10:39-42, 1986.
Wilcox GJ, Barnes A, Mondanlou H: Does transfusion using a syringe infusion pump and small-gauge needle cause hemolysis? *Transfusion* 21(6):750-751, 1981.
Wong EC, Schreiber S, Criss VR, and others: Feasibility of red blood cell transfusion through small bore central venous catheters used in neonates, *Pediatr Crit Care Med* 5(1):69-74, 2004.

*Adapted from the World Health Organization, Geneva, Switzerland; and Centers for Disease Control and Prevention: Managing acute gastroenteritis among children: oral rehydration, maintenance, and nutritional therapy, *MMWR* 52(RR-16):1-16, 2003. For more information on oral rehydration see the Rehydration Project website at *www.rehydrate.org.*

| TABLE 4-9 | Blood Components and Nursing Administration | | |
|---|---|---|---|
| **Components and Indications** | **Dose** | | **Nursing Administration** |
| **Packed red blood cells (PRBCs)**<br>Symptomatic anemia<br>Renal or liver disease<br>Hemolysis<br>Decreased erythropoiesis<br>Thalassemia major<br>Splenic or liver sequestration | Volume packed RBC =<br>weight (kg) × change in<br>hematocrit (Hct) desired | | 1. Regulate infusion rate using microaggregate filter via infusion pump at 5 ml/kg/hr over 1-2 hours (usual rate). Change the filter after 1-2 units of blood are infused or after 4 hours.<br>2. Monitor vital signs before transfusion, 15 minutes after initiation, and every hour until the end of transfusion. |
| **Whole blood (rarely used)**<br>Acute massive blood loss | Volume of whole blood =<br>weight (kg) × change in<br>Hct desired × 2 | | 3. Do not refrigerate blood in the nursing unit. Only the blood bank refrigerator may be used.<br>4. Ensure that each unit is infused in 4 hours or less. If a longer infusion time is needed, the unit must be divided in the blood bank.<br>5. Do not infuse solutions other than normal saline in the line with RBCs. |
| **Fresh frozen plasma (FFP)**<br>Deficiencies of plasma clotting factors in bleeding patients (e.g., disseminated intravascular coagulopathy [DIC]), liver failure, vitamin K deficiency with bleeding, or replacement of antithrombin III (ATIII), protein C, or protein S | 10-15 ml/kg (use within<br>6-24 hours of thawing) | | 1. Use microaggregate filter over 1-2 hours every 12-24 hours until hemorrhage stops at a rate of 20 ml/min.<br>2. Monitor prothrombin time (PT) and partial thromboplastin time (PTT) before and after FFP.<br>3. Monitor levels of other coagulation factors (e.g., fibrinogen, fibrin split products, D-dimer, ATIII, protein C, and protein S). |
| **Platelets (plt)**<br>Active hemorrhage, DIC<br>Thrombocytopenia with bleeding or indicated by clinical status | 1 unit/10 kg or 6 units/m² intravenously (IV) | | 1. Regulate infusion rate using 170 μm microaggregate filter at 10 ml/kg/hr, IV push or over 1 hour or as fast as patient can tolerate.<br>2. Monitor vital signs before transfusion, 15 minutes after initiation, and at the end of infusion.<br>3. Obtain postplatelet count 1 to 24 hours after infusion. |
| **Granulocytes (rarely used)**<br>As an adjunct with other measures in treatment of severe infections in the septic neonate or high-risk patient (e.g., proven bacterial infection in severe neutropenic patient nonresponsive to antibiotic therapy) | 10-15 ml/kg IV usually<br>daily × 4 days | | 1. Monitor vital signs before transfusion, 15 minutes after initiation, and at the end of transfusion.<br>2. Premedicate 1 hour before transfusion, usually antihistamines, acetaminophen, or steroids.<br>3. Infuse at slow rate (2-4 hours) using 170-μm blood filter within a 24-hour period.<br>4. Minimum of 4-6 hours between amphotericin B and granulocyte infusion recommended. |
| **Factor VIII (plasma derived or recombinant)**<br>Hemophilia A<br>Acquired factor VIII deficiency | 1 unit/kg IV of factor VIII =<br>2% of factor activity<br>35-50 units/kg IV of factor VIII every 12-24 hours | | 1. Use reconstituted factor within 3 hours of mixing.<br>2. Inject reconstituted factor over 2-5 minutes.<br>3. Assess for signs of an adverse reaction such as hives, itchy wheals with redness, tightness in chest, wheezing, low blood pressure, or trouble breathing. Notify health care provider immediately if symptoms are present. |
| **Factor IX (plasma derived or recombinant)**<br>Hemophilia B | 1 unit/kg IV of factor IX =<br>1% of factor activity<br>30-50 units/kg IV every 24 hours | | |
| **FEIBA (factor eight inhibitor bypass activity) (plasma-derived)**<br>Hemophilia A or B with inhibitors (antibodies) | 75-100 units/kg IV every 8-24 hours (maximum dose 200 units/kg/day | | |
| **Factor VII a (recombinant)**<br>Hemophilia A or B with inhibitors | 90 mcg/kg IV every 2 hours (35-120 mcg/kg) dosage range | | |
| **Cryoprecipitate (CRYO) (rarely used)**<br>Control bleeding in patients with DIC<br>Hypofibrinogenemia | 4 bags CRYO/10 kg IV | | 1. Monitor closely: PT/PTT, fibrinogen, fibrinogen split products, D-dimer.<br>2. Use a filter needle to draw up and administer within 15-30 minutes. |

| TABLE 4-10 | Nursing Care of the Child Receiving Blood Transfusions | |
|---|---|---|
| **Complication** | **Signs and Symptoms** | **Precautions and Nursing Responsibilities** |
| *Immediate Reactions* | | |
| **Hemolytic Reactions** | | |
| Most severe type, but rare<br>Incompatible blood<br>Incompatibility in multiple transfusions | Chills<br>Shaking<br>Fever<br>Pain at needle site and along venous tract<br>Nausea and vomiting<br>Sensation of tightness in chest<br>Red or black urine<br>Headache<br>Flank pain<br>Progressive signs of shock and/or renal failure<br>Often occur within first 15 minutes | Verify patient identification.<br>Identify donor and recipient blood types and groups before transfusion is begun; verify with another nurse or other practitioner.<br>Transfuse blood slowly for first 15-20 minutes or initial 20% volume of blood; remain with patient.<br>Stop transfusion immediately in event of signs or symptoms, maintain patent intravenous (IV) line, and notify practitioner.<br>Save donor blood to recross-match with patient's blood.<br>Monitor for evidence of shock.<br>Insert urinary catheter, and monitor hourly outputs.<br>Send samples of patient's blood and urine to laboratory for presence of hemoglobin (indicates intravascular hemolysis).<br>Observe for signs of hemorrhage resulting from disseminated intravascular coagulation (DIC).<br>Support medical therapies to reverse shock. |
| **Febrile Reactions** | | |
| Most common reaction<br>Leukocyte or platelet antibodies<br>Plasma protein antibodies | Fever<br>Chills<br>Occur within 1-6 hours after transfusion | May give acetaminophen for prophylaxis.<br>Leukocyte-poor RBCs are less likely to cause reaction.<br>Stop transfusion immediately; report to practitioner for evaluation. |
| **Allergic Reactions** | | |
| Recipient reacts to allergens in donor's blood. | Urticaria<br>Pruritus<br>Flushing<br>Asthmatic wheezing<br>Laryngeal edema | Give antihistamines for prophylaxis to children with tendency toward allergic reactions.<br>Stop transfusion immediately.<br>Administer epinephrine for wheezing or anaphylactic reaction. |
| **Circulatory Overload** | | |
| Too rapid transfusion (even a small quantity)<br>Excessive quantity of blood transfused (even slowly) | Sudden severe headache<br>Precordial pain<br>Tachycardia<br>Dyspnea<br>Rales<br>Cyanosis<br>Dry cough<br>Distended neck veins<br>Hypertension | Transfuse blood slowly.<br>Prevent overload by using PRBCs or administering divided amounts of blood.<br>Use infusion pump to regulate and maintain flow rate.<br>Stop transfusion immediately if signs of overload.<br>Place child upright with feet in dependent position. |
| **Air Emboli** | | |
| May occur when blood is transfused under pressure | Sudden difficulty in breathing<br>Sharp pain in chest<br>Apprehension | Normalize pressure before container is empty when infusing blood under pressure.<br>Clear tubing of air by aspirating air with syringe at nearest Y-connector if air is observed in tubing; disconnect tubing and allow blood to flow until air has escaped only if a Y-connector is not available. |
| **Hypothermia** | | |
| | Chills<br>Low temperature<br>Irregular heart rate<br>Possible cardiac arrest | Use approved mechanical blood warmer or electric warming coil to rapidly warm blood; never use microwave oven.<br>Take temperature if patient complains of chills; if subnormal, stop transfusion. |

| TABLE 4-10 | Nursing Care of the Child Receiving Blood Transfusions—cont'd | |
|---|---|---|
| **Complication** | **Signs and Symptoms** | **Precautions and Nursing Responsibilities** |
| *Immediate Reactions* | | |
| **Electrolyte Disturbances** | | |
| Hyperkalemia (in massive transfusions or in patients with renal problems) | Nausea, diarrhea<br>Muscular weakness<br>Flaccid paralysis<br>Paresthesia of extremities<br>Bradycardia<br>Apprehension<br>Cardiac arrest | Use washed RBCs or fresh blood if patient is at risk. |
| *Delayed Reactions* | | |
| **Transmission of Infection** | | |
| | Signs of infection (e.g., jaundice)<br>Toxic reaction: high fever, severe headache or substernal pain, hypotension, intense flushing, vomiting/diarrhea | Blood is tested for antibodies to human immunodeficiency virus (HIV), hepatitis C virus, and hepatitis B core antigen; in addition, blood is tested for hepatitis B surface antigen (HBsAg) and alanine aminotransferase (ALT), and a serology test is performed for syphilis; positive units are destroyed; individuals at risk for carrying certain viruses are deferred from donation.<br>Report any sign of infection and, if occurring during transfusion, stop transfusion immediately, send sample for culture and sensitivity tests, and notify physician. |
| **Alloimmunization** | | |
| (Antibody formation)<br>Occurs in patients receiving multiple transfusions | Increased risk of hemolytic, febrile, and allergic reactions | Use limited number of donors.<br>Observe carefully for signs of reactions. |
| **Delayed Hemolytic Reaction** | | |
| | Destruction of RBCs and fever 2-10 days after transfusion (anemia, jaundice, dark urine) | Observe for posttransfusion anemia and decreasing benefit from successive transfusions. |

# Peripherally Inserted Central Catheters

### Description
Single or multiple lumen available
Inserted into antecubital fossa and passed through basilic or cephalic vein into superior vena cava (SVC)
Positioning of tip in SVC maximizes hemodilution and reduces likelihood of vessel wall damage, phlebitis, or thrombus formation

### Benefits
Do not require operating room placement
Can be inserted by specially trained RNs
Can use small insertion needles
Fast placement

### Care Considerations
Sometimes difficult to thread into SVC
Reports of resistance to removal
Not suitable for rapid fluid replacement because of small lumen size
Five- to 10-ml syringe is used for flushing to prevent catheter wall rupture

# Long-Term Central Venous Access Devices

## Tunneled Catheter (e.g., Hickman/ Broviac Catheter)
### Description
One or two Dacron cuffs or Vitacuffs (biosynthetic material impregnated with silver ions) on catheter(s) enhance tissue ingrowth.

May have more than one lumen (Figure 4-18)

### Benefits
Reduced risk of bacterial migration after tissue adheres to Dacron cuff or Vitacuff

Easy to use for self-administered infusions

### Care Considerations
Requires daily heparin flushes

Must be clamped or have clamp nearby at all times

Must keep exit site dry

Heavy activity restricted until tissue adheres to cuff

Risk of infection still present

Protrudes outside body; susceptible to damage from sharp instruments and may be pulled out; may affect body image

More difficult to repair

Patient and family must learn catheter care

### Dressings for Tunneled Catheters
A dressing may not be required to prevent infection for catheters that have been in place for prolonged periods. However, dressings may be used to secure the catheter from dislodgement or breakage. Typically, a clear, transparent dressing will be used that allows visualization of the skin around the tube at least daily.

Removal of old dressings may be facilitated by applying adhesive remover. Gently peel off one edge of the dressing at a time. Another technique that is more comfortable to some children is to grasp opposite corners and pull them away from each other to stretch and loosen the dressing, then grasp the two remaining corners and pull.

Cleansing technique is specific to the cleanser used. See Evidence-Based Practice: Central Venous Catheter Site Care for a discussion of cleansers. ChloraPrep™ is applied using a back and forth motion and requires at least 30 seconds to dry. Povidone iodine is applied in a circular motion, beginning at the catheter and moving outward; it requires at least two minutes drying time.

The catheter is looped around the entry site and under the dressing (Figure 4-19). Secure the end of the tube with tape to prevent dangling and dislodgement or damage.

## Implanted Ports (e.g., Port-A-Cath, Infusaport, Mediport, Norport)
### Description
Totally implantable metal or plastic device that consists of self-sealing injection port with top or side access with preconnected or attachable silicone catheter that is placed in large blood vessel

### Benefits
Reduced risk of infection

Placed completely under the skin; therefore cannot be pulled out or damaged

Heparinized monthly and after each infusion to maintain patency

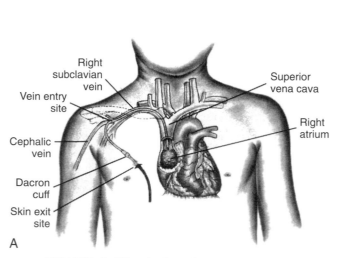

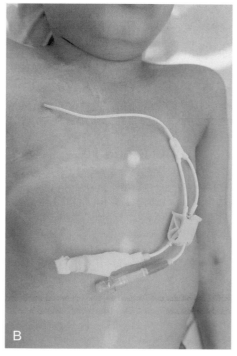

FIGURE **4-18** A, Central venous catheter insertion and exit site. B, External venous catheter.

Can remain in place for years

No limitations on regular physical activity, including swimming

Dressing needed only when Huber needle is in place

No or only slight change in body appearance (slight bulge on chest)

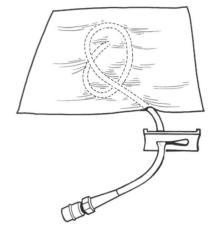

FIGURE **4-19**    Tunneled catheter dressing.

### *Care Considerations*

Must pierce skin for access; pain with insertion of needle; can use local anesthetic (EMLA, LMX, buffered lidocaine, or vapocoolant) before accessing port

Special noncoring needle (Huber) with straight or angled design must be used to inject into port (Figure 4-20).

Hard to manipulate for self-administered infusions

Catheter may dislodge from port, especially if child plays with port site.

Vigorous contact sports generally not allowed

Overlying skin should be protected from irritation by avoiding clothing, straps, and seat belts placing pressure on the port area.

## Family Education: Central Venous Catheters

- Signs of infection: fever, chills, pain or redness, site drainage, shortness of breath, chest pain
- Maintaining catheter patency via flushing
- Keep skin dry around the insertion site when bathing using special shower dressings or plastic wrap
- What to do if the catheter breaks (most require clamping; the Groshong does not)
- Site/needle protection during infusions through implanted ports

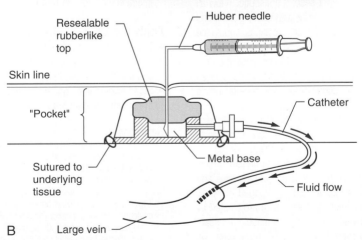

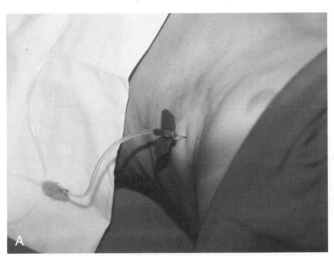

FIGURE **4-20**    A, Implanted venous access device with Huber placement. B, Side view of the implanted port.

## Central Venous Catheter Site Care

Brandi Horvath

### Ask the Question

In children with central venous catheters (CVC), is chlorhexidine gluconate a more effective antiseptic solution than povidone-iodine in preventing CVC-related site infections and bacteremia?

### Search the Evidence
#### Search Strategies
Search selection criteria included English language publications within the past 10 years and research-based articles on catheter site care and chlorhexidine.

#### Databases Used
The National Guideline Clearinghouse (AHRQ), Centers for Disease Control and Prevention (CDC), Cochrane Collaboration, Joanna Briggs Institute, PubMed, Infusion Nurses Society, Oncology Nurses Society, MD Consult, BestBETs, TRIP Database Plus

### Critically Analyze the Evidence
**Grade criteria:** Evidence quality moderate; recommendation strong (Guyatt, Oxman, Vist, and others, 2008)

The CDC (O'Grady, Alexander, Dellinger, and others, 2002) recommends the use of 2% chlorhexidine for disinfecting catheter site before insertion (allow to dry), but tincture of iodine, an iodophor, or 70% alcohol can be used. Iodine needs to remain on the skin for at least 2 minutes or until dry. No recommendations can be made for the use of chlorhexidine in infants younger than 2 months of age. No recommendations can be made regarding the use of topical antibiotic ointments or creams due to the potential to promote fungal infections and antimicrobial resistance. No recommendations are made for the use of impregnated catheters and chlorhexidine sponge dressings to reduce the incidence of infection. Avoid use of sponges in infants less than 7 days old and less than 26 weeks' gestation. Replace the catheter-site dressing when it becomes damp, loosened, or soiled or when inspection of the site is necessary. Replace dressings used on short-term CVC sites every 2 days for gauze dressings and at least every 7 days for transparent dressings, except in those pediatric patients in whom the risk for dislodging the catheter outweighs the benefit of changing the dressing.

The Infusion Nurses Society (2006) recommends the use of alcohol, chlorhexidine gluconate, povidone-iodine, and tincture of iodine. If using povidone-iodine, do not apply alcohol as a second antiseptic. Allow all antiseptics to air dry. Dress vascular access site with sterile gauze, and cover with sterile transparent dressings. Gauze dressings should be changed every 48 hours. Semipermeable transparent dressings should be changed at least every 7 days, and the interval is dependent on the dressing material, age and condition of the patient, infection rate reported by the organization, environmental conditions, and manufacturer's labeled uses and directions.

The Oncology Nursing Society (Camp-Sorrell, 2004) finds chlorhexidine for preinsertion and postinsertion site catheter care superior to alcohol and povidone-iodine. No recommendations are made for the use of chlorhexidine sponge dressing. Routine application of antibiotic ointment is not recommended because of the risk of fungal infections and antimicrobial resistance. Gauze dressings should be changed every 48 hours. Semipermeable transparent dressings over gauze are treated as gauze dressings and changed every 48 hours. Semipermeable transparent dressings should be changed every 5 to 7 days or more often, as indicated.

Three evidence-based systematic reviews were found regarding CVC site care.

- In a nursing evidence-based review by Carson (2004), most studies found chlorhexidine to be superior to povidone-iodine for preventing microbial colonization of the CVC insertion site and catheter tip and for decreasing the risk of local site infection. However, there is still conflicting evidence regarding the efficacy of chlorhexidine versus povidone-iodine for preventing CVC-related bacteremia.
- In a metaanalysis of eight studies by Chaiyakunapruk, Veenstra, Lipsky, and colleagues (2002), chlorhexidine reduced the risk of catheter-related bloodstream infections by 49% compared with povidone-iodine. In a follow-up review (Chaiyakunapruk, Veenstra, Lipsky, and others, 2003), the use of chlorhexidine rather than povidone-iodine for site care led to a cost savings of $113 for each catheter used.
- In a systematic review focused on bone marrow transplant recipients, chlorhexidine is the recommended antisepsis for prevention of catheter-related infection (Zitella, 2003).

Four randomized, controlled trials were found comparing chlorhexidine and povidone-iodine in various populations.

- Chambers, Sanders, Patton, and others (2005) found that chlorhexidine sponge dressings (Biopatch) reduced the incidence of exit-site or tunnel infections of central venous catheters in adult neutropenic patients.
- In the study conducted by Garland, Alex, Mueller, and colleagues (2001), 705 neonates and infants in the Biopatch group had a substantial decrease in colonized catheter tips compared with the group that used standard dressings but no difference in rates of catheter-related bloodstream infections or bloodstream infections without a source between the two groups. However, Biopatch was associated with localized contact dermatitis in infants of very low birth weight.
- In the study conducted by Langgartner, Linde, Lehn, and colleagues (2004), skin disinfection before CVC insertion and daily with dressing changes with propanol-chlorhexidine followed by povidone-iodine was associated with the lowest rate of microbial catheter colonization.
- In a study conducted by Levy, Katz, Solter, and colleagues (2005) in a pediatric cardiovascular intensive care unit, patients with chlorhexidine-impregnated CVC dressing (Biopatch) had a significantly reduced risk of CVC colonization compared with patients with transparent dressing alone. Occurrence of catheter-related bloodstream infection was not different in the two groups.

### Apply the Evidence: Nursing Implications
- Two percent chlorhexidine should be used for catheter site antisepsis.
- Two percent chlorhexidine should be used with caution in premature and low-birth-weight infants.
- Chlorhexidine-impregnated sponges (Biopatch) should be used around the catheter site except in patients older than 2 months of age.

### References
Camp-Sorrell D, editor: *Access device guidelines: recommendations for nursing practice and education*, ed 2, Pittsburgh, 2004, Oncology Nursing Society.

Carson S: Chlorhexidine versus povidone-iodine for central venous catheter site care in children, *J Pediatr Nurs* 19(1):74-80, 2004.

Chaiyakunapruk N, Veenstra D, Lipsky B, and others: Vascular catheter site care: The clinical and economic benefits of chlorhexidine gluconate compared with povidone iodine, *Clin Infect Dis* 37(6):764-771, 2003.

Chaiyakunapruk N, Veenstra D, Lipsky B, and others: Chlorhexidine compared with povidone-iodine solution for vascular catheter-site care: A meta-analysis, *Ann Intern Med* 136(11):792-801, 2002.

## EVIDENCE-BASED PRACTICE

### Central Venous Catheter Site Care—cont'd

Chambers S, Sanders J, Patton W, and others: Reduction of exit-site infections of tunneled intravascular catheters among neutropenic patients by sustained-release chlorhexidine dressings: Results from a prospective randomized controlled trial, *J Hosp Infect* 61(1):53-61, 2005.

Garland J, Alex C, Mueller C, and others: A randomized trial comparing povidone-iodine to a chlorhexidine-impregnated dressing for prevention of central venous catheter infections in neonates, *Pediatrics* 107(6):1431-1436, 2001.

Guyatt GH, Oxman AD, Vist GE, and others: GRADE: An emerging consensus on rating quality of evidence and strength of recommendations, *BMJ* 336(7650):924-926, 2008.

Infusion Nurses Society: *Policies and procedures for infusion nursing*, ed 3, South Norwood, Mass, 2006, The Society.

Langgartner J, Linde H, Lehn N, and others: Combined skin disinfection with chlorhexidine/propanol and aqueous povidone-iodine reduces bacterial colonisation of central venous catheters, *Intensive Care Med* 30(6):1081-1088, 2004.

Levy I, Katz J, Solter E, and others: Chlorhexidine-impregnated dressing for prevention of colonization of central venous catheters in infants and children: A randomized controlled study, *Pediatr Infect Dis J* 24(8):676-679, 2005.

O'Grady N, Alexander M, Dellinger EP, and others: Guidelines for the prevention of intravascular catheter-related infections, *MMWR Morb Mortal Wkly Rep* 51(RR-10):1-29, 2002.

Zitella L: Central venous catheter site care for blood and marrow transplant recipients, *Clin J Oncol Nurs* 7(3):289-298, 2003.

## EVIDENCE-BASED PRACTICE

### Obtaining Blood Specimens from Central Venous Catheters in Children

**Joy Hesselgrave**

### Ask the Question

In children, do blood specimens obtained from central venous catheters using the discard, reinfusion, or push-pull method yield more accurate samples?

### Search for Evidence

#### Search Strategies

Search selection criteria included English language research-based publications on pediatric blood specimen collection from central venous access.

#### Databases Used

National Guideline Clearinghouse (AHRQ), Cochrane Collaboration, Joanna Briggs Institute, PubMed, TRIP database Plus, MD Consult, PedsCCM, BestBETs

### Critically Analyze the Evidence

**Grade criteria:** Evidence quality low; recommendation strong (Guyatt, Oxman, Vist, and others, 2008)

Limited scientific research exists that describes the optimal method for drawing blood samples from CVADs in the pediatric patient.

A convenience sample of paired specimens compared blood drawn from central lines via push-pull method and discard method on 28 pediatric patients ages 6 months to 12 years. Of the 438 pairs of measurements that were compared, 420 or 95.9% were within limits of agreement for hemograms, electrolytes, and glucose. The push-pull method eliminates loss of blood and decreases the amount of times the central line is accessed (Barton, Chase, Latham, and others, 2004).

Forty-two nonneutropenic pediatric patients aged 2 to 20 years were randomly assigned to one of two syringe-handling methods for blood sampling. The discard specimen, routinely reinfused, was collected using the usual clean procedure and an exaggerated unclean alternative procedure. Neither the sterile specimens nor the unclean specimens grew organisms, thus suggesting that the reinfusion of the blood specimen would be safe. This study did not evaluate for clots in the discard specimen (Hinds, Wentz, Hughes, and others, 1991).

Thirty bone marrow transplant units were surveyed to evaluate how blood samples were drawn from CVADs. The average patient age was 5 to 16 years. Seventy-five percent of the units used the discard method, with the volume of discard ranging from 0.5 to 10 ml and an average of 4 to 6 ml. Fourteen percent used the reinfusion method, and 11% used the push-pull or mixing method (Keller, 1994).

The Infusion Nurses Society (2011) recommends that the discard method be used when drawing blood samples from CVADs.

The discard volume should be 1.5 to 2 times the fill volume of the CVAD.

Frey (2003) summarizes evidence for the practice of all three blood sampling methods. The discard method is most widely reported, with disadvantages including blood loss, blood exposure risk for clinicians, and the potential to confuse the discard specimen for the blood sample. The reinfusion method does not deplete blood volume but risks blood exposure for clinician and potential to reinfuse a contaminated specimen or clots in the discard volume. The push-pull or mixing method demonstrates accuracy for other than coagulation and drug levels and reduces blood loss and clinician exposure risk.

### Apply the Evidence: Nursing Implications

- There is limited pediatric research that clearly supports any particular central line blood sampling method as being superior. All three methods yield accurate results and appear safe. The discard method is the most frequently reported in the literature and benchmarking. However, if there is a concern about blood volume, the push-pull or reinfusion method should be considered.
- If the catheter has multiple lumens, use the distal lumen for laboratory specimen collection.
- Infusions should be stopped and lumens clamped before blood sampling.
- Cleanse the injection cap with antiseptic agent, and allow to dry before drawing laboratory specimens.
- Attach a syringe or stopcock depending on specimen method selected, to the injection cap, not directly to the catheter hub. The injection cap at the catheter hub should be removed only if blood cultures are drawn.

### References

Barton S, Chase T, Latham B, and others: Comparing two methods to obtain blood specimens from pediatric central venous catheters, *J Pediatr Oncol Nurs* 21(6):320-326, 2004.

Frey M: Drawing blood samples from vascular access devices, *J Infus Nurs* 26(5):285-293, 2003.

Guyatt GH, Oxman AD, Vist GE, and others: GRADE: An emerging consensus on rating quality of evidence and strength of recommendations, *BMJ* 336(7650):924-926, 2008.

Hinds PS, Wentz T, Hughes W, and others: An investigation of the safety of the blood reinfusion step used with tunneled venous access devices in children with cancer, *J Pediatr Oncol Nurs* 8(4):59-64, 1991.

Infusion Nursing Standards of Practice. *J Infusion Nurs* 34(15), 2011.

Keller CA: Methods of drawing blood samples through central venous catheters in pediatric patients undergoing bone marrow transplant: Results of a national survey, *Oncol Nurs Forum* 21(5):879-884, 1994.

**4 - EVIDENCE-BASED PEDIATRIC NURSING INTERVENTIONS**

# Tube Feeding

The purpose of tube feeding is to supply gastrointestinal feeding for the child who is unable to take nourishment by mouth because of anomalies of the throat or esophagus, impaired swallowing capacity, severe debilitation, respiratory distress, or unconsciousness.

## Procedure: Placement of a Nasogastric or Orogastric Tube

1. Place the child supine with the head slightly hyperflexed or in a sniffing position (nose pointed toward ceiling).
2. Measure from tip of nose to earlobe, then to a point midway between the end of xiphoid process and umbilicus for approximate length of insertion (Figure 4-21), and mark the point with a small piece of tape.
3. Lubricate the tube with sterile water or water-soluble lubricant, and insert through one of the nares or the mouth to the predetermined mark. In older infants and children, the tube is passed through the nose and the position alternated between nostrils. An indwelling tube is almost always placed through the nose. Because most young infants are obligatory nose breathers, insertion through the mouth may be used for intermittent gavage feedings because it causes less distress and also helps to stimulate sucking.
   - When using the nose, slip the tube along the base of the nose and direct it straight back toward the occiput.
   - When entering through the mouth, direct the tube toward the back of the throat.
   - If the child is able to swallow on command, synchronize passing the tube with swallowing.
4. Confirm placement by x-ray if available. Document pH and color of aspirate with initial placement and ongoing placement checks (see Evidence-Based Practice box).
5. Stabilize the tube by holding or taping it to the cheek, not to the forehead because of possible damage to the nostril (Figure 4-22). To assist in maintaining correct placement, measure and record the amount of tubing

extending from the nose or mouth to the distal port when the tube is first positioned. Recheck position before each feeding. A hydrocolloid barrier (DuoDerm or Coloplast) may be placed on the cheeks to protect the skin from tape irritation.

## Procedure: Feeding through the Tube

1. Verify placement of the tube.
2. Check residual. For most infant feedings, any amount of residual fluid aspirated from the stomach is refed to prevent electrolyte imbalance, and the amount is

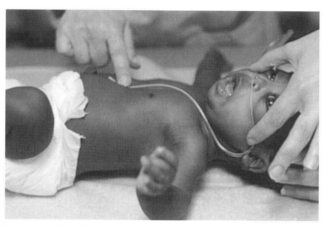

FIGURE **4-21**   Measuring tube for orogastric feeding from tip of nose to earlobe and to midpoint between end of xiphoid process and umbilicus.

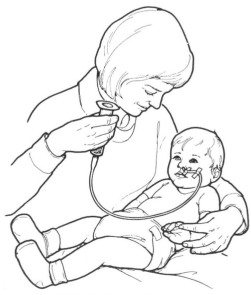

FIGURE **4-22**   Tube securement.

*Text continued on p. 264.*

> ## ! NURSING ALERT
>
> Studies evaluating NG/OG tube length in infants and children found that age-specific methods for predicting the distance based on height is a more accurate prediction of internal distance to the stomach (Beckstrand, Ellett, and McDaniel, 2007; Klasner, Luke, and Scalzo, 2002). The morphologic measure most commonly used by clinicians (nose-ear-xiphoid distance) is often too short to locate the entire tube pore span in the stomach. However, the nose-ear-mid xiphoid umbilicus span approached the accuracy of the age-specific prediction equations and is easier to use in a clinical setting. The best option is to adopt the nose-ear-mid xiphoid umbilicus measurement for NG/OG tube length.

# EVIDENCE-BASED PRACTICE

## Assessing Correct Placement of Nasogastric or Orogastric Tubes in Children

### Marilyn Hockenberry

## Ask the Question

1. What is the most reliable method of predicting correct NG/OG tube placement in infants and children?
2. What steps should be taken when pH testing does not confirm NG/OG correct placement?
3. What pediatric conditions decrease the reliability of gastric pH assessment?
4. How frequently should NG/OG tube placement be verified during intermittent and continuous feedings?
5. What is the most effective method for obtaining NG/OG aspirate for pH testing?

## Search the Evidence

### Search Strategies

English language research studies published in the last 20 years on NG placement verification in infants and children age 0 to 18 years

### Databases Used

Cochrane Collaboration, Agency for Healthcare Research and Quality, PubMed, CINAHL, Up-To-Date, Trip, BestBETS, American Academy of Pediatrics, American Association of Critical-Care Nurses, National Patient Safety Agency—United Kingdom, Association of Women's Health, Obstetric and Neonatal Nurses, National Association of Neonatal Nurses, Joint Commission

### Placement Verification

Observation methods should be combined to confirm tube placement (Ellett, 2004; 2006; Ellett, Croffie, Cohen, and others, 2005; Metheny, Schnelker, McGinnis, and others, 2005; Huffman, Piper, Jarczyk, and others, 2004; Metheny and Stewart, 2002).

#### pH/Color

- Placement should be determined at the bedside by aspirating fluid to examine color and testing the pH. If the pH is <5, then the tube can be presumed in the stomach. Color of gastric aspirate is grassy green, clear and colorless or cloudy white (residual formula). Postpyloric tube aspirate color usually appears golden-yellow, yellow-brown or greenish-brown with a pH >6.

#### Tube Marking

- Once the tube is in place, use an indelible pen to mark the point or document the cm marking where the tube exits the nose/mouth. Compare the marked point on the tube with each NG tube placement evaluation.

#### Physical Symptoms

- Observe for presence of respiratory symptoms (coughing, cyanosis, dyspnea), restlessness/irritability, pallor, mottling, severe discomfort, hoarseness, weak cry, inability to cry. Assessing the patient's physical symptoms remains the most essential component to assuring the tube is properly positioned.

### When pH Does Not Confirm Placement

There is controversy as to whether a chest x-ray (CXR) should be obtained if the pH is >5 to verify proper placement. However, this is often unnecessary if a careful evaluation is completed. If the pH is >5, then continue the assessment of tube placement: evaluate the NG/OG tube marking, and the child's physical symptoms. Evaluate current medications that may be interfering with gastric pH. Determine whether a recent x-ray exists to use as a reference. A risk assessment guideline should be established that provides clear decision points to decide whether a CXR should be ordered (Wilkes-Holmes, 2006; Richardson, Branowicki, Zeidman-Rogers and others, 2006; Huffman, Piper, Jarczyk and others, 2004).

### Conditions That Decrease the Reliability of Gastric Ph Assessment

Gastric fluid volume in infants is small, and obtaining aspirate can be difficult. Newborns have a transient raised gastric pH due to swallowing amniotic fluid. Preterm infants have a reduced ability to produce gastric acid. The benefit of using pH assessment is obvious: If an aspirate can be obtained, a pH <5 will exclude 100% of placements in the lung and 93.9% of placements in the small intestine (Ellett, 2004). Researchers are currently evaluating gastric pH in NICU settings and are finding that while it is difficult to gain aspirate, the pH is almost always <5 in neonates who have been NPO for 2 to 3 hours between bolus feedings and <6 for continuous feedings. Administration of acid inhibiting medications and $H_2$-receptor blockers elevate gastric pH and decrease acid secretion. Researchers support the use of pH testing with a cutoff of 5.9 to 6.0 to assess NG/OG tubes in patients receiving acid inhibitors and $H_2$-receptor blockers (Khair, 2005; Metheny, Stewart, Smith, and others, 1999; Metheny, Reed, Wiersema, and others, 1993). Three studies were specific to children (Ellett, Croffie, Cohen, and others, 2005; Westhus, 2004; Gharpure, Meert, Sarnaik, and others, 2000).

### Frequency of Placement Verification

Tube placement should be verified upon insertion, before intermittent feeds and medication administration, during continuous feeds (frequency not evaluated), and whenever there is concern regarding tube placement.

- Intermittent feedings should have pH, color, and tube marking assessment **prior** to each feeding. If pH >5, wait 30 minutes to 1 hour for gastric pH to reduce, and then retest; (National Patient Safety Agency, 2005; Stevenson, 2005).
- Continuous feedings—Assure tube marking unchanged; pH can be assessed and if <6, it is an appropriate cutoff for patients on continuous feeding regimens (Metheny and Stewart, 2002; Metheny and Titler, 2001). Frequency of assessment is not addressed in these studies.

### Method for Obtaining NG/OG Aspirate for pH Testing

- Aspirate 0.2 to 1 ml of fluid using a 10-ml syringe.
- If unable to obtain aspirate, reposition patient on one side, then the other, and inject 1 to 2 ml of air into the tube using a 10-ml syringe; then try to aspirate fluid again.
- If still unable to obtain aspirate, advance the tube 1 cm and try again.
- Inject 1 to 2 ml of air again, and then try again to aspirate fluid.

*Continued*

**4 - EVIDENCE-BASED PEDIATRIC NURSING INTERVENTIONS**

## EVIDENCE-BASED PRACTICE

### Assessing Correct Placement of Nasogastric or Orogastric Tubes in Children—cont'd

#### References

Ellett M: Important facts about intestinal feeding tube placement, *Gastroenterology Nursing* 29(2):112-124, 2006.

Ellett M: What I know about methods of correctly placing gastric tubes in adults and children, *Gastroenterology Nursing* 27(6):253-259, 2004.

Ellett M, Croffie JM, Cohen MD, and others: Gastric tube placement in young children, *Clinical Nursing Research* 14(3):238-252, 2005.

Gharpure V, Meert KL, Sarnaik AP, and others: Indicators of postpyloric feeding tube placement in children, *Crit Care Med* 28(8):2962-2966, 2000.

Huffman S, Piper P, Jarczyk KS, and others: Methods to confirm feeding tube placement: Application of research in practice, *Pediatr Nurs* 30(1):10-13, 2004.

Khair J: Guidelines for testing the placing of nasogastric tubes, *Nurs Times* 101(20):26-27, 2005.

Metheny NA, Schnelker R, McGinnis J, and others: Indicators of tube site during feedings, *J Neurosci Nurs* 37(6):320, 2005.

Metheny NA, Stewart BJ: Testing feeding tube placement during continuous tube feedings, *Appl Nurs Res* 15(4):254-258, 2002.

Metheny NA, Titler MG: Assessing placement of feeding tubes, *AJN* 101(5):36-45, 2001.

Metheny NA, Stewart BJ, Smith L, and others: pH and concentration of bilirubin in feeding tube aspirates as predictors of tube placement, *Nurs Res* 48(4):189-197, 1999.

Metheny N, Reed L, Wiersema L, and others: Effectiveness of pH measurements in predicting feeding tube placement: An update, *Nurs Res* 42(6):324-331, 1993.

National Patient Safety Agency: Reducing the harm caused by misplaced nasogastric feeding tubes retrieved from www.nrls.npsa.nhs.uk. 2005.

Richardson DS, Branowicki PA, Zeidman-Rogers L, and others: An evidence-based approach to nasogastric tube management: Special considerations, *J Pediatr Nurs* 21(5):388-393, 2006.

Stevenson E: *How to confirm the correct position of naso and orogastric feeding tubes in babies under the care of neonatal units.* London: UK, 2005, National Patient Safety Agency.

Westhus N: Methods to test feeding tube placement in children, *Am J MCN* 29(5):282-287, 2004.

Wilkes-Holmes C: Safe placement of nasogastric tubes in children, *Paediatr Nurs* 18(9):14-17, 2006.

*Procedure: Feeding through the Tube (continued from p. 262).*

subtracted from the prescribed amount of feeding. For example, if the infant is to receive 30 ml and 10 ml is aspirated from the stomach before the feeding, the 10 ml of aspirated stomach contents is refed along with 20 ml of feeding. Another method can be used in children. If residual fluid is more than one fourth of the last feeding, return the aspirate and recheck in 30 to 60 minutes. When residual fluid is less than one fourth of the last feeding, give the scheduled feeding. If large amounts of aspirated fluid persist and the child is due for another feeding, notify the practitioner.

3. Warm the formula to room temperature. Do not microwave.

4. Provide a pacifier for infants to suck on during the feeding. Whenever possible, hold the infant or young child during the feeding to associate the comfort of physical contact with the procedure (Figure 4-23). When this is not possible, place the infant or child supine or slightly toward the right side with head and chest slightly elevated.
   • Use a folded blanket under the head and shoulders for infants and a pillow for small children.
   • Raise the head of the bed for larger children.
   • If possible, allow infant to suck on a pacifier during feeding for association of suck and satiation (feeling satisfied).

5. For feedings delivered by mechanical pump, pour formula into bag or syringe, and prime tubing. Connect to patient and set desired rate.

6. For gravity feedings via syringe, pour formula into the barrel of the syringe attached to the feeding tube. To start the flow, give a gentle push with the plunger, but

then remove the plunger and allow the fluid to flow into the stomach by gravity. To prevent nausea and regurgitation, the rate of flow should not exceed 5 ml every 5 to 10 minutes in preterm and very small infants and 10 ml/min in older infants and children. The rate is determined by the diameter of the tubing and the

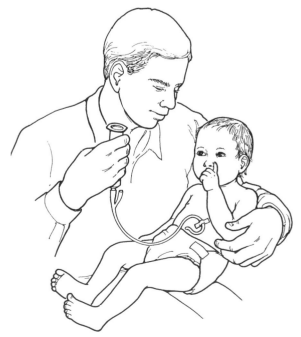

FIGURE **4-23** Comforting child during feeding.

height of the reservoir containing the feeding. The rate is regulated by adjusting the height of the syringe. A typical feeding may take 15 to 30 minutes to complete.

7. Flush the tube with sterile water: 1 or 2 ml for small tubes; 5 to 15 ml or more for large ones.

8. Cap or clamp indwelling tubes to prevent loss of feeding. If the tube is to be removed, first pinch it firmly to prevent escape of fluid as the tube is withdrawn, then withdraw the tube quickly.

9. Position the child with the head elevated about 30 to 45 degrees or on the right side for 30 to 60 minutes in the same manner as following any infant feeding to minimize the possibility of regurgitation and aspiration. If the child's condition permits, bubble the youngster after the feeding.

10. Record the feeding, including the type and amount of residual, the type and amount of formula, and the manner in which it was tolerated. For most infant feedings, any amount of residual fluid aspirated from the stomach is refed to prevent electrolyte imbalance. The amount is subtracted from the prescribed amount of feeding. For example, if the infant or child is to receive 30 ml, and 10 ml is aspirated from the stomach before the feeding, the 10 ml of aspirated stomach contents are refed, plus 20 ml of feeding. Another method in children is that if residual is more than one fourth of the last feeding, then aspirate is returned and rechecked in 30 to 60 minutes. When residual is less than one fourth of last feeding, give scheduled feeding. If high aspirates persist and the child is due for another feeding, notify the practitioner.

11. Between feedings, give infants pacifiers to satisfy oral needs.

## Family Education: NG/OG Tube Feedings

- Insertion technique
- Placement verification
- Call health care provider for: vomiting, change in color of stomach contents, increased amount of stomach contents before feeding, increased bowel movements, irritability, inability to insert tube, or missing two meals because of too much food in the stomach

## Nasoduodenal and Nasojejunal Tubes

Children at high risk for regurgitation or aspiration such as those with gastroparesis, mechanical ventilation, or brain injuries may require placement of a postpyloric feeding tube. Insertion of a nasoduodenal or nasojejunal tube is done by a trained practitioner because of the risk of misplacement and potential for perforation in tubes requiring a stylet. Accurate placement is verified by radiography. Small-bore tubes may easily clog. Flush tube when feeding is interrupted, before and after medication administration, and routinely every 4 hours or as directed by institutional policy. Tube replacement should be considered monthly to ensure optimal tube patency.

### *Feeding Procedure*

Continuous feedings are delivered by mechanical pump to regulate volume and rate. Bolus feeds are contraindicated. Tube displacement is suspected in the child showing signs of feeding intolerance such as vomiting. Stop feedings and notify practitioner.

## Gastrostomy Tubes

The gastrostomy tube is placed with the patient under general anesthesia or percutaneously using an endoscope with the patient under local anesthesia (typically known as percutaneous endoscopic gastrostomy [PEG]). The tube can be a Foley, skin level wing tip, or mushroom catheter G-button. Skin level/G-button devices are cosmetically pleasing in appearance (Figure 4-24), afford increased comfort and mobility to the child, are easy to care for, are fully immersible in water, and have a one-way valve that minimizes reflux and eliminates the need for clamping. Gastrostomy tubes need to be changed periodically.

To prevent tube clogging, medication tablets should be crushed well and mixed with water or food before instillation. Thick liquids can be mixed with warm water to make them thinner. Periodically, flush devices used for continuous feedings with 5 to 10 ml water.

Clean the skin around the gastrostomy each day with mild soap and water. G-buttons should be turned around in a complete circle to ensure that they are clean and without encrusted formula. Small amounts of leakage (less than 5 ml) may occur upon occasion; continual leaking, leaking large amounts, or skin breakdown around the site should be reported. Skin barriers may be used. Balloon inflation should be checked weekly to ensure that correct amount of water is in the balloon. Dress the child in loose-fitting clothing that does not press the gastrostomy tube against the skin. Bib-type overalls cover the tube, making it less likely that the child or other children will play with the tube.

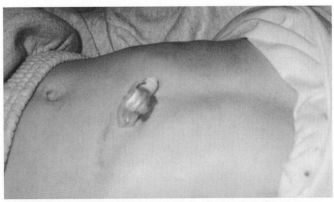

FIGURE **4-24**    Example of skin level device (G-button).

### Feeding Procedure

Positioning and feeding of water, formula, and pureed foods are carried out in the same manner and rate as NG feedings. A mechanical pump may be used to regulate the volume and rate of feeding. With some skin-level devices that do not lock, the child must remain fairly still, because the tubing may easily disconnect from the device if the child moves. Some devices require a tube other than the feeding tube to be used for stomach decompression; some do not. After feedings, the infant or child is positioned on the right side or in Fowler position; the tube may be clamped or left open between feedings, depending on the child's condition.

If the skin-level device is used, insert the extension tube (or decompression tube, in some devices) to remove air in the stomach. This will reduce leaking.

If a Foley catheter is used as the gastrostomy tube, very slight tension is applied and the tube securely taped to maintain the balloon at the gastrostomy opening. This prevents leakage of gastric contents and the tube's progression toward the pyloric sphincter, where it may occlude the stomach outlet. As a precaution, the length of the tube should be measured postoperatively and remeasured each shift to be sure it has not slipped. A mark can be made above the skin level to further ensure its placement. Tube holders are available commercially to assist with tube stabilization.

# Ostomy Care Procedures

This is a brief overview of ostomy care procedures. Consult a Wound/Ostomy/Continence (WOC) nurse for more information, or see the resource list later in this chapter for additional literature.

## Changing Ostomy Pouch

### Materials Needed

Ostomy pouch—One- or two-piece pouches of appropriate type and size and indication (fecal ostomy versus urostomy). A urostomy pouch has a spout opening at the bottom and is appropriate for urine and liquid stool. A drainable ostomy pouch has a large opening at the bottom for thicker stool.

Ostomy closure—Disposable closure provided in box of pouches or reusable clamp to close pouch. Some pouches have a built-in closure so that no additional closure is needed.

Ostomy pattern or measuring guide and marker—This can be a paper backing from a previous pouch that was cut out or a measuring guide found in a box of pouches.

Curved ostomy scissors—Can also use manicure scissors if there is not a starter hole in the pouch wafer.

Barrier paste/strips/rings—Caulking pectin barrier that fills in crevices and skin folds to flatten pouching surface or is placed around the stoma to prevent leaking. Stoma paste usually contains alcohol and may sting if skin is irritated; paste strips and rings may not contain alcohol.

Liquid skin barrier—Skin sealant or barrier wipes protect the peristomal skin from epidermal stripping by applying a clear film to the skin and may improve pouch adhesion in high humidity. Many contain alcohol and can sting denuded skin. Use an alcohol-free skin sealant for infants.

Washcloth or soft paper towel—To cleanse skin with warm water. Do not use a baby wipe to cleanse the skin because many of these contain lanolin, which interferes with the pouch adhering.

Mild soap—Use a mild soap that does not contain moisturizers, lotions, or deodorizers, which can leave a film on the skin and interfere with the pouch adhering.

Stoma powder (optional)—Apply only if peristomal skin is broken, reddened, or denuded. Dust off excess amount before pouching, leaving a thin layer of powder. May use a liquid skin barrier to pat over the powder to assist pouch to seal.

### Procedure

Place child supine, and empty pouch.

If the pouch is leaking, note where the leak is coming from under the wafer.

Using a warm cloth, gently *push* down on the child's abdomen and *pull* up a corner of the pouch. Work your way circumferentially around the stoma, removing the pouch.

Discard the pouch, saving the ostomy closure if it is a plastic reusable type clamp.

Gently cleanse the peristomal skin with warm water and soap if needed. It is normal for the stoma to bleed a little when the cloth rubs against it; this does *not* hurt the child. Allow area to dry thoroughly.

Assess the stoma for color, edema, retraction, bleeding, and prolapse. Assess the peristomal skin to decide what additional products are needed to treat any sign of irritation.

Measure the stoma with a previous pattern or measuring guide, and place the pattern on the pouch wafer to trace. The stoma opening can be cut off-center to move the pouch away from umbilicus or an incision if needed. Do not cut beyond the cutting guide printed on the pouch wafer. The stoma's measurements may change for up to 6 weeks after surgery.

Cut out the pouch wafer, taking care to lay it over the stoma repeatedly until the wafer fits completely and easily over the stoma without more than ⅛ inch of peristomal skin exposed.

If skin is reddened or denuded, apply stoma powder to dry peristomal skin and dust off excess.

Apply a liquid skin barrier to protect peristomal skin, and let dry.

Peel pouch wafer paper, and apply barrier paste, strips, and rings directly around opening cut out for stoma. A syringe may be used to deliver the stoma paste in a thin bead closely around the opening on an infant or toddler ostomy pouch. Barrier paste and strips may also be placed directly on the child's skin to fill in deep crevices, skin folds, or problematic areas for leakage.

Turn the pouch over, and place the pouch on the skin. Ensure that the skin is clean and dry. If stool has seeped onto the skin, clean off with a moist cloth and let dry. It is helpful to apply the pouch at an angle away from the body with the opening down toward the feet if the child is in diapers. If the child is up walking, the pouch can be placed straight down or angled inward for ease in emptying between the legs into the toilet.

Press the wafer down around the stoma to ensure that it is sealed, and place your hand over the wafer for 1 to 2 minutes to warm it and allow it to melt into the skin. The pouch can also be warmed between the hands before peeling off the paper backing and applying.

Apply the pouch closure, and put supplies away. If using a disposable bendable closure, wrap pouch end around the closure three or four times and bend ends tightly. If using a plastic reusable clamp, fold end of pouch *one time* over the smooth end of the clip and snap closed. Save new paper pattern from pouch wafer if needed.

## Pouching Tips

Empty the child's pouch when it is ⅓ to ½ full to prevent it from becoming too heavy and pulling off or leaking.

Choose a quiet time to change an infant's ostomy pouch, such as when the infant is sleepy, or have someone hold the infant's hands while the pouch is changed.

Release gas (flatus) build-up in pouch by opening bottom of pouch, or apply filter to pouch. If pouch gets too taut, it may pull away and leak.

Deodorizing ostomy drops and powders may be placed inside the pouch. Do *not* spray a nonstomy deodorizer inside the pouch, but it can be used in the room away from the child's face.

If the child has a candidal (yeast) rash around the stoma, apply an antifungal powder in place of a stoma powder. Remove pouch every 48 hours, and retreat for 7 to 10 days.

Warm soapy water may be placed inside a small squirt bottle and flushed up inside the pouch to cleanse the pouch of its contents.

Cuffing the bottom of the pouch before emptying the pouch will help keep the ends clean and free of odor. Clean the pouch ends with toilet paper or moist toilet cloths or baby wipes. The pouches are odor proof.

Pediatric ostomy pouches are designed to adhere for 2 to 3 days. Adult ostomy pouches usually adhere for 5 to 7 days.

Incorporate the child in his or her own care as much as possible, as appropriate for age.

Measure a growing child's stoma weekly or whenever a previous pattern is no longer effective.

Urostomy pouches can be attached to a urinary collection container at night.

## Bathing and Hygiene

The child can bathe with the ostomy pouch on or off. If the pouch is left on, ensure that the edges are dried thoroughly when the bathing is finished. If the pouch is taken off, soap and water will not harm the stoma. The stoma may become active during the bath, but to limit this occurrence, bathe 1 hour before or 2 hours after the child eats. Dry the skin thoroughly before replacing the pouch.

## Clothing

There are no restrictions regarding types of clothing. The child can wear items that are form-fitting or loose. Tighter clothing that contains Spandex or Lycra and nylons do not harm the stoma nor hinder the stool output. Do make sure belts and elastic waistbands do not rub across the stoma. One-piece bathing suits with skirts are flattering for girls, and one-piece wetsuits work well for boys. Onesies for infants, overalls for toddlers, and one-piece sleepers keep hands away from pouches and prevent pouches from getting pulled off. Place pouch inside diaper to help keep pouch secure and prevent it from catching on clothing or getting pulled off.

## Diet and Medications

There are no diet restrictions for an infant. There are no diet restrictions for an older child if he or she has a colostomy.

If an older child has an ileostomy, there are specific foods that are fibrous and difficult to digest that can cause a blockage. Instruct the child to eat slowly and chew well, cut food up into small pieces, and encourage plenty of fluids to help prevent blockages.

Foods that commonly cause blockages include the following:

- Raw fruits and vegetables, especially celery
- Peelings of apples and potatoes
- Mcat with casing (bologna, sausage)
- Popcorn
- Seeds in fruit and vegetables
- Peanuts and other nuts

Consult a WOC nurse regarding additional information on foods that cause blockages, how to treat a blockage, and foods that cause excess gas and odors.

Children with an ileostomy are at risk for becoming dehydrated because they do not have a colon to reabsorb water back into the body. Instruct parents on signs and symptoms of dehydration that can occur from diarrhea, vomiting, or sweating and when to call the doctor or go to the emergency room. Encourage plenty of fluids that replenish sodium and potassium, such as oral rehydration solutions and sports drinks.

Time-released medications may not be absorbed if the child has an ileostomy. Encourage parents to let their pharmacist know that their child has an ileostomy each time they fill a new prescription.

## Activities and School

There are no activity restrictions for infants with ostomies. Infants can lie and play on their stomach and can be hugged and held against an adult without concern of harming the stoma. Keep the pouch tucked into a diaper or under clothing so it is not pulled off while the child is crawling.

All activities including swimming and playing sports are generally allowed for children after obtaining a release from the surgeon. A WOC nurse can be consulted for more information about extra protective gear (stoma cups and pouch belts) during contact sports. Waterproof ostomy tape can be used to "picture frame" the edges of the wafer for extra security when swimming or during sports.

Carry extra pouching supplies in a diaper bag, fanny pack, or small backpack, and store in a cool, dry place. The extra supplies should include a pouch that is already cut out to fit and a plastic bag to dispose of the soiled pouch. Pouches cannot be flushed!

Encourage the family to meet with the school nurse to discuss the child's ostomy. The family should find out if there is a private bathroom at school available for the child to use if the pouch needs to be changed or emptied. Have the child keep an extra change of clothes in a backpack, a school locker, or the nurse's office for emergencies.

## Discharge

Ensure that the family has information regarding how to reorder ostomy supplies once the child is discharged from the hospital. The family should reorder pouches when they open the last box so they will not run out of supplies.

## Family Education: When to Call for Help with a Colostomy

- Bleeding from stoma more than usual when cleaning stoma
- Bleeding from skin around stoma
- Change in bowel pattern
- Change in size of stoma
- Change in color of stoma
- Temperature above 100.4° F

## Family Education: Ostomy Care

In addition to the General Principles of Family Education on p. 212, families need to know the following:

- Emptying pouch
- Changing pouch
- Skin care
- Clothing
- Activities

## Resources

Pull-Thru Network—Quarterly newsletter for parents and families with children who have had ostomies
2312 Savoy St.
Hoover AL 35226-1528
205-978-2930
*www.pullthrough.org*
NIDDK—National Institute of Diabetes and Digestive and Kidney Disease
*www.digestive.niddk.nih.gov*
Coloplast—Pediatric ostomy literature, Tipster coloring books: "When I met Tipster ... A child's story about living with an ostomy"

800-533-0464
Hollister—Pediatric ostomy literature and ostomy "Shadow Buddies" dolls for teaching
800-323-4060
Convatec—Pediatric ostomy literature
800-442-8811
WOCN—Pediatric Ostomy Care: Best Practice Guideline
4700 W. Lake Ave.
Glenview, IL 60025-1485
800-224-9626
*www.wocn.org*

# Procedures Related to Maintaining Cardiorespiratory Function

## Oxygen Therapy

Methods include use of a mask, hood, nasal cannula, or face tent.
Method is selected on the basis of the following:
- Concentration of inspired oxygen needed
- Ability of the child to cooperate in its use

Oxygen is a drug and is administered only as prescribed by dose.
Concentration is regulated according to the needs of the child.

Oxygen is dry; therefore it must be humidified.
Use the following precautions with an oxygen hood:
- Do not allow oxygen to blow directly on the infant's face.
- Position hood to avoid rubbing against the infant's neck, chin, or shoulders.

Provide comfort and reassurance to the child. Make sure the child is able to see someone nearby.

## Invasive and Noninvasive Oxygen Monitoring

An essential goal in managing sick or injured children is to ensure the continuous delivery of adequate oxygen to vital organs. Although life-saving, oxygen therapy can cause a number of serious sequelae. To monitor oxygen therapy, blood oxygen levels are routinely measured.

### Arterial Blood Gas

Direct sampling of the blood's oxygen content (measured as partial pressure of oxygen [PO2]) can be done on blood obtained from an indwelling arterial catheter or from arterial puncture (Atraumatic Care box).

Arterial blood gases may also be drawn via an umbilical arterial catheter in neonates, and a radial arterial catheter is sometimes used for blood sampling. These arterial catheters have inherent dangers, and sampling for arterial blood gases must follow stringent institutional policy to minimize complications.*

 **ATRAUMATIC CARE**

**Blood Gas Monitoring**

For continuous monitoring of blood gases, noninvasive measurements are used whenever possible. Oximetry should be used before arterial punctures are performed when information about O₂ saturation is sufficient to evaluate the child's condition.

### *Arterial Blood Gas Analysis*

Subtle and extreme changes in a patient's status need evaluation by a tool that helps give the "big picture" quickly. Arterial blood gas (ABG) analysis results are rapidly available and provide a baseline to determine a patient's current respiratory and metabolic status and needs.

Interpretation of these variables allows the practitioner to assess the degree to which the patient is able to maintain the

*For specific guidelines, see Webster HF: Bioinstrumentation: principles and techniques. In Hazinski MF: *Nursing care of the critically ill child,* ed 2, St Louis, 1992, Mosby.

4 - EVIDENCE-BASED PEDIATRIC NURSING INTERVENTIONS

most essential of bodily functions: airway and breathing (how well the body provides oxygen to the lungs and eliminates carbon dioxide end-products) and circulation (how well the body carries that oxygen to vital end-organs). Interpretation of ABGs is directed at determining whether the blood pH value—an important determinant of how effectively cellular processes occur—has been affected by a lung problem (respiratory acidosis or alkalosis) or kidney problem (metabolic acidosis or alkalosis).

Blood gases are obtained from an artery either via arterial puncture or from an indwelling arterial line. Ice is used to preserve the blood sample for accurate analysis if it cannot be processed within 15 minutes. Delays in analysis may cause inaccuracies owing to separation of blood cells from plasma.

Blood gas interpretation is based on assessing the arterial serum levels of the variables in Table 4-11.

## Consistent Approach Is Key

In order to make an interpretation based on the individual ABG values, a consistent sequence of steps should be followed:

1. Evaluate pH to determine presence of acidosis or alkalosis. The lungs and kidneys regulate the hydrogen ion status within the plasma. Alterations in these systems affect the acid-base balance, causing pH changes that affect multiple body systems.
   - Within normal limits (WNL) indicates normal or compensated state
   - Outside normal limits
     - <7.35: Acidosis—Acidosis may cause pulmonary vasoconstriction leading to decreased pulmonary blood flow. Acidosis may also cause vasoconstriction to cerebral blood vessels.
     - >7.45: Alkalosis—Alkalosis may diminish cellular metabolism, depress myocardial function, and dilate pulmonary blood vessels.
2. Evaluate $PaCO_2$ to assess the alveolar ventilation status. In an uncompensated acidosis or alkalosis, an abnormal $PaCO_2$ level will generally indicate that origin of the pH imbalance is respiratory rather than metabolic.
   - Within normal limits—Adequate ventilation
   - Outside normal limits
     - >45: Hypercarbia—Hypoventilation leads to an increase in $PaCO_2$, which in turn lowers the pH, resulting in a respiratory acidosis.
     - <30: Hypocarbia—Hyperventilation leads to decreased $PaCO_2$, which in turn raises the pH, resulting in a respiratory alkalosis.
3. Evaluate $HCO_3$ to assess the effectiveness of renal regulation of blood pH. In an uncompensated acidosis or alkalosis, an abnormal $HCO_3$ level will generally indicate that origin of the pH imbalance is metabolic rather than respiratory.
   - Within normal limits—Normal renal function
   - Outside normal limits

| TABLE 4-11 | ABG Values for Interpretation | | |
|---|---|---|---|
| Interpretation | pH | PaCO₂ | HCO₃ |
| **Normal Values** | **7.35-7.45** | **35-45** | **22-26** |
| **Acidosis** | | | |
| Respiratory | <7.35 | >45 | WNL |
| Compensated respiratory | WNL | >45 | >29 |
| Metabolic | <7.35 | WNL | <22 |
| Compensated metabolic | WNL | <30 | <22 |
| **Alkalosis** | | | |
| Respiratory | >7.45 | <30 | WNL |
| Compensated respiratory | WNL | <30 | <22 |
| Metabolic | >7.45 | WNl | >29 |
| Compensated metabolic | WNL | >45 | >29 |

WNL, Within normal limits.

- <22: Decreased bicarbonate—Renal mechanisms lead to increased excretion of bicarbonate and a lower serum bicarbonate level. Owing to the absence of normal levels of bicarbonate to buffer serum H+ (acid), the pH lowers and metabolic acidosis is the result.
- >29: Increased bicarbonate—Renal mechanisms lead to increased retention of bicarbonate. Owing to the higher levels of bicarbonate, more serum H+ (acid) is buffered, the pH increases, and metabolic alkalosis is the result.

4. Look for signs of compensation—With prolonged abnormalities in pH, the body tries to return the pH to normal through respiratory compensation (adjusting $PaCO_2$ levels) or metabolic compensation (adjusting $HCO_3$ levels). In a compensated acidosis or alkalosis, the pH will be normal, but the $PaCO_2$ and $HCO_3$ will both be abnormal in the same "direction" (increased or decreased). Table 4-14 may be used to assist with differentiation of respiratory versus metabolic acid-base imbalances, including presence of compensation.
5. Evaluate $PaO_2$ to assess the oxygenation status. It is important to be aware of a patient's specific "normal" values. Patients with certain cardiac or pulmonary conditions may have an "acceptable" $PaO_2$ that is below normal limits. Assess each patient's unique needs and treat accordingly.
   - Within normal limits—Adequate oxygenation
   - Outside normal limits
     - 55-85: Mild hypoxemia
     - 40-55: Moderate hypoxemia
     - <40: Severe hypoxemia

## Pulse Oximetry

Measures arterial hemoglobin oxygen saturation ($SaO_2$) by passage of two different wavelengths of light through blood-perfused tissues to a photodetector. $SaO_2$ and heart rate are displayed on digital readout.

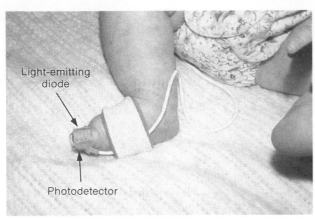

FIGURE **4-25** Oximeter sensor on great toe. Note that sensor is positioned with light-emitting diode opposite photodetector. Cord is secured to foot with self-adhering band (not tape) to minimize movement of sensor.

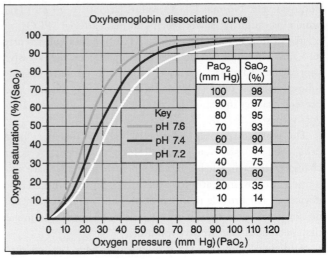

FIGURE **4-26** Oxyhemoglobin dissociation curve. Changes in the affinity of hemoglobin for oxygen shift the position of the oxyhemoglobin dissociation curve. Standard curve *(middle curve):* Assumes normal pH (7.4), temperature, $PCO_2$, and 2,3-DPG levels. Shift to left *(left curve):* Increases $O_2$ affinity of Hb; decreased pH; and increased temperature, $PCO_2$, and 2,3-DPG. Shift to right *(right curve):* Decreases $O_2$ affinity of Hb; decreased pH, and increased temperature, $PCO_2$, and 2,3-DPG.

Attach sensor to earlobe, finger, or toe (Figure 4-25); make certain light source and photodetector are in opposition.

Avoid sites with restricted blood flow (e.g., distal to a blood pressure cuff or indwelling arterial catheter).

Secure sensor cord with self-adhering wrap or tape to avoid interference by patient movement. Shield sensor from bright light. Keep extremity warm (e.g., use a sock over foot or hand if extremity is cool).

Avoid IV dyes; green, purple, or black nail polish; nonopaque synthetic nails; and possibly footprint ink, which may cause erroneous readings.

Change placement of sensor every 4 to 8 hours. Inspect skin at sensor site in compromised children, and change sensor more frequently if needed to prevent pressure necrosis.

Advantages:
- Noninvasive technique
- No complicated preparation or calibration of sensor
- No special skin care needed
- Convenient sites can be used

Disadvantages:
- Requires peripheral arterial pulsation
- Limited use in hypotension or with vasoconstricting drugs
- Sensor affected by movement (Safety Alert)

 **SAFETY ALERT**

**For the Infant**

Attach the sensor securely to the great toe. Do not apply additional tape to the disposable sensors because it can cause a false reading if the sensor becomes disconnected but remains unnoticed. Place a snugly fitting sock over the foot.

**For the Child**

Attach the sensor securely to the index finger, and tape the cable to the back of the hand.

$SaO_2$ is related to $PO_2$, but the values are not the same. As a rule of thumb, an $SaO_2$ of:
- 98% = $PO_2$ of 100 mm Hg or greater
- 90% = $PO_2$ of 60 mm Hg
- 80% = $PO_2$ of 45 mm Hg
- 60% = $PO_2$ of 30 mm Hg
- See Figure 4-26.
- In general, normal range is 95% to 99%. A consistent $SaO_2$ less than 95% should be investigated, and an $SaO_2$ of 90% signifies developing hypoxia.

## End-Tidal Carbon Dioxide ($CO_2$) Monitoring

End-tidal $CO_2$ ($ETCO_2$) monitoring measures exhaled carbon dioxide noninvasively. Capnometry provides a numeric display, and capnography provides a graph over time. Continuous capnometry is available in many bedside physiologic monitors as well as stand-alone monitors. $ETCO_2$ differs from pulse oximetry in that it is more sensitive to the mechanics of ventilation rather than oxygenation. Hypoxic episodes can be prevented through the early detection of hypoventilation, apnea, or airway obstruction.

Children who are experiencing an asthma exacerbation, receiving procedural sedation, or who are mechanically ventilated may have $ETCO_2$ monitoring. Special sampling cannulas are used for nonintubated patients, and a small device is placed between the endotracheal tube and the ventilator tubing in intubated patients. While $ETCO_2$ monitoring is not a substitute for arterial blood gases, it does have the information of providing ventilation information continuously and noninvasively. Normal $ETCO_2$ values are 30 to 43 mm Hg, which is slightly lower than normal arterial $PCO_2$ of 35 to 45 mm Hg. During CPR, $ETCO_2$ values consistently <15 mm Hg indicate ineffective compressions or excessive ventilation. Changes in wave form and numeric display follow changes in ventilation by a very few seconds and precede changes in respiratory rate, skin color, and pulse oximetry values.

For years, disposable colormetric $ETCO_2$ detectors have been used to assess endotracheal tube placement. A color change with each exhaled breath when there is adequate systemic perfusion indicates that the tube is in the lungs. These devices do not provide numbers or graphic representation and do not provide the same early detection of hypoventilation as the continuous quantitative monitors.

Additional uses of $ETCO_2$ monitoring have limited supporting research. While wave form analysis does not yet have standardized nomenclature, some clinicians utilize the angles of the waveform coupled with the quantitative value of $ETCO_2$ to classify the severity of asthma exacerbations. The severity of diabetic ketoacidosis (Fearon and Steele, 2002) and acidosis from gastroenteritis (Nagler, Wright, and Krauss, 2006) has also been researched in children and is used in some facilities.

When there is a change in the $ETCO_2$ value or waveform, assess the patient quickly for adequate airway, breathing, and circulation. Sedated patients may be hypoventilating and need stimulation. Intubated patients may need suctioning, have self-extubated or dislodged the tube, or have equipment failure/disconnection. Asthmatic patients may have a worsening condition. Problems with the $ETCO_2$ monitoring system can include a kink in the sample line or disconnection. In general, check the patient first, then the equipment.

# Suctioning

Indications for suctioning include the following:
- The child is having difficulty breathing.
- The child appears very restless.
- The child has difficulty eating or sucking.
- The child's color becomes paler.
- The child's nostrils flare (spread out).
- You hear the sound of air bubbling through the mucus.

## Nasal Aspirator (Bulb Syringe)
Young infants are obligatory nose breathers and need clear nares. Young children may also benefit from nasal suctioning at times. The aspirator can remove excessive runny mucus or dry, crusted mucus. Nose drops must first be used to moisten dry mucus; saline nose drops are safest.

1. Squeeze the rounded end of the bulb to remove air (Figure 4-27, A).
2. Place the tip of the bulb snugly into one nostril.
3. Let go of the bulb slowly; the bulb will suck the mucus out of the nose (Figure 4-27, B).
4. When the bulb is reinflated, remove it from the nose.
5. Squeeze the bulb into a tissue to get rid of the mucus.
6. Repeat steps 1 through 5 for the other side of the nose.
7. Repeat this process as often as needed to keep the nose clear.
8. When used in the home, clean the nasal aspirator by filling it with tap water. Then squeeze the bulb to remove the water and the mucus. Refill the bulb with water and boil for 10 minutes. Let the bulb cool, and squeeze out the water before using it again.

## Nasopharyngeal Suctioning
### Equipment
Suction regulator or machine with tubing
Suction catheters
Saline or water (cool)
Clean container for rinsing catheter

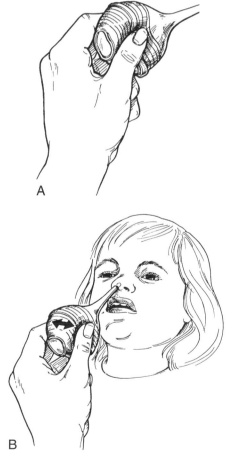

FIGURE **4-27**   A, Squeezing nasal aspirator to remove air. B, Releasing grasp to suck mucus from nose.

### Procedure

1. Turn on the suction regulator/machine.
2. Open the suction catheter package, put on gloves, and connect the catheter to the suction regulator/machine.
3. Measure the tube for the insertion distance. Place the tip of the catheter at the child's earlobe, and mark the distance to the tip of the child's nose. Hold the catheter at this mark.
4. Wet the tip of the catheter by placing the tip of the catheter in the sterile saline, and place your thumb over the opening to obtain suction.
5. Tell the child to take a deep breath.
6. With your thumb off the opening (no suction), insert the suction catheter in one nostril up to the measured distance.
7. Place your thumb on the suction port to obtain suction.

8. Rotate or twist the catheter as you remove it with a slow steady motion. Both inserting the catheter and suctioning should take no longer than 5 seconds. Remember, the child may not breathe while you are suctioning.
9. Look at the mucus. Check the color, smell, and consistency for any change.
10. Rinse the suction catheter in the sterile saline or water with your thumb on the suction port.
11. Allow the child to take a few deep breaths.
12. Repeat steps 5 through 10 up to two times if needed (for large amounts of mucus), then repeat for the other nostril.
13. After suctioning the nose, you can use the same catheter to clear the child's mouth up to three times if needed.

## Tracheostomy Care

Tracheostomy is a surgical opening in the trachea between the second and fourth tracheal rings (Figure 4-28). Congenital or acquired structural defects, such as subglottic stenosis, tracheomalacia, and vocal cord paralysis, account for many long-term tracheostomies. A tracheostomy may be required in an emergency situation for epiglottitis, croup, or foreign body aspiration. These tracheostomies remain in place for a short time. An infant or child requiring long-term ventilatory support may also have a tracheostomy.

Pediatric tracheostomy tubes are usually made of plastic or Silastic (Figure 4-29). The most common types are the Hollinger, Jackson, Aberdeen, and Shiley tubes. These tubes are constructed with a more acute angle than adult tubes, and they soften at body temperature, conforming to the contours of the trachea. Because these materials resist the formation of crusted respiratory secretions, they are made without an inner cannula. Some children require a metal tracheostomy tube (usually made of sterling silver or stainless steel), which contains an inner cannula. The principal advantages of metal tubes are their nonreactivity and decreased chance for an allergic reaction. Tracheostomy tubes are secured using either a Velcro tube holder or twill tape ties; twill tape is more prone to abrading the neck and takes longer to secure (Sherman, Davis, Albamonte-Petrick, and others, 2000).

### Tracheostomy Suctioning

The practice of instilling sterile saline in the tracheostomy tube before suctioning is not supported by research and is no longer recommended by many institutions. Suctioning should require no more than 5 seconds. Counting 1, one thousand, 2, one thousand, 3, one thousand, and so on while suctioning is a simple means for monitoring the time. Without a safeguard, the airway may be obstructed for too long. Hyperventilating the child with 100% $O_2$ before and after suctioning (using a bag-valve-mask or increasing the $FiO_2$ ventilator setting) is

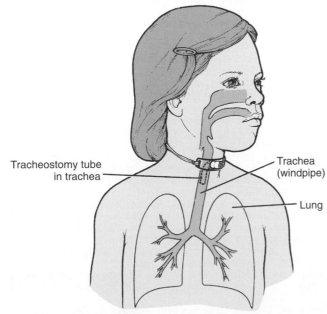

Tracheostomy tube in trachea

Trachea (windpipe)

Lung

FIGURE **4-28** Secured tracheostomy tube.

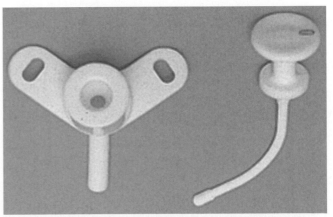

FIGURE **4-29** Silastic pediatric tracheostomy tube and obturator.

also performed to prevent hypoxia. Closed tracheal suctioning systems that allow for uninterrupted $O_2$ delivery may also be used. In a closed suction system, a suction catheter is directly attached to the ventilator tubing. This system has several advantages. First, there is no need to disconnect the patient from the ventilator, which allows for better oxygenation. Second, the suction catheter is enclosed in a plastic sheath, which reduces the risk of exposure to the patient's secretions.

In the acute care setting, aseptic technique is used during care of the tracheostomy. Secondary infection is a major concern because the air entering the lower airway bypasses the natural defenses of the upper airway. Standard Precautions are recommended, and the nurse should wear gloves during the suctioning procedure, although a sterile glove is needed only on the hand touching the catheter. It is recommended that the nurse follows institution protocols for the use of nonsterile and sterile gloves during suctioning. Use a new sterile suction catheter and sterile gloves each time in the acute care setting. In the home care setting nonsterile gloves may be worn, and the suction catheter may be rinsed with water internally and cleansed with alcohol on the external surface (Sherman, Davis, Albamonte-Petrick, and others, 2000).

---

## EVIDENCE-BASED PRACTICE

## Normal Saline Instillation Before Endotracheal or Tracheostomy Suctioning—Helpful or Harmful?

### Ask the Question
In intubated children and those with tracheostomy, is normal saline instillation before suctioning helpful or harmful?

### Search the Evidence
**Search Strategies**
Searched all literature from 1980 to 2009

**Databases Used**
PubMed, Cochrane Collaboration, MDConsult, BestBETs, PedsCCM

### Critically Analyze the Evidence
**Grade criteria:** Evidence quality moderate; recommendation strong (Guyatt, Oxman, Vist, and others, 2008)

- Instillation of normal saline before endotracheal (ET) tube suctioning has been used for years to loosen and dilute secretions, lubricate the suction catheter, and promote cough. In recent years, the possible adverse effects of this procedure have been explored. Adult studies have found decreased oxygen saturation, increased frequency of nosocomial pneumonia, and increased intracranial pressure after instillation of normal saline before suctioning (O'Neal, Grap, Thompson, and others, 2001; Kinlock, 1999; Ackerman, 1998; Hagler and Traver, 1994; Reynolds, Hoffman, Schlichtig, and others, 1990; Ackerman, 1993; Bostick and Wendelgass, 1987).

- Two of the first research studies evaluating the effect of normal saline instillation before suctioning in neonates found no deleterious effects. Shorten, Byrne, and Jones (1991) found no significant differences in oxygenation, heart rate, or blood pressure before or after suctioning in a group of 27 intubated neonates.

- In a second study of nine neonates acting as their own controls, no adverse effects on lung mechanics were found after normal saline instillation and suctioning (Beeram and Dhanireddy, 1992).

- A study evaluating the effects of normal saline instillation before suctioning in children found results similar to those in the previously published adult studies. Ridling, Martin, and Bratton (2003) evaluated the effects of normal saline instillation before suctioning in a group of 24 critically ill children, ages 10 weeks to 14 years (level 1 evidence). A total of 104 suctioning episodes were analyzed. Children experienced significantly greater oxygen desaturation after suctioning if normal saline was instilled.

- The American Thoracic Society's (2005) official position statement on the care of children with tracheostomies now states that normal saline should not be instilled before suctioning.

- Gardner and Shirland (2009) evaluated 10 studies on the effects of instilling NS in intubated neonates. They concluded that the evidence does not support routine instillation of NS, however the evidence indicating adverse effects of NS instillation are abundant.

- Morrow and Argent (2008) suggest that despite evidence indicating the detriment of the use of saline for suctioning in adults, evidence is lacking in the pediatric population. They conclude, however, that saline should not be routinely used for suctioning infants and children.

### Apply the Evidence: Nursing Implications
Studies support the contention that the adverse effects of normal saline instillation before suctioning in children are similar to those found for adults. This technique causes a significant reduction in oxygen saturation that can last up to 2 minutes after suctioning. The evidence does not support the use of normal saline instillation before ET suctioning in children.

### References
Ackerman MH: Instillation of normal saline before suctioning in patients with pulmonary infections: A prospective randomized controlled trial, *Am J Crit Care* 7(4): 261-266, 1998.

Ackerman MH: The effect of saline lavage prior to suctioning, *Am J Crit Care* 2(4):326-330, 1993.

Ackerman MH, Gugerty B: The effect of normal saline bolus instillation in artificial airways, *J Soc Otorhinolaryngol Head Neck Nurs* 8:14-17, 1990.

American Thoracic Society: Care of the child with a chronic tracheostomy, 2005, available at *www.thoracic.org/sections/publications/statements/pages/respiratory-disease-pediatric/childtrach1-12.html* (accessed April 17, 2006).

Beeram MR, Dhanireddy R: Effects of saline instillation during tracheal suction on lung mechanics in newborn infants, *J Perinatol* 12(2):120-123, 1992.

Bostick J, Wendelgass ST: Normal saline instillation as part of the suctioning procedure: Effects of $PaO_2$ and amount of secretions, *Heart Lung* 16(5):532-537, 1987.

Gardner DL, Shirland L: Evidence-based guideline for suctioning the intubated neonate and infant, *Neonatal Netw* 28(5): 281-302, 2009.

Guyatt GH, Oxman AD, Vist GE, and others: GRADE: An emerging consensus on rating quality of evidence and strength of recommendations, *BMJ* 336(7650): 924-926, 2008.

Hagler DA, Traver GA: Endotracheal saline and suction catheters: Sources of lower airway contamination, *Am J Crit Care* 3(6):444-447, 1994.

Kinlock D: Instillation of normal saline during endotracheal suctioning: Effects on mixed venous oxygen saturation, *Am J Crit Care* 8(4):231-240, 1999.

Morrow BM, Argent AC: A comprehensive review of pediatric endotracheal suctioning: Effects, indications, and clinical practice, *Pediatr Crit Care Med* 9(5):465-477, 2008.

O'Neal PV, Grap MJ, Thompson C, and others: Level of dyspnoea experienced in mechanically ventilated adults with and without saline instillation prior to endotracheal suctioning, *Intensive Crit Care Nurs* 17(6):356-363, 2001.

Reynolds P, Hoffman LA, Schlichtig R, and others: Effects of normal saline instillation on secretion volume, dynamic compliance, and oxygen saturation (abstract), *Am Rev Respir Dis* 141:A574, 1990.

Ridling DA, Martin LD, Bratton SL: Endotracheal suctioning with or without instillation of isotonic sodium chloride in critically ill children, *Am J Crit Care* 12(3):212-219, 2003.

Shorten DR, Byrne PJ, Jones RL: Infant responses to saline instillations and endotracheal suctioning, *J Obstet Gynecol Neonatal Nurs* 20(6):464-469, 1991.

## Suction Catheter Length

Traditional technique for suctioning ET or tracheostomy tubes recommends advancing a suction catheter into the tube until it meets resistance, then withdrawing it slightly and applying suction. However, studies indicate that this approach causes trauma to the tracheobronchial wall. This trauma can be avoided by inserting the catheter and advancing it to the premeasured depth of just to the tip (especially in infants) or no more than 0.5 cm beyond the tube (Kleiber, Krutzfield, and Rose, 1988) (Figure 4-30).

Calibrated catheters are easier to use for premeasured suctioning technique, but unmarked catheters can also be used. To measure the length for catheter insertion, place the catheter near a sample ET or tracheostomy tube (same size as child's tube), with the end of the catheter at the correct position. Grasp the catheter with a sterile-gloved hand to mark the length, and insert the catheter until the hand reaches the stoma.

## Changing the Tracheostomy Tube

Tracheostomy tubes are changed monthly or when a mucus plug is suspected of obstructing airflow and cannot be cleared by suctioning.

Non-emergent changes should be done 2 to 3 hours after meals to avoid any chance of the child vomiting. Assess the skin around the tracheostomy for any redness, swelling, cuts, or bruises.

### Procedure for Changing the Tracheostomy Tube

1. Place the child in an infant seat or sitting upright.
2. If the child is unable to help, have someone hold the child's arms while the tube is being changed.
3. Suction the tracheostomy until it is clear.
4. Remove the old tracheostomy tube holder or ties.
5. Remove the tracheostomy tube.
6. Quickly check the skin.
7. Quickly dip the clean tracheostomy tube in sterile saline, and shake to remove excess water.
8. Insert the clean tracheostomy tube (with or without an obturator) into the opening (stoma).
9. Remove obturator if used.
10. Secure the tracheostomy tube. If ties requiring a knot are used, change the position of the knot each time the tube or ties are changed. Make sure that the holder is snug enough to let you put only one finger underneath.
11. If you are unable to put the new tube in, reposition the child's neck, dip the tube into the saline, and try again. If you still cannot get the tube in, seek additional help. If the child is having difficulty breathing, begin rescue breathing if necessary.

## Skin Care

Keep the area around the tracheostomy clean and dry to prevent skin irritation and infection. Wash the skin with soap and water, and dry well. Change the tracheostomy tube holder each day or if it becomes wet or dirty. Dressings should of a material free of lint (e.g., gauze or foam) and fenestrated (pre-slit); cutting the dressing will allow fraying and unraveling. Lint can be irritating to the stoma and may enter the respiratory tract. Dressings, if used, should be changed when soiled and when routine skin care is performed.

Do not apply any ointments or other medications on the skin unless specifically ordered. Barrier creams or ointments (e.g., Desitin, Vaseline, Ilex) or barrier wafers, wipes, or dressings (e.g., Cavilon No Sting barrier film, AllKare Protective Barrier Wipe, Stomahesive Skin Barrier, Coloplast Skin Barrier) can be used to protect the skin around the tube if leaking occurs.

## Safety

Careful adult supervision is needed when the child is near water. Tub baths can be given, but be careful not to allow water into the tracheostomy. Swimming and boating must be avoided; however, the child can use a wading pool with supervision.

Any smoke, aerosol sprays, powder, or dust can irritate the lining of the child's trachea. Therefore the child should not be in the same room with anyone who is smoking or where aerosol sprays (e.g., hairspray, antiperspirants) are being used.

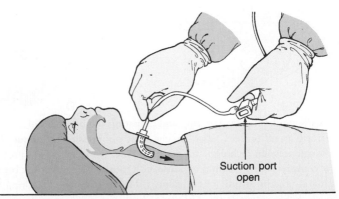

FIGURE **4-30**    Tracheostomy suction catheter insertion. Note that catheter is inserted just to the end of the tracheostomy tube.

4 - EVIDENCE-BASED PEDIATRIC NURSING INTERVENTIONS

Strong cleaning liquids such as ammonia are also irritating. Hair from animals that shed can clog the child's trachea. Avoid stuffed animals and toys with small parts that can be removed and put into the tracheostomy by a curious child.

All the people who provide care for the child must be aware of how to suction the tracheostomy. Anyone caring for the child alone must also know cardiopulmonary resuscitation (CPR).

## Family Education: Traveling Outside the Home with a Tracheostomy

Keep the following supplies in a to-go bag that is ready at all times for when you are outside the house:

- Suction catheters, suction source, a mucus trap that can be used when the suction machine is not available
- Sterile saline
- Water-soluble lubricant
- Tracheostomy tube of current size with tube holder or ties attached, tracheostomy tube one size smaller, extra ties
- Towel or blanket for shoulder roll
- Scissors
- Ambu bag
- Emergency phone numbers, brief description of medical history

In hot, dry, or cold weather or on very windy days, wrap a handkerchief or scarf around the child's neck since inspired air is no longer warmed, moistened or filters through the nose and mouth prior to entering the lungs.

# Cardiopulmonary Resuscitation

## Procedures for Cardiopulmonary Resuscitation

Methods of cardiopulmonary resuscitation (CPR) for health care workers are discussed in Figure 4-31. Several changes were made in 2010 by the American Heart Association (AHA, 2010), including an emphasis on faster and deeper chest compression and a change in sequence to Chest compressions, Airway, and Breathing (C-A-B). "Look, listen, and feel" has

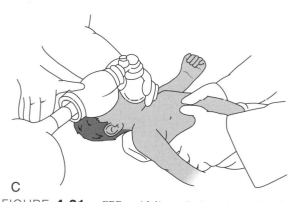

A

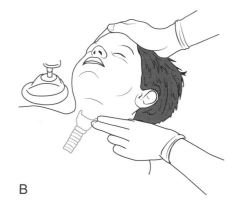

B

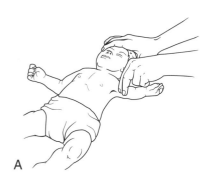

C

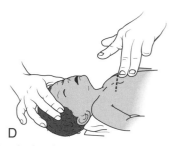

D

FIGURE **4-31**   CPR guidelines. A, Locating and palpating the brachial pulse. B, Locating and palpating the carotid artery pulse. C, Two-rescuer chest compression technique in infant. D. One-rescuer chest compression technique in infant. E, One-handed chest compressions in a child. F, Two-handed chest compressions in a child or adult. G. Open airway and check breathing. H, Mouth-to-mouth-and-nose breathing for an infant. I, Mouth-to-barrier breathing for child; mask covers nose and mouth. J, Placement of the AED on a child.

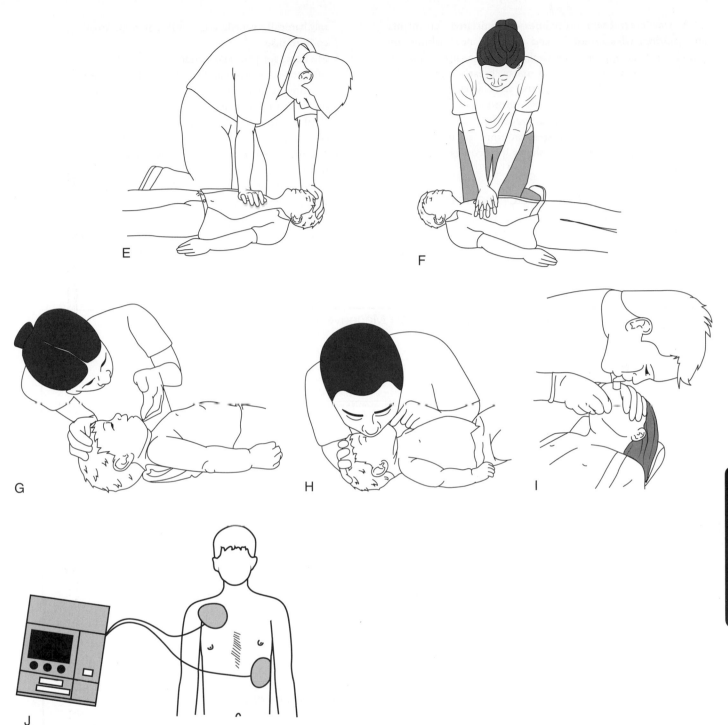

FIGURE **4-31, cont'd.** For legend, see opposite page.

been discontinued; pause no longer than 10 seconds to check for a pulse. Continuous end tidal carbon dioxide monitoring (via a change in color, numeric value, or waveform) is recommended for confirming tracheal tube placement, monitoring the quality of CPR, and detecting spontaneous circulation.

Automated external defibrillators (AEDs) are now supported for infant use if a manual defibrillator is not immediately available. A summary of basic life support maneuvers for infants, children, and adults are shown in Table 4-12. Medications used during CPR in children are summarized in Table 4-13.

Airway obstruction procedures are initiated for infants and children who are awake and alert but not making any sounds or cries, appear to be choking, have a dusky color or bluish lips, have high-pitched noisy breathing, or make the choking sign of clutching the neck with both hands. Should the infant or child become unconscious, begin CPR. Each time the rescuer opens the airway, check to see if a foreign object can be visualized; if seen, attempt to remove with a finger sweep. Figure 4-32 shows procedures for airway obstruction.

## Postrescuscitation Stabilization

Preserving brain function, avoiding secondary organ injury, and treating the underlying cause are the goals of postresuscitation care.

- Continue supplemental oxygen to maintain an arterial oxyhemoglobin saturation ≥94% but <100%;

mechanically ventilate if significant respiratory compromise.
- Medicate for pain and agitation.
- Monitor respiratory and cardiovascular function. Continuous quantitative capnography is recommended for intubated patients.
- Replace intraosseous access (if used) with venous access.
- Maintain cardiac output with vasoactive medications.
- Brain function preservation efforts include normal ventilatory rate (not hyperventilation), aggressive seizure management, and temperature control. Therapeutic hypothermia may be considered for pediatric patients who remain unresponsive after resuscitation from cardiac arrest; fever is aggressively treated due to its adverse effects on ischemic brain injury.

| TABLE 4-12 | Summary of Basic Life Support Maneuvers for Infants, Children, and Adults* | | |
|---|---|---|---|
| | **RECOMMENDATIONS** | | |
| **Component** | **Adults** | **Children** | **Infants** |
| Recognition | Unresponsive (for all ages) | | |
| | No breathing or no normal breathing (ie, only gasping) | No breathing or only gasping | |
| | No pulse palpated within 10 seconds for all ages (HCP only) | | |
| CPR sequence | C-A-B | | |
| Compression rate | At least 100/min | | |
| Compression depth | At least 2 inches (5 cm) | At least ⅓ AP diameter About 2 inches (5 cm) | At least ⅓ AP diameter About 11/2 inches (4 cm) |
| Chest wall recoil | Allow complete recoil between compressions HCPs rotate compressors every 2 minutes | | |
| Compression interruptions | Minimize interruptions in chest compressions Attempt to limit interrruptions to <10 seconds | | |
| Airway | Head tilt–chin lift (HCP suspected trauma: jaw thrust) | | |
| Compression-to-ventilation ratio (until advanced airway placed) | 30:2 1 or 2 rescuers | 30:2 Single rescuer 15:2 2 HCP rescuers | |
| Ventilations: when rescuer untrained or trained and not proficient | Compressions only | | |
| Ventilations with advanced airway (HCP) | 1 breath every 6-8 seconds (8-10 breaths/min) Asynchronous with chest compressions About 1 second per breath Visible chest rise | | |
| Defibrillation | Attach and use AED as soon as available. Minimize interruptions in chest compressions before and after shock; resume CPR beginning with compressions immediately after each shock. | | |

Abbreviations: AED, automated external defibrillator; AP, anterior-posterior; CPR, cardiopulmonary resuscitation; HCP, healthcare provider.
*Excluding the newly born, in whom the etiology of an arrest is nearly always asphyxial.
*Newborn/neonatal information not included.
From Hazinski, Chameides, Hemphill, Samson, Schexnayder, and Sinz: Highlights of the 2010 American Heart Association guidelines for CPR and ECC available at www. heart.org.

## TABLE 4-13  Drugs for Pediatric Cardiopulmonary Resuscitation

| Drug and Dose | Action | Implication |
|---|---|---|
| **Epinephrine HCl*** IV/IO: 0.01 mg/kg (1:10,000) Maximum single dose: 1 mg Endotracheal tube (ET): 0.1 mg/kg (1:1000) | Adrenergic Acts on both alpha- and beta-receptor sites, especially heart and vascular and other smooth muscle | Most useful drug in cardiac arrest Disappears rapidly from bloodstream after injection; instill 5 ml saline after ET administration May produce renal vessel constriction and decreased urine formation |
| **Atropine sulfate*** 0.02 mg/kg/dose Minimum dose: 0.1 mg Maximum single dose: infants and children, 0.5 mg; adolescents, 1 mg | Anticholinergic-parasympatholytic Increases cardiac output, heart rate by blocking vagal stimulation in heart | Used to treat bradycardia caused by increased vagal tone or cholinergic drug toxicity Always provide adequate ventilation, and monitor oxygen saturation Produces pupillary dilation, which constricts with light |
| **Calcium chloride 10%** 20 mg/kg IV/IO 0.2 mg/kg/dose q 10 min | Electrolyte replacement Needed for maintenance of normal cardiac contractility | Used only for hypocalcemia, calcium blocker overdose, hyperkalemia, or hypermagnesemia Administer slowly; very sclerosing; administer in central vein Incompatible with phosphate solutions |
| **Lidocaine HCl*** 1 mg/kg/dose | Antidysrhythmic Inhibits nerve impulses from sensory nerves | Used for ventricular arrhythmias only |
| **Amiodarone** IV: 5 mg/kg over 30 min followed by continuous infusion Start at 5 mcg/kg/min May increase to maximum 10 mcg/kg/min | Antidysrhythmic agent Inhibits adrenergic stimulation; prolongs action potential and refractory period in myocardial tissues; decreased atrioventricular (AV) conduction and sinus node function | Recommended as first choice for shock-refractory or recurrent ventricular fibrillation or pulseless ventricular tachycardia Contraindicated in severe sinus node dysfunction, marked sinus bradycardia, second- and third-degree AV block Monitor ECG and blood pressure |
| **Adenosine** 0.1-0.2 mg/kg as a rapid IV bolus Maximum single initial dose: 6-12 mg (given over 1-2 sec) May repeat administration: double initial dose (maximum dose = 12 mg) Follow with ≥5 ml normal saline flush | Antidysrhythmic, for supraventricular tachycardia Causes temporary block through AV node and interrupts reentry circuits | Administer by rapid IV push followed by saline flush May cause transient bradycardia |
| **Naloxone (Narcan)*** 0.1 mg/kg/dose† May repeat q 2-3 min | Reverses respiratory arrest caused by excessive opiate administration | Evaluate level of pain after administration because analgesic effects of opioids are reversed with large doses of naloxone |
| **Magnesium sulfate** 25-50 mg/kg IV/IO Maximum: 2 g | Inhibits calcium channels and causes smooth muscle relaxation | Given by rapid IV infusion for suspected hypomagnesemia Have calcium gluconate (IV) available as antidote |

### Infusions

| Drug and Dose | Action | Implication |
|---|---|---|
| **Epinephrine HCl infusion** 0.05 mcg/kg/min | Adrenergic See above | Titrated to desired hemodynamic effect |
| **Dopamine HCl infusion** 2 mcg/kg/min | Agonist Acts on alpha receptors, causing vasoconstriction Increases cardiac output | Titrated to desired hemodynamic response |
| **Dobutamine HCl infusion** 2 mcg/kg/min | Adrenergic direct-acting β₂-agonist Increases contractility and heart rate | Titrated to desired hemodynamic response Little vasoconstriction, even at high rates See above |
| **Lidocaine HCl infusion** 20-50 mcg/kg/min | Antidysrhythmic Increases electrical stimulation threshold of ventricle | Lower infusion dose used in shock |

*ECG*, Electrocardiogram; *IO*, intraosseous; *IV*, intravenous.
Calculate drugs on actual body weight for nonobese pediatric patients. In obese patients, use ideal body weight, estimated from length to avoid drug toxicity.
*These drugs may be administered via ET tube if IV/IO is not available; IV/IO is the preferred route.
†Dose of naloxone to reverse respiratory depression without reversing analgesia from opioids is 0.5 mcg/kg in children <40 kg (88 lb) (American Pain Society, 1999).

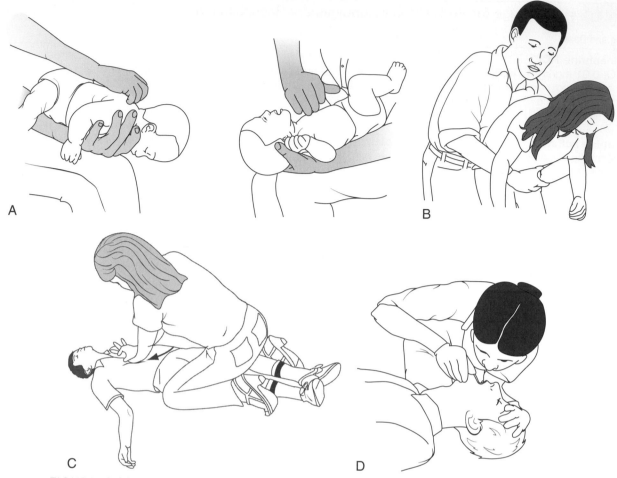

FIGURE **4-32** Procedures for airway obstruction. A, Relief of choking in the infant. *Left,* Back slaps. *Right,* Chest thrusts. B, Abdominal thrusts in standing choking child. C, Abdominal thrusts in supine choking child. D, Open airway and look for object.

## EVIDENCE-BASED PRACTICE

### Family Presence during Resuscitation of a Child

#### Ask the Question
Is family presence at the resuscitation of a child perceived by the family as a positive event?

#### Search the Evidence
##### Search Strategies
The literature between 1994 and 2010 was searched to obtain information regarding the presence of family members during the resuscitation of a child family member.

##### Databases Used
PubMed, CINAHL, Professional Organization Websites

#### Critically Analyze the Evidence
**Grade criteria:** Evidence quality moderate; recommendation strong (Moreland, 2005)
- A number of studies in adult patients indicate that family presence during invasive procedures and resuscitation alleviates the family's

anger about being separated from the patient during a crisis, reduces their anxiety, eliminates doubts about what was done to help the patient, facilitates the grieving process, increases the perception of the patient as an individual and increases respect for the patient, lessens the family's feelings of helplessness, allows closure and a chance to say good-bye, facilitates a relationship between the medical staff and family through increased communication, and helps family understand the gravity or severity of the patient's condition (Mangurten, Scott, Guzzetta, and others, 2006; Meyers, Eichhorn, Guzzetta, and others, 2000; Powers and Rubenstein, 1999; Sacchetti, Lichenstein, Caraccio, and others, 1996; Eichhorn, Meyers, Mitchell, and others, 1996; Tucker, 2002). In many cases family members expressed that it was their right to be present when a family member receives emergent treatment or resuscitation.
- Interviews with 39 English-speaking family members and 96 health care providers who were present in the emergency department (ED) during invasive procedures or cardiopulmonary resuscitation (CPR) revealed that their presence at the procedure was helpful and that

# EVIDENCE-BASED PRACTICE

## Family Presence during Resuscitation of a Child—cont'd

they would do it again (Meyers, Eichhorn, Guzzetta, and others, 2000). Ninety-six percent of the nurses and 79% of the attending physicians supported family presence and thought it should be continued at the hospital. Eighty percent of family members said they wanted to be at the patient's side during an ED visit that involved resuscitation. The sample consisted mostly of adult patients with a mean age of 44.5 (±23.1) years.

- In a survey of parents with children admitted to the ED for invasive procedures and possibly CPR, family members responded favorably to being present if the child was conscious (less favorably if child was unconscious) on admission to the ED, and 83% of the respondents expressed a desire to be present if the child was likely to die (Boie, Moore, Brummett, and others, 1999). The survey consisted of five case scenarios with increasing levels of invasiveness, and the parents were asked whether they would want to be present at the family member's bedside during the procedure.
- Tinsley, Hill, Shah, and others (2008) conducted 40 interviews of guardians or parents who were present during the child's resuscitation in a PICU. Seventy one percent of the parents/guardians surveyed felt that their presence during the resuscitation comforted the child, while 67% of the parents/guardians expressed that their presence helped them adjust to the loss of the child. This study is unique in that all of the children resuscitated died 6 months before the interview.
- Professional organizations support the presence of family members during CPR. The Emergency Nurses Association (2001) has developed national guidelines for family presence during invasive procedures and CPR. These guidelines include recommendations for assessing family members to determine whether family presence is appropriate and the use of a family facilitator (e.g., nurse, child life specialist, social worker, or chaplain) who remains with the family during resuscitation to answer questions, clarify information, and offer comfort.
- The American Heart Association (2005) recommends that providers offer families the option to remain with the loved one during resuscitation. Likewise, the PALS [pediatric advanced life support] Provider Manual (Hazinski, Zaritsky, Nadkarni, and others, 2002) supports the presence of family during the child's CPR with the presence of a family support facilitator. A sample protocol to prepare and support family presence, based on the recommendations of the Association for the Care of Children's Health, can be found in a publication by Meyers, Eichhorn, Guzzetta, and colleagues (2000).
- Some studies addressed health care workers' attitudes about family presence during resuscitation of a child. Health care workers' attitudes about family presence during resuscitation vary considerably. Sixty percent of the health care workers (nurses and physicians) surveyed said they felt comfortable performing resuscitation procedures with a family member present; no distinction was made between adult or child patient (Mangurten, Scott, Guzzetta, and others, 2005). ED staff with previous experience in having family members present during pediatric resuscitation favored the practice, whereas the staff without prior exposure to family presence were against the practice (Sacchetti, Caraccio, Leva, and others, 2000). Tsai (2002) asserted that most physicians and nurses do not favor family members' presence during resuscitation procedures, and in a survey of pediatricians, nurses, and residents, 65% said they would not allow family presence during pediatric CPR (O'Brien, Creamer, Hill, and others, 2002). Dudley, Hansen, Furnival, and others (2009) found that family presence in the

ED did not delay time to CT scan or the resuscitation procedure itself for pediatric patients requiring trauma resuscitation.

- Two critical reviews examined the presence of family members during resuscitation. Moreland's 2005 review of 23 studies on family presence during resuscitation and invasive procedures emphasizes the differing aspects of each study reviewed; mixed research methodologies make it difficult to draw conclusions for the general population, and most were based on sample interviews and questionnaires after the event. Moreland concludes that further research is needed to evaluate the long-term effects of family presence on family members and health care providers. Nibert and Ondrejka (2005) concluded that there is no research supporting the exclusion of family from resuscitation events, that many clinician beliefs and practices on the topic are not evidence based, and that families want to be consulted regarding their presence during the resuscitation of a child.

### Summary of Findings

- The studies reviewed included information regarding family presence during invasive procedures and resuscitation, not solely pediatric resuscitation.
- Only one of these studies evaluated the responses of family members actually present during a pediatric resuscitation in the ED (Dudley, Hansen, Furnival, and others, 2009) but the goal of the study was to evaluate the effect of FP on the procedure itself, therefore minimal family opinions were obtained.
- Most of the studies published to date did not address the issue of family presence during resuscitation in areas other than the ED (general pediatric floor, postanesthesia care unit, PICU, outpatient settings). Three studies identified family presence in the PICU as being important for invasive procedures and end-of-life decisions but did not address family presence during resuscitation and subsequent reactions to the event (Anderson, McCall, Leversha, and others, 1994; Meyer, Burns, Griffith, and others, 2002; Powers and Rubenstein, 1999).
- Studies addressed the reactions and opinions of the health care workers regarding family presence during the resuscitative event. Health care worker beliefs and opinions for or against the practice of family presence during resuscitation were not a significant part of this review.
- There is no evidence to support excluding family members during a child's resuscitation unless a facilitator is unavailable to communicate with the family during the process.
- Further research is needed to validate the effects of family presence in childhood resuscitation events.

### Apply the Evidence: Nursing Implications

- The presence of family at the resuscitation of a child can be beneficial provided that a facilitator is present to communicate with the family.
- Giving the family the option of being present during a pediatric resuscitation may help the family be a part of the decision-making process and help achieve closure in the event of the child's death.
- Health care workers should encourage family presence during resuscitation when appropriate.
- Protocols for family presence during resuscitation should be developed and implemented in institutions where children and families are served.

4 - EVIDENCE-BASED PEDIATRIC NURSING INTERVENTIONS

*Continued*

## EVIDENCE-BASED PRACTICE
### Family Presence during Resuscitation of a Child—cont'd

**References**

American Heart Association: 2005 American Heart Association guidelines for cardiopulmonary resuscitation and emergency cardiovascular care, *Circulation* 112(24, Suppl I):IV-166, 2005.

Anderson B, McCall E, Leversha A, and others: A review of children's dying in a paediatric intensive care unit, *New Zealand Med J* 107(985):345-347, 1994.

Boie T, Moore GP, Brummett C, and others: Do parents want to be present during invasive procedures performed on their children in the emergency department? A survey of 400 parents, *Ann Emerg Med* 34(1):70-74, 1999.

Dudley NC, Hansen KW, Furnival RA, and others: The effect of family presence on the efficacy of pediatric trauma resuscitations, *Ann Emerg Med* 53(6):777-784, 2009.

Eichhorn DJ, Meyers TA, Mitchell TG, and others: Opening the doors: Family presence during resuscitation, *J Cardiovasc Nurs* 10(4):59-70, 1996.

Emergency Nurses Association: Position statement: *Family presence at the bedside during invasive procedures and resuscitation*, 2001, available at www.ena.org/about/position (accessed June 2005).

Hazinski MF, Zaritsky AL, Nadkarni VM, and others: *PALS provider manual*, Dallas, 2002, American Heart Association.

Mangurten J, Scott SH, Guzzetta CE, and others: Effects of family presence during resuscitation and invasive procedures in a pediatric emergency department, *J Emerg Nurs* 32(3):225-233, 2006.

Mangurten JA, Scott SH, Guzzetta CE, and others: Family presence: Making room, *AJN* 105(5):40-48, 2005.

Meyer EC, Burns JP, Griffith JL, and others: Parental perspectives on end-of-life care in the pediatric intensive care unit, *Crit Care Med* 30(1):226-231, 2002.

Meyers TA, Eichhorn DJ, Guzzetta CE, and others: Family presence during invasive procedures and resuscitation, *Am J Nurs* 100(2):32-42, 2000.

Moreland P: Family presence during invasive procedures and resuscitation in the emergency department: A review of the literature, *J Emerg Nurs* 31(1):58-72, 2005.

Nibert L, Ondrejka D: Family presence during pediatric resuscitation: An integrative review of evidence-based practice, *J Pediatr Nurs* 20(2):145-147, 2005.

O'Brien M, Creamer KM, Hill EE, and others: Tolerance of family presence during pediatric cardiopulmonary resuscitation: A snapshot of military and civilian pediatricians, nurses, and residents, *Pediatr Emerg Care* 18(6):409-413, 2002.

Powers KS, Rubenstein JS: Family presence during invasive procedures in the pediatric intensive care unit: A prospective study, *Arch Pediatr Adolesc Med* 153(9):955-958, 1999.

Sacchetti A, Caraccio C, Leva E, and others: Acceptance of family member presence during pediatric resuscitations in the emergency department: Effects of personal experiences, *Pediatr Emerg Care* 16(2):85-87, 2000.

Sacchetti A, Lichenstein R, Caraccio CA, and others: Family member presence during pediatric emergency department procedures, *Pediatr Emerg Care* 12(4):268-271, 1996.

Tinsley C, Hill B, Shah J, and others: Experience of families during cardiopulmonary resuscitation in a pediatric intensive care unit, *Pediatrics* 122(4): e799-e804, 2008.

Tsai E: Should family members be present during cardiopulmonary resuscitation? *N Engl J Med* 346(13):1019-1021, 2002.

Tucker T: Family presence during resuscitation, *Crit Care Clin North Am* 14(2):177-185, 2002.

## Intubation Procedures

### Rapid Sequence Intubation

*Rapid sequence intubation* (RSI) is commonly performed in pediatric (and some neonatal) patients to induce an unconscious, neuromuscular blocked condition to avoid the use of positive pressure ventilation and the risk of possible aspiration (Bottor, 2009). Atropine, fentanyl, and vecuronium or rocuronium are drugs commonly used during RSI. In neonates, endotracheal intubation is often a stressful event, and hypoxia and pain are commonly associated with routine intubation; RSI in neonates may serve to prevent such adverse events (Bottor, 2009).

### Indications for Intubation

Respiratory failure or arrest, agonal or gasping respirations, apnea

Upper airway obstruction

Significant increase in work of breathing, use of accessory muscles

Potential for developing partial or complete airway obstruction—respiratory effort with no breath sounds, facial trauma, and inhalation injuries

Potential for or actual loss of airway protection, increased risk for aspiration

Anticipated need for mechanical ventilation related to chest trauma, shock, increased intracranial pressure

Hypoxemia despite supplemental oxygen

Inadequate ventilation

### Intubation Procedure

Gather supplies needed for intubation.

- Suction, large bore tonsil tip or Yankauer, and sterile suction catheter
- ET tube of appropriate size plus 0.5 mm larger and 0.5 mm smaller. Length-based charts are most reliable for determining appropriate ET size. Estimation formulas for children >2 years of age are as follows:
  - Uncuffed ET tube size in mm = (age in years/4) + 4
  - Cuffed ET tube size in mm = (age in years/4) + 3.5
- Stylet to fit the selected ET
- Laryngoscope and blade
- Light source (ensure that it is functioning)
- Bag and mask
- Oxygen source
- Adhesive tape and skin barrier or securement device
- End-tidal carbon dioxide detector
- NG tube and catheter tip syringe
- Gloves and eye protection for universal precautions
- Emergency cardiopulmonary resuscitation equipment including medications
- RSI medications

Monitor cardiac rhythm, heart rate, and pulse oximetry continuously with audible tones.

Preoxygenate with 100% oxygen using appropriately sized bag and mask.

Administer RSI medications.
- Sedative, if conscious
- Short-acting muscle relaxant
- Muscarinic anticholinergic

Assist with intubation by providing supplies and monitoring patient.

Verify placement by at least one clinical sign and at least one confirmatory technology:
- Visualization of bilateral chest expansion
- Auscultation over the epigastrium (breath sounds should not be heard) and the lung fields bilaterally in the axillary region (breath sounds should be equal and adequate)
- Water vapor in the tube (helpful; not definitive)
- Color change on end-tidal carbon dioxide detector during exhalation after at least 3 to 6 breaths or waveform/value verification with continuous capnography
- Chest radiograph

Apply protective skin barrier, and secure ET tube with tape or securement device.

Insert NG tube, and verify placement.

## Ongoing Assessment

Chest rise and fall, symmetry

Bilateral breath sounds

Pulse oximetry

End-tidal carbon dioxide

Vital signs
- Heart rate too fast or too slow is a possible indication of hypoxemia, air leak, or low cardiac output.
- Hypotension or hypertension may be indicative of hypoxemia or hypovolemia.

Capillary refill and skin color

Level of consciousness

Intake and output

Blood gas

ET tube stabilization and patency

Skin integrity

If sudden deterioration of an intubated patient occurs, consider the following (DOPE*):

Displacement—tube is not in trachea or has moved into a bronchus (right mainstream most common)

Obstruction—secretions or kinking of the tube

Pneumothorax—chest trauma, barotraumas, or non-compliant lung disease

Equipment failure—check oxygen source, ambu bag, and ventilator

Verify placement again during each transport and when patients are moved to different beds.

## Patient Comfort and Safety Procedures

### Skin Integrity

Reposition at least every 2 hours, as patient condition tolerates.

Apply a hydrocolloid barrier to protect facial cheeks.

Place gel pillows under pressure points such as occiput, heels, elbows, and shoulders.

Allow no tubes, lines, wires, or wrinkles in bedding under patient.

Provide meticulous skin care.

### Comfort

Provide analgesia and sedation as needed.

Use a system for communication including sign boards, pointing, opening and closing eyes.

Provide oral care every 2 hours.

### Safety

Use soft restraints if necessary to maintain a critical airway.

Continuously assess for complications:
- Tube dislodgment caused by position change, agitation, or transport
- Tube occlusion caused by excessive secretions or biting on ET tube
- Pneumothorax or other air leaks
- Equipment failure or disconnection from ventilator

## Procedures to Prevent Ventilator-Associated Pneumonia

Use aggressive hand hygiene.

Provide enteral nutrition to decrease risk of bacterial translocation.

Minimize aspiration potential with enteral feeds.

Elevate the head of the bed between 30 and 45 degrees unless contraindicated.

Routinely verify the appropriate placement of the feeding tube.

Routinely assess the patient's intestinal motility (e.g., by auscultating for bowel sounds and measuring residual gastric volume or abdominal girth), and adjust the rate and volume of enteral feeding to avoid regurgitation.

Use postpyloric (duodenal or jejunal) feeding in high-risk patients (decreased gag reflex, delayed gastric emptying, gastroesophageal reflux, severe bronchospasm).

Provide aggressive oral care every 2 hours with an approved oral care regimen.

To prevent the aspiration of pooled secretions, suction hypopharynx before suctioning the ET tube, before repositioning the ET tube, and before repositioning the patient.
- Use closed endotracheal suctioning.
- Do not instill saline.

Prevent ventilator circuits' condensate from entering ET tube or in-line medication nebulizers.

Use orotracheal or orogastric tubes to prevent nosocomial sinusitis.

If cuffed ET tubes are used, inflate them to maintain cuff pressure no greater than 20 cm $H_2O$.

Provide peptic ulcer prophylaxis, as ordered.

*American Heart Association, 2005.

Avoid neuromuscular blockade.

Assess readiness to extubate daily.

- Underlying condition improved
- Hemodynamically stable
- Able to clear and maintain secretions
- Mechanical support no longer necessary

## Extubation Procedure

Assess level of consciousness and ability to maintain a patent airway by mobilizing pulmonary secretions through effective coughing.

Maintain nothing by mouth (NPO) status 4 hours before extubation.

Preoxygenate.

Place patient in a semi-Fowler position.

Suction the ET tube and the oropharynx. Suction down to the cuff when using a cuffed ET tube.

Remove tape or ET tube securement device.

If cuff is present, deflate and ask the patient to cough if developmentally appropriate.

Remove ET tube.

Provide oxygen via facemask or nasal cannula.

Perform chest x-ray examination after extubation as ordered.

Monitor for postextubation respiratory distress, which could develop within minutes or hours after extubation:

- Unstable vital signs
- Desaturations
- Stridor
- Hoarseness
- Increased work of breathing

# Pericardiocentesis

Pericardiocentesis is a procedure performed to remove the fluid of a pericardial effusion (PCE). A PCE is an accumulation of fluid in the pericardial space that surrounds the heart. Therapeutic indications for pericardiocentesis include the relief of cardiac tamponade or the prevention of cardiac compression by a moderate to large PCE. Pericardiocentesis is also performed to assist in diagnosis of neoplasms, rheumatologic conditions, and infections.

Sedatives and analgesics are administered before the procedure. The xyphoid area is prepped with antiseptic, a needle is introduced into the pericardial space by a physician, and the catheter is then placed. Pericardial fluid is aspirated via the

catheter until most of the fluid has been evacuated. The catheter is then secured to the skin with sutures, and the drainage bag is attached. In emergent situations, a 60-ml Luer-Lok syringe attached to a stopcock and an 18-gauge Angiocath may be used to tap the pericardial space and aspirate fluid (Figure 4-33).

## Preparation for Procedure

Gather supplies. Many institutions stock prepackaged pericardiocentesis kits that will include the supplies needed for the procedure. Be familiar with these kits so that items not included can be obtained from floor stock supplies.

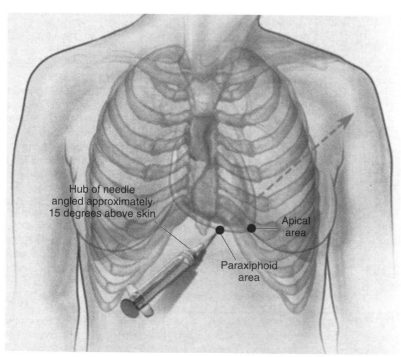

FIGURE **4-33**   Pericardiocentesis.

- Sterile gloves, mask, gown, and cap
- Sterile drapes and towels
- Sterile gauze (variety of sizes)
- Sterile drainage bag
- Sterile saline flush
- Sterile specimen container
- Skin antiseptic, per hospital policy
- Three- or four-way stopcock
- Luer-Lok syringes in a variety of sizes (10, 15, 30, 60 ml)
- Straight or pigtail catheter with side holes (request style and size from physician)
- 18-gauge needle (6 inches long) or 18-gauge Angiocath (physician preference)
- 1% or 2% lidocaine for local anesthesia
- Suture material (physician preference)
- Scalpel blade
- Fluid for volume resuscitation as needed
- Emergency equipment nearby

Ensure that the patient has well-functioning venous access.

Administer pain and sedation medication as ordered.

Attach patient to monitoring equipment (electrocardiogram [ECG] at a minimum).

## Procedural Support

Position the patient with the head of the bed elevated 30 to 45 degrees.

Assist physician with preparation of the sterile field as directed.

Provide sterile supplies to the physician as directed.

Monitor airway, breathing, circulation, and cardiac rhythm throughout the procedure.

Send specimens to the laboratory as ordered. Ask the physician before discarding fluid.

Place dressing over catheter insertion site per hospital policy.

Obtain chest radiograph to confirm placement of catheter.

## After the Procedure

Ensure that daily chest radiographs are scheduled to monitor placement of the pericardial drain.

Assess for signs and symptoms of infection around the catheter insertion site throughout the duration of pericardial drain placement.

Assess drainage for color, consistency, and quantity. If quantity of drainage significantly decreases, assess area around the insertion site for drainage.

Notify the physician of any changes in quality or quantity of drainage.

# Chest Tube Procedures

A chest tube is placed to remove fluid or air from the pleural or pericardial space. Chest tube drainage systems collect air and fluid while inhibiting backflow into the pleural or pericardial space. Indications for chest tube placement include pneumothorax, hemothorax, chylothorax, empyema, pleural or pericardial effusion, and prevention of accumulation of fluid in the pleural and pericardial space after cardiothoracic surgery. Nursing responsibilities include assisting with chest tube placement, managing chest tubes, and assisting with chest tube removal.

## Chest Tube Insertion

Before procedure, assess hematologic and coagulation studies for any risk of bleeding during the procedure. Notify the physician of abnormal findings.

Gather supplies.

- Appropriately sized chest tube with or without trocar, as desired by inserter
- Disposable chest drainage system (pediatric or adult size)
- Connecting tubing
- Vacuum suction
- Skin antiseptic such as chlorhexidine or povidone-iodine, per hospital policy
- Scalpel, blade, suture, needle driver, clamps
- 1% or 2% lidocaine for local anesthesia
- Selection of syringes and needles
- Tape
- Sterile gloves, mask, gown, and cap
- Sterile drapes and towels
- Sterile gauze (variety of sizes)
- Sterile specimen container
- Sterile water

Attach monitoring equipment (pulse oximeter at a minimum) to patient.

Administer pain and sedation medications as ordered.

Follow Universal Protocol for Preventing Wrong Site, Wrong Procedure, Wrong Person Surgery (Time-Out Procedure) as guided by hospital policy.

Prepare drainage system with sterile water as described in package insert (some systems may not require this step).

Monitor airway, breathing, and circulation throughout the procedure.

Once the chest tube is inserted and secured, hand the physician the drainage system tubing while keeping the open end sterile. The physician will join the chest tube to the drainage system with the patient tube connector. Secure tubing so it does not become disconnected.

If suction is required, use connection tubing to join the drainage system to a wall suction adapter, and adjust suction on drainage system as ordered (usually $-10$ to $-20$ cm $H_2O$). There should be gentle, continuous bubbling in the suction control chamber.

Place occlusive dressing over chest tube insertion site per hospital policy. Note date, time, and your initials on the dressing. If gauze is used, use presplit gauze; "homemade" split gauze may leave loose threads in the wound.

Ensure that the drainage system is positioned below the patient's chest.

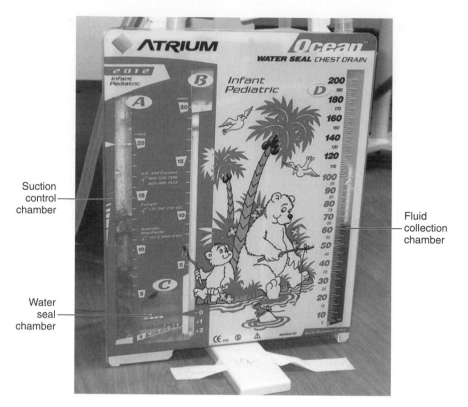

FIGURE **4-34**   Chest tube drainage system.

Obtain a chest radiograph to confirm placement of the chest tube. Ensure that daily chest radiographs are scheduled to monitor placement of the chest tube as well as the resolution of the pneumothorax or effusion.

## Chest Drainage System Management

Disposable chest drainage systems typically consist of three chambers next to one another in one drainage unit (Figure 4-34). The fluid collection chamber collects drainage from the patient's pleural or pericardial space. The water seal chamber is directly connected to the fluid collection chamber and acts as a one-way valve, protecting patients from air returning to the pleural or pericardial space. The suction chamber may be a dry suction or calibrated water chamber. It is connected to external vacuum suction set to the amount of suction ordered and controls the amount of suction patients experience.

Closely monitor the patient's cardiorespiratory status.

Provide adequate analgesia.

Secure the drainage system to the floor or bed.

Ensure that all connections are tight.

Keep drainage tubing free of dependent loops.

Assess for blood clots and fibrin strands in tubes with sanguinous or serosanguineous drainage, and ensure that there are no obstructions to drainage in the tube.

Maintain chest tube clearance per hospital policy. Milking or stripping of chest tubes is not recommended for chest tube clearance because of the high negative intrathoracic pressure that is created. However, there are special circumstances that warrant chest tube clearance with these methods, such as maintaining chest tube patency while a patient is bleeding. Notify the physician immediately if chest tube obstruction is suspected.

Generally, chest tubes should not be clamped. However, it may be necessary to clamp a chest tube when exchanging the collection chamber or to determine the site of an air leak.

Assess the drainage in the collection chamber.

- Type (sanguinous, serosanguineous, serous, chylous, empyemic), color, amount, consistency. If there is a marked decrease in the amount of drainage, assess for drainage around the chest tube insertion site.
- Notify the physician of any changes in the quantity or quality of drainage.
- If 3 ml/kg/hr or greater of sanguinous drainage occurs for 2 to 3 consecutive hours after cardiothoracic surgery, it may indicate active hemorrhaging and warrants immediate attention of the physician.
- If the collection chamber is almost full, exchange existing drainage system with a new one per manufacturer's instructions using sterile technique.

Assess the suction control chamber.

- Ensure that the prescribed amount of suction is being applied to the patient.

Assess the water seal chamber.

- Water level is at 2 cm. If the water column is too high, the flow of air from the chest may be impeded.

To lower the water column, depress the manual vent on the back of the unit until the water level reaches 2 cm. *Do not depress the filtered manual vent when the suction is not functioning or connected.*

- Bubbling in the water seal chamber is normal if the chest tube was placed to evacuate a pneumothorax. The bubbling will stop when the pneumothorax has resolved.
- If evacuation of a pneumothorax was not the indication for placement of the chest tube, bubbling in the water seal chamber may be the result of a break in the chest drainage system. Identify the break in the system by briefly clamping the system between the drainage unit and the patient. When the clamp is placed between the unit and the break in the system, the bubbling will stop. Tighten any loose connections. If the air leak is suspected to be at the patient's chest wall, notify the physician.
- Fluctuations may be seen in the water column because of changes in intrathoracic pressure. Substantial fluctuations may reflect changes in a patient's respiratory status.

Assess and maintain the chest tube insertion site.

- Change dressing and perform site care per hospital policy. Typically a minimal, occlusive dressing is applied.
- Ensure that chest tube sutures are intact.
- Dressing should be clean, dry, and intact.
- Assess skin for signs and symptoms of infection or skin breakdown.
- Palpate for the presence of subcutaneous air.

Encourage patient ambulation. Secure chest tube drainage system to prevent chest tube dislodgment from patient or disconnection from drainage system.

Obtain samples from the chest tube per hospital infection control policy.

Prepare a syringe with a 20-gauge (or smaller) needle.

Form a temporary dependent loop, and, using aseptic technique, insert the needle at an angle into the dependent loop.

Aspirate amount of drainage required.

## Chest Tube Removal

Administer additional pain medication before removal.

Gather supplies: gloves, suture removal kit, sterile gauze (2 × 2 or 4 × 4), and tape.

Assist in removal of the chest tube. The chest tube is removed on patient exhalation to prevent a pneumothorax.

Apply dressing, and perform site care per hospital policy.

Obtain a chest radiograph as ordered to confirm that a pneumothorax has not occurred after chest tube removal.

Closely monitor patient's respiratory status.

# Cardioversion Procedures

Supraventricular tachycardia (SVT) is the most common tachydysrhythmia in children. SVT is a rapid, regular rhythm of over 200 beats per minute. Because cardiac output is a product of heart rate and stroke volume, prolonged SVT can cause hemodynamic compromise. Signs and symptoms of SVT in infants include irritability, poor feeding, sweating, and pallor. Older children may complain of dizziness, chest pain, or a feeling that their heart is racing.

Whenever SVT is suspected, assess the adequacy of the patient's airway and ventilatory effort. Check for a pulse. If the patient does not have a pulse or adequate respirations, proceed with cardiopulmonary resuscitation. If a patient does have a pulse, assess the patient's perfusion. Notify the physician if SVT is suspected. Choosing the appropriate type of treatment depends on accurate evaluation of the patient's cardiac output and hemodynamic status.

The treatment of SVT is cardioversion, or converting an abnormal heart rhythm into a normal one. A physician should be present for all forms of cardioversion. There are three types of cardioversion:

- *Mechanical* refers to the use of vagal maneuvers such as ice to the face, one-sided carotid massage, or Valsalva maneuvers
- *Chemical* refers to the use of medications
- *Electrical* refers to the use of electrical energy delivered to a patient to convert the tachydysrhythmia to a normal rhythm.

If the patient has adequate perfusion, anticipate the need for a 12-lead ECG and pediatric cardiology consult (if available). Proceed with mechanical cardioversion, then chemical, if needed. Elective synchronized cardioversion may also be required.

If the patient has poor perfusion, mechanical cardioversion may be attempted but should not delay treatment. Chemical cardioversion may be attempted if reliable IV access in a large vein, such as antecubital, is immediately available. Electrical cardioversion should be employed if reliable IV access is not available or chemical cardioversion is unsuccessful. Administer sedation or analgesia before chemical or electrical cardioversion.

## Mechanical Cardioversion

Administer oxygen.

Attach an ECG monitor and pulse oximeter to the patient.

Vagal maneuvers such as ice to the face, one-sided carotid massage, and the Valsalva maneuver may be attempted to cardiovert the patient.

Ice to the face is the most effective vagal maneuver. Place crushed ice in a glove or bag and apply to the patient's face for 10 to 15 seconds, being careful not to obstruct the nose or mouth. If a Valsalva maneuver is desired, one method is to have the child blow into an occluded straw.

Assess the patient's cardiac rhythm, breathing, pulse, and perfusion.

If cardioversion is unsuccessful and the patient remains stable with adequate perfusion, additional attempts at mechanical cardioversion may be considered before advancing to chemical cardioversion.

## Chemical Cardioversion

Adenosine is the drug of choice for chemical conversion of SVT. It works by blocking electrical conduction through the AV node. To be effective, adenosine must be delivered rapidly because it is metabolized quickly in the bloodstream. Verapamil is an alternative in older children, but not infants, Procainamide or amiodarone may be considered for refractory SVT.

Administer oxygen.

Attach the ECG monitor component of a defibrillator to the patient. Also attach a pulse oximeter.

Check patency of IV, or start IV in large vein, such as antecubital.

Have several syringes of saline flush available.

Prepare the dose of adenosine based on the patient's weight.

Rapidly administer adenosine using two syringes connected to a T-connector or stopcock; give adenosine rapidly with one syringe, and immediately flush with 5 ml of NS with the other.

Assess the patient's cardiac rhythm, breathing, pulse, and perfusion.

Because adenosine blocks conduction through the AV node, patients may have asystole for 1 to 2 seconds after adenosine administration. Closely monitor the patient; if asystole does not resolve, proceed with cardiopulmonary resuscitation.

## Electrical Cardioversion

Electrical cardioversion for SVT is *synchronized*. This means that the electrical impulses delivered to the patient are coordinated with the patient's own rhythm. This is very important because delivering electrical impulses that are not synchronized can cause the patient to develop a more dangerous dysrhythmia. Ensure that the "sync mode" is always used.

Administer oxygen, as ordered.

Attach the ECG monitor of a defibrillator to the patient. Attach a pulse oximeter to the patient.

Place appropriately sized pads or paddles on the patient.

Select the sync mode.

Set the appropriate amount of energy to be delivered. The starting dose is 0.5 to 1 joules/kg.

Deliver energy to the patient.

Assess the patient's cardiac rhythm, breathing, pulse, and perfusion.

Advance to 2 joules/kg if the first dose is ineffective.

Assess the patient's cardiac rhythm, breathing, pulse, and perfusion.

Throughout all cardioversion procedures, monitor the patient's airway, breathing, and circulation. Continuously monitor the patient's heart rhythm. Intervene with cardiopulmonary resuscitation if warranted at any point.

# Procedures Related to Maintaining Neurologic Function

## Increased Intracranial Pressure Management

A neurologic pressure monitoring system is used to measure intracranial pressure (ICP). Causes of increased ICP include accidental and abusive head trauma, hydrocephalus, tumor, edema, and subarachnoid or other intracranial hemorrhage. The system may be used to alleviate increased ICP by draining cerebral spinal fluid (CSF) from the ventricular system. A decrease in cerebral oxygen delivery related to hypotension, hypoxemia, cerebral edema, intracranial hypertension, or abnormalities in cerebral blood flow may precipitate a secondary injury. General nursing care activities and environmental stimuli can present a challenge to the patient with increased ICP. If ICP is increasing, then further nursing activities should be delayed if possible. Care must be individualized based on the patient's responses. The optimal rest period is at least 1 hour between nursing care interventions.

### Positioning

Maintain neutral or midline head and neck alignment.

Elevate the head of bed (HOB) 15 to 30 degrees to promote venous drainage.

Closely evaluate the effect of HOB elevation on ICP, cerebral perfusion pressure (CPP), and mean arterial pressure (MAP).

Avoid extreme hip flexion, as this can increase intraabdominal pressure and restrict movement of the diaphragm and impede respiratory effort.

Reposition the patient by using the logrolling technique.

### Endotracheal Suctioning

Preoxygenate per intensive care unit (ICU) routine. Use of hyperventilation is controversial, can reduce cerebral blood flow to ischemic levels, and may cause loss of autoregulation.

Premedicate as ordered. Adequate sedation may prevent movement and coughing during suctioning and prevent decreases in CPP.

Administer lidocaine intravenously or via endotracheal tube to attenuate possible ICP increases that occur with endotracheal suctioning.

Limit each pass of the suction catheter to 10 seconds or less.

## Temperature

Maintain normothermia (37° C). Core temperatures greater than 37.5° C are associated with increased cerebral metabolic rate, increased oxygen consumption, and increased ICP.

Moderate hypothermia is reserved for children with refractory intracranial hypertension that is not responsive to traditional therapies.

## Sedation and Neuromuscular Blocking Agents

Use of sedatives and analgesics should be based on the patient's ICP and response to the sedation being administered. Protocols vary from institution to institution.

Cautious use of neuromuscular blocking agents is recommended. Neuromuscular assessment is altered (with the exception of pupillary response) with the use of neuromuscular blockade, sedation, and analgesia. This is an important consideration when assessing the patient's ICP response and neurologic status. Continuous electroencephalographic (EEG) monitoring may be indicated for patients at risk for seizures and receiving neuromuscular blocking agents. The risk for ventilator-acquired pneumonia is also increased with the use of neuromuscular blocking agents.

When neuromuscular blocking agents are used, sedation and analgesia should always be used.

Eye care should be implemented to prevent corneal abrasions. Polyethylene covers (e.g., Glad wrap) are most effective; ointments and drops are more effective than nothing at all (Joanna Briggs Institute, 2002).

## Touch and Family Visitation

ICP does not generally increase significantly or decrease with family presence or with physical touch.

## Nursing Essentials

### Normal Intracranial Pressure Ranges

ICP: 0 to 15 mm Hg or 0 to 20 mm $H_2O$

CPP represents the pressure drop between the arterial pressure and the venous pressure. Normal CPP is not delineated in the pediatric population. The thought is that if CPP is greater than 50 mm Hg, then there is adequate cerebral perfusion; if CPP is less than 40 mm Hg, cerebral perfusion is compromised. CPP is calculated by subtracting the ICP from the MAP: CPP = MAP − ICP.

### Hemodynamic Monitoring

Arterial line—necessary for consistent blood pressure monitoring and obtaining MAP for calculation of CPP.

Central venous left atrium line—necessary for monitoring of central venous pressure (CVP).

Pulmonary artery pressure monitoring—if indicated.

### Patient and Family Preparation

Placement of ICP monitoring systems may be performed at the bedside or in the operating room.

Family should be aware that the patient may remain intubated for an extended period of time if the neurologic status is compromised.

Explain the monitor and the waveforms and that the patient will be continually monitored for increased ICP.

### Intracranial Pressure Monitoring Systems

Fluid-coupled systems—An intraventricular catheter (IVC) is placed in the anterior horn of the lateral ventricle; this is the most accurate and reliable method of monitoring. This system allows for CSF drainage and measurement of ICP when attached to an external fluid-filled transducer (not simultaneously). Must be zeroed to atmosphere and maintained at a fixed point such as the foramen of Monroe.

Fiberoptic—Placed in intraventricular, intraparenchymal, subarachnoid, and subdural spaces. These catheters are light-sending and light-receiving systems and respond to the movement of a diaphragm at the tip of the catheter. Zeroed to atmospheric pressure just before insertion. No leveling or rezeroing is necessary because the transducer is located in the catheter tip.

Internal strain gauge or microchip transducer—Placed in intraparenchymal, subarachnoid, and subdural spaces. A miniature strain-gauge pressure sensor is positioned at the tip of the catheter; when pressure is exerted, an electrical signal is generated and pressure is measured. Catheter is zeroed to atmosphere before insertion and never rezeroed after the catheter is inserted.

# External Ventricular Drain Procedures

Children with external ventricular drains (EVDs) may be hospitalized in an ICU, step-down unit, or acute care floor. EVDs are used to temporarily control ICP by draining CSF from the ventricles, most often in shunt infections, brain tumors, and intracranial bleeds. The drainage is dependent on gravity, and the level of the flow chamber determines the amount of CSF flow. Proper positioning, maintenance of patency, infection prevention, and patient monitoring are important aspects of care.

## Positioning of External Ventricular Drains

Raising the flow chamber too high results in decreased CSF flow into the external reservoir and increased ICP. Positioning a flow chamber too low will result in too much drainage of CSF and potential collapse of the ventricles. The zero reference point is the foramen of Monro, usually aligned with the external auditory canal. The level of the flow chamber is prescribed by a physician. A level and measure is then used to set the collection device at the prescribed height, often 20 cm $H_2O$. Physicians will lower a chamber to increase drainage and reduce ICP and raise the height as the patient's condition improves. The drain will be removed when normal ICPs have been sustained and a temporary condition has resolved. Internal ventriculoperitoneal shunts are placed when hydrocephaly continues, infection clears, and protein amounts are low enough to maintain shunt tubing patency.

## Patency of External Ventricular Drains

Keep the tubing free from kinks. Observe for oscillation of CSF in the tubing. Do not milk or strip EVD tubing. Keep the air filter on the collection chamber dry. Change the bag when three-quarters full using aseptic technique.

## Infection Prevention: External Ventricular Drain Dressing Changes

Dressings are not used by all practitioners. There is limited evidence on the infection rates of EVDs with and without the use of dressings. When dressings are used, they should be changed when damp, loose, or soiled. Report damp dressings caused by CSF leak immediately. Dressing change frequency is established by each institution.

Clamp ventriculostomy drainage system.

Allow the child to choose a position of comfort as long as head control and sterility of supplies and dressing area can be maintained.

Open sterile dressing kit using sterile technique. Prepare sterile supplies on sterile drape.

Put on clean gloves. Remove all components of the dressing.

Assess insertion site for redness, edema, drainage from site, and intact sutures.

Remove clean gloves, perform hand hygiene, and put on sterile gloves.

Clean skin around ventriculostomy insertion site. Start at the insertion site, making concentric circles around the ventriculostomy 3 inches in diameter. Conclude by cleaning the length of the tubing that was coiled, if applicable. Repeat two times.

A 1-inch antimicrobial disc may be placed around drain at insertion site.

Using forceps, place 2 × 2 split gauze on ventriculostomy with catheter between the split. Place 2 × 2 gauze over split gauze.

Carefully coil remainder of catheter, if applicable, on top of 2 × 2 gauze. Prevent pressure ulcers by padding hub of catheter with additional 2 × 2 gauze.

Place 2 × 2 gauze on top of coiled ventriculostomy tubing. Place 4-inch clear occlusive dressing on top of gauze dressing.

Remove sterile gloves.

Position the patient for comfort. Ensure that the collection chamber is at the level ordered, and unclamp ventriculostomy drainage system.

## Patient Monitoring

Record CSF drainage. Report excessive drainage or a sudden cessation in drainage immediately. Document color, and report any changes in color (milky, cloudy, blood-tinged).

Monitor neurologic status including verbal, motor, and pupillary assessments hourly.

Abnormal findings include irritability, confusion, lethargy, headache, and vomiting. Changes in blood pressure (increased), heart rate (decreased), respiratory pattern (periods of apnea), and pupils (dilated, sluggish, or nonreactive) are later signs of increased intracranial pressure.

## Patient Activity or Clamping of the External Ventricular Drain System

Nurses should assist the child with all position changes and ensure the proper height of the collection chamber at all times the tubing is unclamped.

Clamp for short periods of time, not to exceed 30 minutes. Clamping is generally done to allow position changes, during transport to other areas of the hospital, and during patient ambulation.

# Seizure Precautions

The extent of precautions depends on type, severity, and frequency of seizures. They may include the following:

- Side rails raised when child is sleeping or resting.
- Side rails and other hard objects padded.
- Waterproof mattress or pad on bed or crib.
- Suction and oxygen set up in room.

## Family Education: Safety with Seizures

- Swimming with a companion.
- Showers preferred; bathing only with close supervision.
- Use of protective helmet and padding during bicycle riding, skateboarding, or skating.
- Medical identification with child at all times.
- May not operate hazardous machinery or equipment or drive a vehicle unless seizure free for designated period (varies by state).

## Pediatric Coma Rating Scale

Several scales have been devised in an attempt to standardize the description and interpretation of the degree of depressed consciousness. The most popular of these is the Glasgow Coma Scale (GCS), which consists of a three-part assessment: eye opening, verbal response, and motor response. A pediatric version incorporates developmental principles into the assessment of verbal and motor responses and can be used for infants and children age 6 months and older (see Figure 1-31). In children younger than age 5 years, speech is understood to be any sound at all, even crying. A person with an unaltered level of consciousness would score the highest, 15; a score of 8 or below is generally accepted as a definition of coma; the lowest score, 3, indicates deep coma or death.

# End-of-Life Care Interventions

## Communicating with Families of Dying Children

Listen for an "invitation" to talk about the situation.
- "Sometimes I wonder if I am doing the right thing."
- "What have other parents done in this situation?"

- "Do you know of other children who have survived this?"
- "I think the doctor is not telling me everything."

---

Evidence-Based Practice—Pediatric Pain and Symptom Management at the End of Life

## EVIDENCE-BASED PRACTICE

### Pediatric Pain and Symptom Management at the End of Life

**Ask the Question**

In children, what is the pain and symptom experience at the end of life?

**Search the Evidence**

*Search Strategies*

Published studies from 2005 to 2009 were identified and examined. Retrospective descriptive studies characterizing infants' and children's end-of-life experiences through the use of medical record reviews and provider and parental surveys dominated the findings. Most studies examined the symptom experience of the infant or child with cancer.

*Database Used*

PubMed

**Critically Analyze the Evidence**

**Grade criteria:** Evidence quality moderate; recommendation strong (Guyatt, Oxman, Vist, and others, 2008).

Children experienced an average of nine symptoms near the end of life (Theunissen, Hoogerbrugge, van Achterberg, and others, 2007; Zhukovsky, Herzog, Kaur, and others, 2009. Pain, dyspnea, fatigue, loss of motor function, changes in behavior, changes in appearance, not eating, vomiting, cough, diarrhea, mouth sores, sadness, difficulty talking with others about their feelings, fear, and anxiety were the most frequently acknowledged symptoms experienced by most children at the end of life (Bradshaw, Hinds, Lensing, and others, 2005; Hechler, Blankenburg, Friedrichsdorf, and others, 2008; Hendricks-Ferguson, 2008; Jalmsell, Kreicbergs, Onelov, and others, 2006; Lavy, 2007; Pritchard, Burghen,

Srivastava, and others, 2008; Theunissen, Hoogerbrugge, van Achterberg, and others, 2007; Zhukovsky, Herzog, Kaur, and others, 2009). Children and their parents reported high distress over pain and symptoms at the end of life. Parents reported the child's pain and suffering as one of the most important factors in deciding to withhold or withdraw their child from life support in the pediatric intensive care unit (Sharman, Meert, and Sarnaik, 2005).

Helpful interventions to manage symptoms included physical comfort, time spent with child and family, and pharmacologic agents (Hechler, Blankenburg, Friedrichsdorf, and others, 2008; Hendricks-Ferguson, 2008; Pritchard, Burghen, Srivastava, and others, 2008). Morphine, diamorphine, and fentanyl were the most common pain medication; the most common routes of pain medication administration were oral, intravenous, subcutaneous, rectal, and transdermal (Hewitt, Goldman, Collins, and others, 2008). Most studies reported a lack of documented symptom assessment and intervention, as well as inadequate symptom management (Hechler, Blankenburg, Friedrichsdorf, and others, 2008; Lavy, 2007; Zhukovsky, 2009; Zhukovsky, Herzog, Kaur, and others, 2009), particularly the psychological symptoms of the dying child (Hechler, Blankenburg, Friedrichsdorf, and others, 2008; Theunissen, Hoogerbrugge, van Achterberg, and others, 2007).

### Apply the Evidence: Nursing Implications

Although the philosophy of palliative care encompasses pain and symptom management for infants and children who may not outlive their disease, the provision of that care to ease physical and psychologic suffering and provide comfort to those who will die continues to lag.

4 - EVIDENCE-BASED PEDIATRIC NURSING INTERVENTIONS

Nursing Care Plan—The Child who is Terminally Ill or Dying

*Continued*

**EVIDENCE-BASED PRACTICE**

**⊖ Pediatric Pain and Symptom Management at the End of Life—cont'd**

Studies show that children experience significant pain and other distressing symptoms at the end of life that are not well managed. Discrepancies in the assessment of infant and child pain and suffering continue to exist between providers and parents. Improvements are needed in the management of pain and symptoms at the end of life for infants and children.

**References**

Bradshaw G, Hinds PS, Lensing S, and others: Cancer-related deaths in children and adolescents, *J Palliat Med* 8(1):86-95, 2005.

Guyatt GH, Oxman AD, Vist GE, and others: GRADE: An emerging consensus on rating quality of evidence and strength of recommendations, *BMJ* 336(7650): 924-926, 2008.

Hechler T, Blankenburg M, Friedrichsdorf SJ, and others. Parents' perspective on symptoms, quality of life, characteristics of death and end-of-life decisions for children dying from cancer, *Klin Padiatr* 220(3):166-174, 2008.

Hendricks-Ferguson V: Physical symptoms of children receiving pediatric hospice care at home during the last week of life, *Oncol Nurs Forum* 35(6):E108-E115. 2008.

Hewitt M, Goldman A, Collins GS, and others: Opioid use in palliative care of children and young people with cancer, *J Pediatr* 152(1):39-44, 2008.

Jalmsell L, Kreicbergs U, Onelov E, and others: Symptoms affecting children with malignancies during the last month of life: A nationwide follow-up, *Pediatrics* 117(40):1314-1320, 2006.

Lavy V: Presenting symptoms and signs in children referred for palliative care in Malawi, *Palliat Med* 21(4):333-339, 2007.

Pritchard M, Burghen E, Srivastava DK, and others: Cancer-related symptoms most concerning to parents during the last week and last day of their child's life, *Pediatrics* 212(5):e1301-e1309, 2008.

Sharman M, Meert KL, and Sarnaik AP: What influences parents' decisions to limit or withdraw life support? *Pediatr Crit Care Med* 6(5):513-518, 2005.

Theunissen JM, Hoogerbrugge PM, van Achterberg T, and others: Symptoms in the palliative phase of children with cancer, *Pediatr Blood Cancer* 49(2):160-165, 2007.

Zhukovsky DS: The impact of palliative care consultation on symptom assessment, communication needs, and palliative interventions in pediatric patients with cancer, *J Palliat Med* 12(4):343-349, 2009.

Zhukovsky DS, Herzog CE, Kaur G, and others: Impact of palliative care consultation on symptom assessment, communication needs, and palliative interventions in pediatric patients with cancer, *J Palliat Med* 12(4):333-339, 2009.

Use open-ended, nonjudgmental questions to explore families' wishes.

- "Can you tell me more about how you are feeling?"
- "What questions do you (or your child) have that I can have answered for you?"
- "What are your concerns (or worries, fears) right now?"
- "What is important to you (your child, your family) at this time?"

## Common Symptoms Experienced by Dying Children

### Pain
Visceral
Bone
Neuropathic

### Gastrointestinal
Anorexia
Nausea and vomiting
Constipation
Diarrhea

### Genitourinary
Urinary tract infections
Urinary retention

### Hematologic
Anemia
Bleeding

### Respiratory
Cough
Congestion
Shortness of breath
Wheezing

### Central Nervous System
Fevers and chills
Sleep disturbance
Restlessness, agitation
Seizures

### Integumentary
Dry skin
Rash, itching
Pressure sores
Edema

### Emotional
Fear
Anxiety
Depression

## Physical Signs of Approaching Death

Increased sleeping

Loss of sensation and movement in the lower extremities, progressing toward the upper body

Sensation of heat, although body feels cool

Mottling of skin

Loss of senses:

- Tactile sensation decreases
- Sensitive to light
- Hearing is last sense to fail

Confusion, loss of consciousness, slurred speech

Muscle weakness

Decreased urination, more concentrated urine

Loss of bowel and bladder control

Decreased appetite and thirst

Difficulty swallowing

Change in respiratory pattern:

- Cheyne-Stokes respirations (waxing and waning of depth of breathing with regular periods of apnea)
- "Death rattle" (noisy chest sounds from accumulation of pulmonary and pharyngeal secretions)

## Care During the Terminal Phase

### Physical Support

Provide frequent mouth care to prevent drying, cracking, and bleeding of lips and mucous membranes.

Maintain good hygiene by giving bed baths and using skin lotion as tolerated.

Continue necessary medications to manage symptoms and maintain comfort using IV (if access is easily established) or subcutaneous infusion.

Discontinue unnecessary medications and procedures (e.g., vital signs).

See Table 4-14 for common ethical dilemmas in caring for terminally ill children.

---

### GUIDELINES

### Supporting Grieving Families*

#### General

Stay with the family; sit quietly if they prefer not to talk; cry with them if desired.

Accept the family's grief reactions; avoid judgmental statements (e.g., "You should be feeling better by now").

Avoid offering rationalizations for the child's death (e.g., "You should be glad your child isn't suffering anymore").

Avoid artificial consolation (e.g., "I know how you feel," or "You are still young enough to have another baby").

Deal openly with feelings such as guilt, anger, and loss of self-esteem.

Focus on feelings by using a feeling word in the statement (e.g., "You're still feeling all the pain of losing a child").

Refer the family to an appropriate self-help group or for professional help if needed.

#### At the Time of Death

Reassure the family that everything possible is being done for the child, if they wish lifesaving interventions.

Do everything possible to ensure the child's comfort, especially relief of pain.

Provide the child and family the opportunity to review special experiences or memories in their lives.

Express personal feelings of loss or frustration (e.g., "We will miss him so much," or "We tried everything; we feel so sorry that we couldn't save him").

Provide information that the family requests, and be honest.

Respect the emotional needs of family members, such as siblings, who may need brief respites from the dying child.

Make every effort to arrange for family members, especially parents, to be with the child at the moment of death, if they wish to be present.

Allow the family to stay with the dead child for as long as they wish and to rock, hold, or bathe the child.

Provide practical help when possible, such as collecting the child's belongings.

Arrange for spiritual support, such as clergy; pray with the family if no one else can stay with them.

#### After the Death

Attend the funeral or visitation if there was a special closeness with the family.

Initiate and maintain contact (e.g., sending cards, telephoning, inviting them back to the unit, or making a home visit).

Refer to the dead child by name; discuss shared memories with the family.

Discourage the use of drugs or alcohol as a method of escaping grief.

Encourage all family members to communicate their feelings rather than remaining silent to avoid upsetting another member.

Emphasize that grieving is a painful process that often takes years to resolve.

*"Family" refers to all significant persons involved in the child's life, such as parents, siblings, grandparents, or other close relatives or friends.

| TABLE 4-14 | Common Ethical Dilemmas in Caring for Terminally Ill Children |
|---|---|
| **Rationale for Providing to Patient** | **Rationale for Withholding from Patient** |
| **Pain Control** | |
| Comfort (the primary goal)<br>Improved quality of life<br>Easier dying process if child is pain-free | Side effects of opioids<br>Decreased level of cognition<br>Fear of addiction (unfounded in terminally ill patients) |
| **Chemotherapy or Experimental Therapy** | |
| Prolonged life span<br>Possible increase in quality of life<br>Provision of sense that family has done everything they can to save the child | Decreased blood counts, increased risk of infection, bleeding<br>Side effects of treatment may be painful, uncomfortable |
| **Supplemental Nutrition and Hydration (Intravenous, Nasogastric, Gastrostomy Tube)** | |
| Belief that the child is hungry or thirsty<br>Inability or unwillingness of child to eat<br>Fear that child will "starve" to death<br>Primary role of parent to feed and nourish child<br>Parental guilt | Supplemental feedings beyond what child can ingest may actually cause nausea or vomiting<br>Increase in tumor growth (feeding the tumor)<br>Increase in fluid volume may result in congestive heart failure, increased respiratory secretions, and/or pulmonary congestion, which leads to questions of whether or not to implement diuresis<br>Increased urine output leads to increased risk of skin breakdown if child is incontinent<br>Risk of third spacing<br>More comfortable and natural death<br>Complaint of thirst is associated with dying process, not level of hydration (Zerwekh, 1997) |
| **Resuscitation** | |
| Unwillingness of family to give up<br>Conflicts with cultural or religious beliefs<br>Denial that child is actually going to die | Allowing nature to take its course<br>Family believes child has suffered enough, does not want aggressive intervention<br>Relieves family of responsibility to stop interventions that might prolong life |
| **Autopsy** | |
| Research to help other children<br>Ability to check genetic link | Religious, cultural belief<br>Family emotions<br>Belief that body will be desecrated for funeral viewing (an unfounded fear) |

## Emotional Support

See Table 4-15.

Encourage family to discuss impending death openly with child and other family members.

Encourage family to continue to speak to child in calm, reassuring voice.

Provide familiar surroundings or objects.

Encourage caregivers to provide one another with periods of respite.

Allow the performance of spiritual and cultural rituals as desired.

Allow family time with child after the death and participation in the preparation of the body if they choose.

| TABLE 4-15 | Communicating with Dying Children |
|---|---|
| **Approach** | **Effective Technique** |
| Discuss at the child's level | Gear information to the child's developmental age, remembering that younger children tend to be concrete thinkers, whereas older children are capable of abstract thought.<br>Begin with the child's experiences: "You've told us how tired you've been lately." |
| Let the child's questions guide | Begin the conversation with basic information, and let the child's questions direct the conversation. |
| Provide opportunities for the child to express feelings | Look for clues that child is open to communication.<br>Be accepting of whatever emotion is expressed. |
| Encourage feedback | Ask the child to summarize what has been heard. This provides the opportunity to clarify misunderstandings. |
| Use other resources | Use books and movies to encourage dialogue.<br>Ask the child to name the people with whom he or she can discuss problems. |
| Use the child's natural expressive means to stimulate dialogue | Use books, games, art, play, and music to provide a means of expression. |

## Strategies for Intervention with Survivors after Sudden Childhood Death*

### Arrival of the Family

Meet the family immediately and escort to a private area.

A health care worker with bereavement training should remain with the family.

Provide information about the extent of illness or injury and treatment efforts (Table 4-16).

If the health care worker must leave the family or if the family requests privacy, return in 15 minutes so the family does not feel forgotten.

Provide tissues and a telephone. Offer coffee, water, and a Bible.

### Pronouncement of Death

When available, the family's own physician should inform the family of the child's death.

Alternatively, the physician or nurse should introduce himself or herself and establish calm, reassuring eye contact with the parents.

Honest, clear communication that avoids misinterpretation is essential.

Nonverbal communication such as hugging, touching, or remaining with the family in silence may be most empathetic.

Acknowledge the family's guilt, attempt to alleviate it, and deal openly and nonjudgmentally with anger.

Provide information, answer questions, and offer reassurance that everything possible was done for the child.

### Viewing the Body

Offer the family the opportunity to see the body; repeat the offer later if they decline.

Before viewing, inform the family of bodily changes they should expect (tubes, injuries, cold skin).

A single staff member should accompany the family but remain inconspicuous.

Offer the opportunity to hold the child.

Allow the family as much time as they need.

Offer parents the opportunity for siblings to view the body.

**4 - EVIDENCE-BASED PEDIATRIC NURSING INTERVENTIONS**

*Modified from Back K: Sudden, unexpected pediatric death: caring for the parents, *Pediatr Nurs* 17(6):571-574, 1991.

| TABLE 4-16 | Communicating Bad News to Families |
|---|---|
| **Approach** | **Effective Techniques** |
| Provide a setting conducive to communication | Ensure privacy; use appropriate body language; make eye contact. Have parents choose who will attend. |
| Determine what the family knows | Ask questions (e.g., "What have you made of all this?" or "What were you told?"). Listen to the vocabulary and comprehension of the family. Recognize denial, but do not acknowledge it at this stage. |
| Determine what the family wants to know | Obtain a clear invitation to share information (if this is what the family wants). Use questions such as, "Are you the sort of person who likes to know every detail, or just the basic facts?" |
| Give information (aligning and educating) | Start at level of family's comprehension, and use the same vocabulary. Give information slowly, concisely, and in simple language. Avoid medical jargon. Check regularly to be certain that content is understood. |
| Respond to family's reactions | Acknowledge all reactions and feelings, particularly using the emphatic response technique (identifying emotion, identifying cause of emotion, and responding appropriately). Expect tears, anger, and other strong emotions. |
| Close | Briefly summarize major areas discussed. Ask parents if they have other important issues to discuss at this time. Make an appointment for the next meeting. |

## Formal Concluding Process

Discuss and answer questions concerning autopsy and funeral arrangements; obtain signatures on the body release and autopsy forms.

Provide anticipatory guidance regarding symptoms of grief response and their normalcy.

Provide written materials about grief symptoms.

Escort the family to the exit or to their car if necessary.

Provide a follow-up phone call in 24 to 48 hours to answer questions and provide support.

Provide referral for community health nursing visit.

Provide referrals to local support and resource groups (e.g., bereavement groups, bereavement counselors, SIDS groups, Parents of Murdered Children, Mothers Against Drunk Driving).

## REFERENCES

Abo A, Chen L, Johnston P, Santucci K: Positioning for lumbar puncture in children evaluated by bedside ultrasound, *Pediatrics* 125: e1149-e1153, 2010.

American Heart Association: 2010 American Heart Association guidelines for CPR and ECC, *Circulation* 122(Suppl 2), 2001.

Baranoski S, Ayello E: *Wound care essentials: Practice principles*, Philadelphia, 2004, Lippincott Williams & Wilkins.

Bennett L, Rosenblum R, Perlov C, and others: In vivo comparison of topical agents on wound repair, *Plast Reconstr Surg* 108(3):675-687, 2001.

Beckstrand J, Ellett MLC, McDaniel A: Predicting internal distance to the stomach for positioning NG and OG feeding tubes in children, *J Adv Nurs* 59(3):274-289, 2007.

Bottor LT: Rapid sequence intubation in the neonate, *Adv Neonat Care* 9(3):111-117, 2009.

Bryant R: *Acute and chronic wounds: Nursing management*, ed 2, St Louis, 2002, Mosby.

Fearon DM, Steele DW: End-tidal carbon dioxide predicts the presence and severity of acidosis in children with diabetes, *Acad Emerg Med* 9(12): 1373-1379, 2002.

Fernandez R, Griffiths R, Ussia C: Water for wound cleansing. In *Cochrane Database Syst Rev* 2002, Issue 4. Article No. CD003861. DOI: 10.1002/14651858.CD003861.

Foster H, Ritchey M, Bloom D: Adventitious knots in urethral catheters: report of 5 cases, *J Urol* 148(5):1496-1498, 1992.

Gonzalez CM, Palmer LS: Double-knotted feeding tube in a child's bladder, *Urology* 49(5):772. 1997.

Hazinski MF, Chameides L, Hemphill R, Samson R, Schexnayder SM, and Sinz E: Highlights of the 2010 American Heart Association guidelines for CPR and ECC available at *www.heart.org* (accessed December 1, 2010).

Joanna Briggs Institute: Eye care for intensive care patients [electronic version]. *Best Practice*, 6(1), 2002, Blackwell Publishing, Australia, available at *www.joannabriggs.edu.au/pdf/BPISEng_6_1.pdf* (accessed July 7, 2010).

Kilbane BJ: Images in emergency medicine. Knotting of a urinary catheter, *Ann Emerg Med* 53(5):e3-4, 2009.

Klasner AE, Luke DA, Scalzo AJ: Pediatric orogastric and nasogastric tubes: A new formula evaluated, *Ann Emerg Med* 39(3):268-272, 2002.

Kleiber C, Krutzfield N, Rose EF: Acute histologic changes in tracheobronchial tree associated with different suction catheter insertion techniques, *Heart Lung* 17(1):10-14, 1988.

Krasner D, Rodeheaver G, Sibbald G: *Chronic wound care: A clinical source book for healthcare professionals*, ed 3, Wayne, Penn, 2001, Health Management Publications.

Levison J, Wojtulewicz J: Adventitious knot formation complicating catheterization of the infant bladder, *J Paediatr Child Health* 40(8):493-494, 2004.

Lineweaver W, Howard R, Soucy D, and others: Topical antimicrobial toxicity, *Arch Surg* 120(3):267, 1985.

Lodha A, Ly L, Brindle M, Daneman A, McNamara PJ: Intraurethral knot in a very-low-birth-weight infant: Radiological recognition, surgical management and prevention, *Pediatr Radiol* 35(7):713-716, 2005.

Lund C, Kuller J, Lane A, and others: Neonatal skin care: The scientific basis for practice, *Neonatal Netw* 18(4):241-254, 1999.

Moore ZEH, Cowman S: Wound cleansing for pressure ulcers. In *Cochrane Database Syst Rev* 2005, Issue 4. Article No. CD004983. DOI: 10.1002/14651858.CD004983.pub2.

Nagler J, Wright R, Krauss B: End-tidal carbon dioxide as a measure of acidosis among children with gastroenteritis, *Pediatrics* 118(1):260-267, 2006.

North American Society for Pediatric Gastroenterology, Hepatology, and Nutrition: Evaluation and treatment of constipation in children: Recommendations of the North American Society for Pediatric Gastroenterology, Hepatology, and Nutrition, *J Pediatr Gastroenterol Nutr* 43(4):e1-e13, 2006.

Schechter NL, Zempsky WT, Cohen LL, and others: Pain reduction during pediatric immunizations: Evidence-based review and recommendations, *Pediatrics* 119(5):e1184-1198, 2007.

Selekman J, Snyder B: Institutional policies on the use of physical restraints on children, *Pediatr Nurs* 23(5):531-537, 1997.

Sherman JM, Davis S, Albamonte-Petrick S, and others: Care of the child with a tracheostomy: Official statement of the American Thoracic Society, *Am J Respir Crit Care Med* 161(1):297-308, 2000.

Turner TW: Intravesical catheter knotting: An uncommon complication of urinary catheterization, *Pediatr Emerg Care* 20(2):115-117, 2004.

Zerwekh JV: Do dying patients really need IV fluids? *Am J Nurs* 97(3):26-30, 1997.

4 - EVIDENCE-BASED PEDIATRIC NURSING INTERVENTIONS

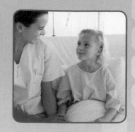

# Nursing Care Plans

## ⊖volve WEBSITE

# The Process of Nursing Infants and Children

## Nursing Diagnoses and the Nursing Process

The nursing process is a theory of how nurses organize the care of individuals, families, and communities. The nursing process involves the implementation of cognitive and operational skills across five phases:

1. **Assessment**—The analysis and synthesis of data obtained from a comprehensive and focused health history and physical examination of the child and family

## BOX 5-1 | NANDA-International Nursing Diagnoses 2009-2011

Activity Intolerance
Risk for Activity Intolerance
Ineffective Activity Planning
Ineffective Airway Clearance
Latex Allergy Response
Risk for Latex Allergy Response
Anxiety
Death Anxiety
Risk for Aspiration
Risk for Impaired Parent/Infant/Child Attachment
Autonomic Dysreflexia
Risk for Autonomic Dysreflexia
Risk Prone Health Behavior
Risk for Bleeding
Disturbed Body Image
Risk for Imbalanced Body Temperature
Bowel Incontinence
Effective Breastfeeding
Ineffective Breastfeeding
Interrupted Breastfeeding
Ineffective Breathing Pattern
Decreased Cardiac Output
Risk for Decreased Cardiac Perfusion
Risk for Ineffective Cardiac Tissue Perfusion
Caregiver Role Strain
Risk for Caregiver Role Strain
Risk for Ineffective Cerebral Tissue Perfusion

Readiness for Enhanced Childbearing Process
Readiness for Enhanced Comfort
Impaired Comfort
Impaired Verbal Communication
Readiness for Enhanced Communication
Decisional Conflict
Parental Role Conflict
Acute Confusion
Chronic Confusion
Risk for Acute Confusion
Constipation
Perceived Constipation
Risk for Constipation
Contamination
Risk for Contamination
Compromised Family Coping
Defensive Coping
Disabled Family Coping
Ineffective Coping
Ineffective Community Coping
Readiness for Enhanced Coping
Readiness for Enhanced Community Coping
Readiness for Enhanced Family Coping
Risk for Sudden Infant Death Syndrome
Readiness for Enhanced Decision Making
Ineffective Denial
Impaired Dentition

*Continued*

2. **Problem identification or diagnosis**—The determination of actual or potential health problems stated as a nursing diagnosis
3. **Plan formulation**—A set of nursing interventions planned to prioritize the health care needs of the child and family. Patient-centered outcomes may be formulated in this phase.
4. **Implementation**—The performance or execution of the plan
5. **Evaluation**—A measure of the outcome of nursing action(s) that either completes the nursing process or serves as a basis for reassessment

The American Nurses Association has established Standards of Practice (use of the nursing process):

1. **Assessment**—The nurse collects comprehensive data pertinent to the patient's health or the situation.
2. **Diagnosis**—The nurse analyzes assessment data to determine the diagnoses or issues.

3. **Outcomes identification**—The nurse identifies expected outcomes for a plan individualized to the patient or the situation.
4. **Planning**—The nurse develops a plan of care that prescribes strategies and alternatives to attain expected outcomes.
5. **Implementation**—The nurse implements the identified plan.
6. **Evaluation**—The nurse evaluates progress toward attainment of outcomes.*

The North American Nursing Diagnosis Associations-International† defines nursing diagnosis as a clinical judgment about individual, family, or community responses to actual and potential health problems. The nursing diagnoses used in this manual are taken from the North American Nursing Diagnosis Association-International (Box 5-1). Nursing diagnoses are suggested for select health system dysfunctions. Included is the **Nursing Intervention Classification (NIC)**

*Adapted from American Nurses Association: The nursing process: a common thread amongst all nurses. American Nurses Association, 2011, Sliver Springs, MD. Available at http://www.nursingworld.org/EspeciallyForYou/StudentNurses/Thenursingprocess.aspx. Accessed March 21, 2011.
†From North American Nursing Diagnosis Association International: Nursing diagnoses: definitions and classification 2009-2011. Copyright 2009, 2007, 2005, 2003, 2001, 1998, 1996, 1994 by NANDA International. Used in arrangement with Wiley-Blackwell Publishing, a company of John Wiley & Sons, Inc. In order to make safe and effective judgments using NANDA-I nursing diagnoses, it is essential that nurses refer to the definitions and defining characteristics of the diagnoses listed in this work.

5 - NURSING CARE PLANS

| BOX 5-1 | NANDA-International Nursing Diagnoses 2009-2011—cont'd |

Risk for Delayed Development
Diarrhea
Risk for Compromised Human Dignity
Moral Distress
Risk for Disuse Syndrome
Deficient Diversional Activity
Risk for Electrolyte Imbalance
Disturbed Energy Field
Impaired Environmental Interpretation Syndrome
Adult Failure to Thrive
Risk for Falls
Dysfunctional Family Processes: Alcoholism
Interrupted Family Processes
Readiness for Enhanced Family Processes
Fatigue
Fear
Readiness for Enhanced Fluid Balance
Deficient Fluid Volume
Excess Fluid Volume
Risk for Deficient Fluid Volume
Risk for Imbalanced Fluid Volume
Impaired Gas Exchange
Dysfunctional Gastrointestinal Motility
Risk for Dysfunctional Gastrointestinal Motility
Risk for Ineffective Gastrointestinal Tissue Perfusion
Risk for Unstable Glucose Level
Grieving
Complicated Grieving
Risk for Complicated Grieving
Delayed Growth and Development
Effective Health Management
Risk for Disproportionate Growth
Ineffective Health Maintenance
Effective Self Health Management
Ineffective Self Health Management
Readiness for Enhanced Self Health Management
Health-Seeking Behaviors
Impaired Home Maintenance
Readiness for Enhanced Hope
Hopelessness
Hyperthermia
Hypothermia
Disturbed Personal Identity
Readiness for Enhanced Immunization Status
Functional Urinary Incontinence
Overflow Urinary Incontinence
Reflex Urinary Incontinence
Stress Urinary Incontinence
Urge Urinary Incontinence
Risk for Urge Urinary Incontinence
Disorganized Infant Behavior

Risk for Disorganized Infant Behavior
Readiness for Enhanced Organized Infant Behavior
Ineffective Infant Feeding Pattern
Risk for Infection
Risk for Injury
Risk for Perioperative Positioning Injury
Neonatal Jaundice
Insomnia
Decreased Intracranial Adaptive Capacity
Deficient Knowledge
Readiness for Enhanced Knowledge
Sedentary Lifestyle
Risk for Impaired Liver Function
Risk for Loneliness
Risk for Disturbed Maternal/Fetal Dyad
Impaired Memory
Impaired Bed Mobility
Impaired Physical Mobility
Impaired Wheelchair Mobility
Nausea
Self Neglect
Unilateral Neglect
Noncompliance
Imbalanced Nutrition: Less Than Body Requirements
Imbalanced Nutrition: More Than Body Requirements
Readiness for Enhanced Nutrition
Risk for Imbalanced Nutrition: More Than Body Requirements
Impaired Oral Mucous Membrane
Acute Pain
Chronic Pain
Readiness for Enhanced Parenting
Impaired Parenting
Risk for Impaired Parenting
Risk for Peripheral Neurovascular Dysfunction
Ineffective Peripheral Tissue Perfusion
Risk for Poisoning
Post-Trauma Syndrome
Risk for Post-Trauma Syndrome
Readiness for Enhanced Power
Powerlessness
Risk for Powerlessness
Ineffective Protection
Rape-Trauma Syndrome
Readiness for Enhanced Relationship
Impaired Religiosity
Readiness for Enhanced Religiosity
Risk for Impaired Religiosity
Relocation Stress Syndrome
Risk for Relocation Stress Syndrome
Risk for Ineffective Renal Perfusion
Risk for Compromised Resilience

BOX **5-1** | NANDA-International Nursing Diagnoses 2009-2011—cont'd

Readiness for Enhanced Resilience
Impaired Individual Resilience
Ineffective Role Performance
Readiness for Enhanced Self-Care
Bathing/Hygiene Self-Care Deficit
Dressing/Grooming Self-Care Deficit
Feeding Self-Care Deficit
Toileting Self-Care Deficit
Readiness for Enhanced Self-Concept
Chronic Low Self-Esteem
Situational Low Self-Esteem
Risk for Situational Low Self-Esteem
Self-Mutilation
Risk for Self-Mutilation
Disturbed Sensory Perception
Sexual Dysfunction
Ineffective Sexuality Patterns
Risk for Shock
Impaired Skin Integrity
Risk for Impaired Skin Integrity
Sleep Deprivation
Readiness for Enhanced Sleep
Disturbed Sleep Pattern
Social Isolation
Chronic Sorrow

Spiritual Distress
Risk for Spiritual Distress
Readiness for Enhanced Spiritual Well-Being
Stress Overload
Risk for Suffocation
Risk for Suicide
Delayed Surgical Recovery
Impaired Swallowing
Ineffective Family Therapeutic Regimen Management
Ineffective Thermoregulation
Impaired Tissue Integrity
Ineffective Tissue Perfusion
Impaired Transfer Ability
Risk for Trauma
Impaired Urinary Elimination
Readiness for Enhanced Urinary Elimination
Urinary Retention
Risk for Vascular Trauma
Impaired Spontaneous Ventilation
Dysfunctional Ventilatory Weaning Response
Risk for Other-Directed Violence
Risk for Self-Directed Violence
Impaired Walking
Wandering

From North American Nursing Diagnosis Association International: Nursing diagnoses: definitions and classification 2009-2011. Copyright 2009, 2007, 2005, 2003, 2001, 1998, 1996, 1994 by NANDA International. Used in arrangement with Wiley-Blackwell Publishing, a company of John Wiley & Sons, Inc.
   In order to make safe and effective judgments using NANDA-I nursing diagnoses, it is essential that nurses refer to the definitions and defining characteristics of the diagnoses listed in this work.

for each nursing diagnosis. The NIC is a standardized list of evidence-based nursing care interventions. In addition, the **Nursing Outcomes Classification (NOC)** is included to provide standardized patient outcomes. The selected nursing diagnoses and care interventions serve as general guides for the nursing care of children and families. Other nursing diagnoses and care interventions should be added to individualize care as appropriate.

Interventions to guide nursing care of children and families consist of three types of practice activities: dependent,

interdependent, and independent. Dependent activities hold the nurse accountable for implementing medical interventions that are prescribed by medical providers. Interdependent practice activities require collaboration (labeled *Collaborative* in care plan) between two or more disciplines to implement collaborative medical/nursing interventions. Independent practice activities are nurse-prescribed and implemented nursing interventions.

5 - NURSING CARE PLANS

# Nursing Care of Common Problems of Ill and Hospitalized Children

## NURSING CARE PLAN

### The Child in Pain

| Nursing Diagnosis | Expected Patient Outcomes | Nursing Interventions | Rationale |
|---|---|---|---|
| Pain related to (specify acute or chronic) | Experiences either no pain or a reduction of pain to level acceptable to child (equal to or less than comfort or function goal) when receiving analgesics | Use QUESTT pain assessment: | Child's self-report of pain is the most important factor in assessment. |
| **Child's/Family's Defining Characteristics** | | Question the child. | |
| *Subjective and Objective Data* | | Use pain-rating scales. | |
| • Facial expression changes | | Evaluate behavior and physiologic changes. | |
| • Physiologic changes: Increased heart rate and blood pressure, increased respirations, crying, sweating, decreased oxygen saturation, dilation of pupils, flushing or pallor, nausea, muscle tension in the early onset of acute pain that subsides in continuing and chronic pain, making these symptoms unreliable indicators of persistent acute and chronic pain | **The Following NOC Concepts Apply to These Outcomes:** Comfort Status Pain Control Pain Level Pain: Disruptive Effects | Secure parents' involvement. Take cause of pain into account. Take action and assess its effectiveness. Ask parents about child's behavior when in pain by taking a pain history before pain is expected. Obtain information regarding current pain, such as duration, type, and location. Asses for influencing factors that may include (1) precipitating events (those that cause or increase the pain), (2) relieving events (those that lessen the pain, e.g , medications), (3) temporal events (times when the pain is relieved or increased), (4) positional events (standing, sitting, lying down), and (5) associated events (meals, stress, coughing). Have parent or child describe pain in terms of interruption of daily activities. | To evaluate the child's pain history To collect pain information data for implementation of appropriate nursing interventions to manage pain |
| Occurrence of specific behaviors (e.g., pulling ears, rolling head from side to side, lying on side with legs flexed, limping, refusing to move a body part) that indicate location of body pain | | Use objective, age-appropriate pain assessment scales to promote accurate assessment. Have child locate pain by marking body part on a human figure drawing or pointing to area with one finger on self, doll, stuffed animal, or "where Mommy or Daddy would put a bandage." | To promote accurate assessment To ensure accurate assessment, because children as young as toddler age, or even children who have difficulty understanding pain scales, can usually locate pain on a drawing or on their bodies |
| Occurrence of improvement in behavior when pain medication is given (e.g., less irritability, cessation of crying, or playing) | | Be aware of reasons why children may deny or not tell the truth about pain. | To decrease fear of receiving an injection if they admit to discomfort; belief that suffering is punishment for some misdeed; lack of trust in telling a stranger (but readily admitting to parent that they are hurting) |
| Occurrence of coping strategies child uses during painful procedure (e.g., talking, moaning, lying rigidly still, squeezing hand, yelling) | | | |

| Intervention | Rationale |
|---|---|
| Use a variety of words to describe pain (e.g., "ouch," "owie," "boo-boo," "hurt," "ow ow") and use appropriate foreign-language words. | To assess pain in a young child who may not know what the word *pain* means and may need to describe pain using familiar language |
| Select a scale that is suitable to the child's developmental or cognitive age, abilities, and preference. | To promote accuracy, because some scales are more appropriate for younger children than other scales |
| Use a pain assessment record or adapt existing form to include pain assessment to document effectiveness of interventions. | To give practitioners objective documentation of pain, rather than opinion, is more likely to lead to favorable change in analgesic orders. |
| Encourage parents to participate in assessing current pain by using the pain assessment record. | To involve parents in their child's care |
| Anticipate administration of analgesic before painful procedure. | To ensure that the peak effect coincides with painful event |
| Plan preventive schedule of medication around the clock (ATC) or, if analgesic is ordered PRN, administer it at regular intervals when pain is continuous and predictable (e.g., postoperatively). | To maintain steady blood levels of analgesic |
| Administer analgesia by least traumatic route whenever possible; avoid intramuscular or subcutaneous injections. | To avoid causing additional pain |
| Prepare child for administration of analgesia by using supportive statements (e.g., "This medicine I am putting in the IV will make you feel better in a few minutes"). | To minimize fear and anxiety |
| Reinforce the effect of the analgesic by telling the child that he or she will begin to feel better in the appropriate amount of time, according to drug used; use a clock or timer to measure onset of relief with the child; reinforce the cause and effect of pain-analgesic. | To promote expectations of pain relief |
| If an injection must be given, avoid saying, "I am going to give you an injection for pain"; if the child refuses an injection, explain that the little hurt from the needle will take away the bigger hurt for a long time. | To minimize fear and anxiety, because an injection causes pain |
| Give the child control whenever possible (e.g., using patient-controlled analgesia, choosing which arm for a venipuncture, taking bandages off, or holding the tape or other equipment). | To promote participation in self-care |
| Administer prescribed analgesic. | To treat pain at the peripheral nervous system and at the central nervous system and provide increased analgesia without increased side effects |

*Continued*

# NURSING CARE PLAN

## The Child in Pain—cont'd

| Nursing Diagnosis | Expected Patient Outcomes | Nursing Interventions | Rationale |
|---|---|---|---|
| Risk for Injury related to sensitivity (to medication), excessive dose, decreased gastrointestinal motility, respiratory depression | Child will not develop constipation and will receive treatment for other opioid-related side effects. | After intervention, assess child's response to pain relief measures. | To evaluate response to pain medication |
| | | Titrate (adjust) dosage for maximum pain relief with minimal side effects.(Collaborative) | To promote maximum pain relief |
| **Child's/Family's Defining Characteristics** | Child will feel less distress about the painful experience by using appropriate nonpharmacologic strategies. | Increase dosage and/or decrease interval between dosages if pain relief is inadequate.(Collaborative) | To manage pain most effectively |
| *Subjective and Objective Data* | | If using parenteral route, request change to oral route as soon as possible using equianalgesic (equal analgesic effect) dosages. (Collaborative) | To consider the first-pass effect (an oral opioid is rapidly absorbed from the gastrointestinal tract and enters the portal or hepatic circulation, where it is partially metabolized before reaching the systemic circulation; therefore oral dosages must be larger) |
| Behavioral or physiologic changes may indicate physical conditions or emotions other than pain (e.g., respiratory distress, fear, anxiety, constipation) | | | To ensure adequate pain management |
| | **The Following NOC Concepts Apply to These Outcomes:** | | |
| | Pain: Adverse Psychological Response | | |
| | Bowel Elimination | | |
| | Depression Self-Control | | |
| | Risk Detection | | |
| | Risk Control | | |
| | Child will exhibit normal respiratory function | Avoid combining opioids with so-called *potentiators*. (Collaborative) | To prevent risk of sedation and respiratory depression without increasing analgesia by combining drugs such as promethazine (Phenergan) and chlorpromazine (Thorazine) |
| | | Avoid use of placebos in the assessment or treatment of pain. (Collaborative) | To prevent use of placebos, because they do not provide useful information about the presence or severity of pain, can cause side effects similar to those of opioids, and can destroy child's and family's trust in the health care staff |
| | | Monitor rate and depth of respirations as well as level of sedation. | To prevent depression of these functions, which can lead to apnea |
| | | Have emergency drugs, narcotic reversal agent, and equipment ready in case of respiratory depression from opioids. | To prevent apnea |
| | | Administer laxative (with or without stool softener). | To begin therapy as soon as needed |
| | | Encourage activity such as sitting in a bedside chair, ambulation | To prevent constipation |
| | | | To promote peristalsis and prevent constipation |

| Interventions | Rationale |
| --- | --- |
| Observe for occurrence of rash urticaria). Recommend administration of antipruretic in the event of pruritis. (Collaborative) | To minimize histamine release from opioids such as morphine and intervene to minimize effects of urticaria |
| Administer prescribed antipruritic. | To decrease pruritus |
| Administer prescribed antiemetic. | To decrease/avoid nausea and vomiting |
| Encourage child to lie quietly until nausea subsides. | To decrease nausea and vomiting |
| Recognize signs of tolerance (e.g., decreasing pain relief, decreasing duration of pain relief). | To ensure adequate pain management |
| Recognize signs of withdrawal after discontinuation of drug (physical dependence). | To ensure adequate management, because these signs and symptoms are involuntary, physiologic responses that occur from prolonged use of opioids |
| Assess the appropriateness of using nonpharmacologic interventions; used alone, they are not appropriate for moderate to severe pain. | To emphasize that they are most useful for mild pain and when pain is reasonably well controlled with analgesics |
| Employ nonpharmacologic strategies to help child manage pain. | To encourage techniques such as relaxation, rhythmic breathing, guided imagery, and distraction, which can make pain more tolerable |
| Use nonpharmacologic strategy that is familiar to child, or describe several strategies and let child select one. | To facilitate the child's learning and use of strategy |
| Involve parent in selection and implementation of strategy. | To promote family involvement |
| Teach child to use specific nonpharmacologic strategies before pain occurs or before it becomes severe. | To prevent pain when possible |

## The Following NIC Concepts Apply to These Interventions:

Airway Management
Analgesic Administration
Respiratory Monitoring
Fluid Management
Constipation/Impaction Management
Pain Management
Distraction
Behavior Management
Coping Enhancement
Art Therapy
Music Therapy
Active Listening
Medication Management
Risk Identification

# Nursing Care of the Newborn

## NURSING CARE PLAN

### The Newborn with Jaundice

| Nursing Diagnosis | Expected Patient Outcomes | Nursing Interventions | Rationale |
|---|---|---|---|
| Neonatal Jaundice related to abnormal blood profile (increased breakdown of products of red blood cells), developmental age (immature blood-brain barrier and immature liver function) | Newborn will receive appropriate therapy to enhance bilirubin excretion. Newborn will remain injury-free. | Initiate breast-feeding within first hour of life in delivery room. | To promote breast milk intake and stooling |
| | | If formula feeding, assist parents in initiation of early feeding. | To promote milk intake and stooling |
| **Child's/Family's Defining Characteristics** | | Assess skin for jaundice every 4 hours. | To detect evidence of clinical jaundice and rising bilirubin levels |
| *Subjective and Objective Data* | **The Following NOC Concept Applies to These Outcomes:** | Observe for development of jaundice, especially within 24 hours of birth. | To institute treatment and prevent complications |
| • Skin jaundice evident within 24 hours of birth | Risk Control | Monitor transcutaneous bilirubin levels per institution protocol or at least every 6 to 8 hours. | To detect rising levels of bilirubin for institution of appropriate therapy |
| • Altered breast-feeding (ineffective latch-on, nurses less than 6 to 8 times in a 24-hour period) | Risk Detection Nutritional status: food and fluid intake | Monitor fluid intake and output with each occurrence. | To evaluate effectiveness of breast-feeding or formula intake by measuring urinary and stool output |
| • Altered stooling pattern (less than one stool in 24 hours) in first 3 days of life | | Obtain hour-specific predischarge total serum bilirubin (Collaborative) | To obtain a baseline total serum bilirubin measurement |
| • Yellow-orange skin color | | Note risk level on hour-specific nomogram, and inform practitioner of results. | To determine risk for development of hyperbilirubinemia postdischarge |
| • Total serum bilirubin in high intermediate of high-risk zone on hour-specific nomogram in first 48 to 72 hours of life | | Maintain accurate record of urine and stool output, and assist parents in same. | To provide accurate record of output to evaluate effectiveness of feedings |
| | | Monitor vital signs per unit protocol or at least every 8 hours. Report signs of poor transition to extrauterine life. | To evaluate transitional events and ensure that infant is making an effective transition without cardiorespiratory, metabolic, thermoregulatory, or other physiologic problems |

Instruct parents regarding newborn care, including jaundiced appearance, its significance, importance of follow-up visit to practitioner within 2 to 3 days of discharge, feeding methods, and noting stooling and voiding patterns.

To promote physical care of newborn and decrease parents' anxiety related to home care

**The Following NIC Concepts Apply to These Interventions:**
Risk Identification
Nutrition Management
Breast-feeding Assistance
Lactation Counseling
Newborn Monitoring
Newborn Care
Fluid Monitoring
Family Support

Initiate skin-to-skin contact between mother and newborn and father and newborn in delivery room within first hour of birth.

To enhance parent-infant interaction and acquaintance with newborn

Encourage early breast-feeding in first hour of birth.

To enhance breast-feeding and parent-infant interaction and to promote early stooling and bilirubin clearance

Perform physical assessment with parents present, and show typical newborn characteristics. Point out state traits such as quiet awake and cues to feeding readiness.

To promote parents' knowledge of infant physical characteristics and behavior

Encourage parent participation in care behaviors such as diapering, formula feeding (as applicable), and bathing.

To promote familiarity with behaviors and decrease parental anxiety

To enhance parental feeling of contribution as newborn's primary caretakers

Encourage sibling visitation and participation in care and holding of newborn as age-appropriate.

To promote sibling participation in care and acceptance of new family member

**The Following NIC Concepts Apply to These Interventions:**
Anxiety Reduction
Family Support
Family Process Maintenance
Parent Education: Infant

---

**Readiness for Enhanced Parenting** related to birth of a new family member

**Child's/Family's Defining Characteristics**
*Subjective and Objective Data*
• Parent(s) express willingness to enhance parenting
• Emotional support of child is evident; bonding or attachment is evident

Parent(s) of newborn assume responsibility for emotional and physical care and well-being of the new family member

**The Following NOC Concepts Apply to These Outcomes:**
Parent-Infant Attachment
Parenting: Psychosocial Safety
Caregiver Home Care Readiness

# Nursing Care of the Child with Respiratory Dysfunction

## NURSING CARE PLAN

### The Child with Acute Respiratory Infection

| Nursing Diagnosis | Expected Patient Outcomes | Nursing Interventions | Rationale |
|---|---|---|---|
| Ineffective Breathing Pattern related to inflammatory process | Child's ventilatory status is adequate for oxygenation. | Position for maximal ventilatory efficiency and airway patency. | To allow increased chest expansion |
| **Child's/Family's Defining Characteristics** | **The Following NOC Concepts Apply to These Outcomes:** | Position to facilitate drainage of secretions. | To maintain patent airway and prevent airway obstruction |
| *Subjective and Objective Data* | Respiratory Status: Airway Patency | Provide humidified oxygen as necessary. | To improve oxygenation |
| • Use of accessory muscles to breathe | Respiratory Status: Ventilation | Monitor oxygenation status, including vital signs for changes in condition. | To determine need for additional interventions |
| • Dyspnea | | Suction airway (nose, trachea) as necessary. | To remove secretions and maintain airway patency |
| • Shortness of breath | | | To facilitate secretion removal |
| • Nasal flaring | | Provide gentle chest percussion and physiotherapy as necessary. | |
| • Altered chest excursion | | Administer bronchodilator medications. | To promote bronchodilation and improve ventilation |
| • Assumption of three-point position (tripod) | | Administer antiinflammatory medications. | To decrease airway inflammation |
| • Respiratory rate is outside normal parameter for child's age (increased or decreased rate) | | Administer antibiotics (if bacterial). | To decrease inflammatory response |
| | | **The Following NIC Concepts Apply to These Interventions:** | |
| | | Aspiration Precautions | |
| | | Positioning | |
| | | Respiratory Monitoring | |
| | | Surveillance | |
| | | Oxygen Therapy | |
| | | Airway Suctioning | |
| | | Vital Signs Monitoring | |
| | | Cough Enhancement | |
| | | Medication Administration. | |

| Nursing Diagnosis / Characteristics | Interventions | Rationale |
|---|---|---|
| **Ineffective Airway Clearance** related to inflammation, mechanical obstruction, increased secretions<br><br>**Child's/Family's Defining Characteristics**<br>*Subjective and Objective Data*<br>• Dyspnea<br>• Difficulty vocalizing<br>• Orthopnea<br>• Adventitious breath sounds (crackles, wheezing, rhonchi)<br>• Cough ineffective or absent<br>• Restlessness<br>• Changes in respiratory rate and rhythm | Child's airway remains patent<br>**The Following NOC Concepts Apply to These Outcomes:**<br>Aspiration Prevention<br>Respiratory Status: Airway Patency<br><br>Position to facilitate drainage of secretions.<br>Perform chest physiotherapy.<br>Suction airway as necessary.<br>Provide humidified oxygen as necessary.<br><br>Assist with coughing (as developmentally or age-appropriate).<br>Avoid throat examination if epiglottitis is suspected.<br>Assure child (as appropriate) that all measures will be taken to ensure that adequate airway is maintained.<br>Implement comfort measures such as allowing parental presence, parental holding, favorite blanket or stuffed animal at side; explain all procedures beforehand.<br><br>**The Following NIC Concepts Apply to These Interventions:**<br>Cough Enhancement<br>Positioning<br>Chest Physiotherapy<br>Vital Signs Monitoring<br>Anxiety Reduction | To prevent airway obstruction<br>To loosen and remove secretions<br>To remove secretions<br>To moisten secretions and prevent airway drying<br>To remove secretions<br><br>To prevent airway compromise<br>To allay anxiety<br>To promote anxiety reduction and decrease effects of medical therapy, including hospitalization if required |
| **Risk for Injury** related to presence (only as indicated) of infective organisms<br><br>**Child's/Family's Defining Characteristics**<br>*Subjective and Objective Data*<br>• Tissue hypoxia<br>• Abnormal blood profile<br>• People or provider (nosocomial agents)<br>• Mode of transport<br>• Developmental age | Child remains free from complications of infection<br>**The Following NOC Concept Applies to These Outcomes:**<br>Risk Control<br><br>Maintain aseptic environment using sterile suction equipment and technique.<br>Implement and practice Standard Precautions.<br>Implement contact and/or airborne precautions as necessary.<br>Obtain (secretion, tissue, or blood) specimen as indicated.<br>Encourage child and family contacts to practice frequent hand-washing and to avoid hand-to-eye and hand-to-mouth contact.<br>Teach child (as age-appropriate) and family how to decrease spread of organisms by covering mouth when coughing and disposing of secretions to avoid cross-contamination.<br>Administer antibiotic or antiviral medications.<br>Administer fever-reduction medication(s) as appropriate.<br>Monitor and assess for signs and symptoms of secondary complications: hypoxia, skin breakdown, poor nutrient and fluid intake, increased work of breathing, deteriorating cardiorespiratory status.<br><br>**The Following NIC Concepts Apply to These Interventions:**<br>Risk Identification<br>Environmental Management<br>Infection Control<br>Parent Education: Childrearing Family<br>Medication Administration | To prevent spread of infectious organisms in child and family<br>To prevent spread of infection<br>To prevent spread of infection<br>To identify infective organism<br>To prevent spread of infection<br><br>To prevent spread of infection<br><br>To treat infection source<br>To promote comfort.<br>To implement therapy for prevention of secondary complications |

*Continued*

5 - NURSING CARE PLANS

# NURSING CARE PLAN

## The Child with Acute Respiratory Infection—cont'd

| Nursing Diagnosis | Expected Patient Outcomes | Nursing Interventions | Rationale |
|---|---|---|---|
| Interrupted Family Processes related to child's illness and/or hospitalization, medical therapeutic regimen<br><br>**Child's/Family's Defining Characteristics**<br>*Subjective and Objective Data*<br>• Communication patterns<br>• Participation in decision making<br>• Availability for emotional support<br>• Expressions of conflict within family<br>• Patterns and rituals | Family demonstrates ability to cope with child's illness.<br><br>**The Following NOC Concepts Apply to These Outcomes:**<br>Family Integrity<br>Family Support during Treatment<br>Family Functioning | Allow family to remain with child.<br>Promote family-centered care.<br>Explain procedures and therapeutic regimen to family.<br>Keep family informed of child's status.<br>Encourage family involvement in child's care.<br>Provide support and referral for continued support as necessary.<br><br>**The Following NIC Concepts Apply to These Interventions:**<br>Caregiver Support<br>Family Support<br>Coping Enhancement<br>Emotional Support<br>Financial Resource Assistance<br>Family Integrity Promotion | To decrease effects of separation<br>To provide accurate information regarding therapy and child's condition<br>To promote family's sense of control and involvement in care |

# NURSING CARE PLAN

## The Child with Asthma

| Nursing Diagnosis | Expected Patient Outcomes | Nursing Interventions | Rationale |
|---|---|---|---|
| Risk for Suffocation related to interaction between individual and triggering factors (allergens, respiratory infection, exercise, irritants, emotions, temperature changes)<br><br>**Child's/Family's Defining Characteristics**<br>*Subjective and Objective Data*<br>• Wheezing<br>• Dry cough<br>• Labored respirations<br>• Dyspnea | Child will have adequate air exchange.<br>Family and child assume responsibility for asthma symptom management.<br><br>**The Following NOC Concepts Apply to These Outcomes:**<br>Asthma Self-Management<br>Anxiety Self-Control<br>Knowledge: Child Physical Safety<br>Symptom control<br>Knowledge: asthma management<br>Risk control | Educate child and family to recognize factors such as allergens, irritants, temperature changes, exercise, and upper respiratory infections (URIs) that trigger asthma symptoms.<br>Assist child (according to developmental age) and family to recognize early signs of an asthmatic exacerbation (use peak expiratory flow meter [PEFM]). For example, if PEF is 50% to 79% of personal best, use quick-relief medication and consider contacting practitioner (NAEPP, 2007).<br>Educate child and family regarding proper use of asthma medications such as inhaled corticosteroids and bronchodilator.<br>Educate child and family regarding proper use of rescue asthma medications such as inhaled corticosteroids and bronchodilator in case of illness exacerbation.* | To avoid asthma exacerbations<br>To control symptoms with medication<br>To control symptoms and minimize shortness of breath<br>To prevent illness exacerbations and hospitalization; to prevent side effects from improper use of certain asthma drugs |

*According to the 2007 National Asthma Education and Prevention Program (NAEPP) guidelines for medication administration using the stepwise approach to asthma management (according to the diagnosed asthma severity). Institutes of Health: *Expert Panel Report 3: Guidelines for the diagnosis and management of asthma,* available at www.nhlbi.nih.gov/guidelines/asthma/asthgdln.htm (accessed September 10, 2010).

- Intercostal retractions
- Complains of tightness in chest, shortness of breath
- Bronchial inflammation and airway constriction

Educate child and family regarding proper use of MDI inhaler with spacer, aerosolized nebulizer, and PEFM (know child's personal best).

**The Following NIC Concepts Apply to These Interventions:**
Respiratory Monitoring
Medication Administration: Inhalation, Oral
Risk Identification
Family Integrity Promotion
Energy Management
Coping Enhancement
Environmental Management
Allergy management

To help child and family effectively manage asthma symptoms independently

---

**Interrupted Family Processes** related to child with a chronic illness

**Child's/Family's Defining Characteristics**

*Subjective and Objective Data*
- Anxiety
- Family interactions with child and members are disrupted
- Family conflicts
- Inadequate child support
- Child's health status is ignored
- Family ignores other members' needs for those of the child with asthma

Family copes with effects of the disease
Family provides child an appropriate protective environment

**The Following NOC Concepts Apply to These Outcomes:**
Family Functioning
Family Normalization

Educate child and family (as age appropriate) about asthma and management of the condition.†

Collaborate with child and family to develop a written action plan for asthma management.

Discuss facilitators and barriers to effective asthma management (e.g., ensuring that bronchodilator inhalers are readily available for the child's use; prescriptions for bronchodilators are renewed in a timely manner; exposure to asthma triggers is avoided; primary care is adhered to on a regular basis for evaluation of asthma).

Discuss impact of illness on the family's lifestyle.

Evaluate family resources for asthma management in relation to the following:
- Access to health care
- Medication availability in home and at school (or daycare, as appropriate)
- Allergen exposure control and eradication

**The Following NIC Concepts Apply to These Interventions:**
Emotional Support
Anticipatory Guidance
Family Involvement Promotion
Financial Resource Assistance
Decision-Making Support
Mutual Goal Setting

To provide adequate knowledge for management of asthma symptoms
To provide realistic expectations about requirements for managing the condition
To provide family and child sense of control
To proactively manage asthma symptoms
To assist family members in understanding their role as being vital in the management of asthma

To provide opportunity to verbalize frustrations and challenges of having a child with a chronic illness
To enhance family coping with chronic illness

---

†According to the 2007 NAEPP, the four components of asthma management are: assessment and monitoring, education of child and family, control of environmental and comorbid factors, and pharmacologic therapy. Family education in these areas according to the child's asthma classification is essential.

**5 - NURSING CARE PLANS**

# Nursing Care of the Child with Cardiovascular Dysfunction

## NURSING CARE PLAN

### The Child with Heart Failure (HF)

| Nursing Diagnosis | Expected Patient Outcomes | Nursing Interventions | Rationale |
|---|---|---|---|
| Decreased Cardiac Output related to structural defect, myocardial dysfunction, altered hemodynamics | Child will have adequate cardiac output as evidenced by: | Assess and record heart rate (HR), respiratory rate (RR), blood pressure (BP), and any signs and symptoms of decreased cardiac output (listed under defining characteristics) every 2 to 4 hours and as needed (PRN). | To assess for changes in vital signs and child's physical status that reflect altered cardiac output |
| **Child's/Family's Defining Characteristics** | • Heart rate within acceptable range (state specific range) | | |
| *Subjective and Objective Data* | • Respiratory rate within acceptable range (state specific range) | Administer cardiac drugs (e.g., digoxin, ACE inhibitor) on schedule. | To improve heart function. |
| • Tachycardia | • Skin warm to touch | Assess for and record any side effects or any signs or symptoms of toxicity to cardiac drugs. | To maximize drug effectiveness |
| • Tachypnea | • Strong and equal peripheral pulses | Follow hospital protocol for drug administration. | |
| • Ineffective peripheral circulation, cool extremities | • Blood pressure normal for age | Keep accurate record of fluid intake and output. | |
| | • Brisk capillary refill within 2 to 3 seconds | | |
| • Hypotension | • Lack of distended neck veins | Weigh child or infant on same scale at same time of day. Document results and compare with previous weight. | To assess for HF, which causes decreased urinary output |
| • Rapid, weak peripheral pulses | • Normal sinus rhythm | | To observe for weight increase that may indicate excess fluid accumulation |
| • Prolonged capillary refill, longer than 2 to 3 seconds | • Lack of edema | Administer diuretics as prescribed. Assess and record effectiveness and any side effects noted. | To prevent fluid retention. |
| • Narrow pulse pressure | • Adequate urine output (state specific; 1 to 2 ml/kg/hr) | Elevate head of bed at a 30- to 45-degree angle. | To promote maximum chest expansion and ease work of breathing |
| • Distended neck veins in older children | | | |
| • Cardiomegaly (evident on chest radiograph) | Child will have age-appropriate weight gain on standardized growth curve. Infant will demonstrate successful feeding. | | |
| • Gallop rhythm | | | |
| • Edema | | | |
| • Rapid weight gain | | | |
| • Feeding difficulty | | | |
| • Irritability | | | |
| • Decreased urine output | | | |
| | Child and/or family will be able to state at least four characteristics of heart failure such as: | Offer small frequent feedings to infant's or child's tolerance. | To prevent fatigue during feeding. |
| | • Rapid heart rate | Increase caloric density of feedings. | To provide adequate calories for growth |
| | • Fast breathing | Organize nursing care to allow child/infant uninterrupted rest and sleep. | To provide conservation of energy and decrease demands on heart |
| | • Cool extremities | Provide play activities which are nonstressful on heart but appropriate for developmental stimulation | To allow expression of feelings through play activities; to provide for appropriate child development, and to decrease demands on heart |
| | • Puffiness (edema) | | |
| | • Fussiness | | |
| | • Decreased appetite | | |
| | • Decreased feeding ability | | |

*Continued*

| Nursing Diagnosis/Defining Characteristics | Patient/Family Goals & Outcomes | Interventions | Rationale |
|---|---|---|---|
| | Child and/or family will be able to state knowledge of care regarding:<br>• Medication administration<br>• Head-elevated positioning<br>• Sufficient rest periods<br>• Feeding<br>• Monitoring fluid intake and output<br>• When to contact health care provider<br>**The Following NOC Concepts Apply to These Outcomes:**<br>Cardiac Pump Effectiveness<br>Knowledge: Illness Care<br>Tissue Perfusion: Cardiac | Educate child and family about characteristics of HF. Assess and record teaching session.<br>Educate child and family about care such as medication administration.<br>Assess and record results and family's participation in care.<br>**The Following NIC Concepts Apply to These Interventions:**<br>Cardiac Care<br>Fluid Management<br>Medication Administration<br>Positioning<br>Vital Signs Monitoring<br>Respiratory Monitoring | To provide parent education that can promote measures to improve cardiac function and decrease demands on heart<br>To promote safety and family involvement in child's care. |
| **Ineffective Breathing Pattern** related to pulmonary congestion, decreased cardiac output<br>**Child's/Family's Defining Characteristics**<br>*Subjective and Objective Data*<br>• Tachypnea<br>• Dyspnea<br>• Retractions<br>• Crackles<br>• Shortness of breath<br>• Cyanosis<br>• Pallor<br>• Mottling<br>• Nasal flaring<br>• Grunting<br>• Head bobbing<br>• Cough<br>• Use of accessory muscles<br>• Activity intolerance | Child will have effective breathing pattern as evidenced by:<br>• Respiratory rate within acceptable range (state specific range)<br>• Clear and equal breath sounds bilaterally anterior and posterior<br>• Pink oral mucosa<br>• Absence of nasal flaring, retractions, cough, and head bobbing<br>• Unlabored respirations<br>• Tolerance of activities appropriate for age<br><br>Child and/or family will be able to state four characteristics of ineffective breathing pattern such as:<br>• Color change from pink or tan to pale, dusky, or blue<br>• Fast breathing<br>• Change in amount and/or characteristics of secretions<br>• Retractions, head bobbing<br>• Ineffective cough<br>• Decreased or altered activity level | Assess and record respiratory rate, breath sounds, and any signs and symptoms of ineffective pattern (listed under characteristics) every 2 to 4 hours and PRN.<br>Administer humidified oxygen in correct amount using correct route of delivery. Record percent of oxygen and route of delivery. Assess and record child's response to therapy.<br>Keep head of bed elevated at a 30- to 45-degree angle.<br>Suction if child has ineffective cough or is unable to manage secretions.<br>Assess and record amount and characteristics of secretions.<br>Assess and record oxygen saturation every 2 to 4 hours and PRN.<br>Educate child and family about characteristics of ineffective breathing pattern.<br>Assess and record results of teaching.<br>Educate child and family about child's care, including medication administration, feeding, and provision of rest.<br>Assess and record results and family participation in care.<br>**The Following NIC Concepts Apply to These Interventions:**<br>Airway Management<br>Airway Suctioning<br>Chest Physiotherapy<br>Family Involvement Promotion<br>Health Education | To assess for respiratory changes that can be indicators of worsening HF.<br>To improve tissue oxygenation.<br>To promote maximum chest expansion<br>To maintain patent airway to promote respiratory expansion<br>To evaluate respiratory function<br>To provide parent education that can promote measures to improve breathing effort<br>To promote family involvement in child's care. |

## NURSING CARE PLAN

### The Child with Heart Failure (HF)—cont'd

| Nursing Diagnosis | Expected Patient Outcomes | Nursing Interventions | Rationale |
| --- | --- | --- | --- |
| | Child and/or family will be able to state knowledge of care regarding: <br> • Positioning to facilitate respiratory effort <br> • Oxygen administration <br> • When to contact health care provider <br><br> The Following NOC Concepts Apply to These Outcomes: <br> Activity Tolerance <br> Knowledge: Illness Care <br> Respiratory Status: Gas Exchange <br> Tissue Perfusion: Pulmonary | | |

# Nursing Care of the Child with Hematologic/Immunologic Dysfunction

## NURSING CARE PLAN

### The Child with Sickle Cell Disease

| Nursing Diagnosis | Expected Patient Outcomes | Nursing Interventions | Rationale |
| --- | --- | --- | --- |
| Risk for Injury related to abnormal hemoglobin shape, decreased oxygen-carrying capacity. <br><br> Child's/Family's Defining Characteristics <br> *Subjective and Objective Data* <br> • Shortness of breath <br> • Dyspnea <br> • Fatigue <br> • Headache <br> • Pallor <br> • Icteric sclera or jaundice <br> • Systolic murmur <br> • Cyanosis <br> • Increased pulse | Child will avoid situations that reduce tissue oxygenation and will allow for adequate tissue oxygenation <br><br> The Following NOC Concepts Apply to These Outcomes: <br> Risk Control <br> Parenting: Early/Middle Childhood Physical Safety | Explain measures to minimize complications related to physical exertion and emotional stress. <br> Prevent infection. <br> Avoid low-oxygen environment (e.g., high altitudes). <br><br> The Following NIC Concepts Apply to These Interventions: <br> Health Education <br> Behavior Modification | To avoid additional tissue deoxygenation <br> To avoid additional tissue deoxygenation <br> To prevent a decrease in oxygenation |

| Nursing Diagnosis / Defining Characteristics / Outcomes | Interventions | Rationale |
|---|---|---|
| **Risk for Deficient Fluid Volume** related to decreased fluid intake, fluid losses<br><br>**Child's/Family's Defining Characteristics**<br>*Subjective and Objective Data*<br>• Dry mucous membranes<br>• Loss of skin turgor<br>• Sunken eyes, absent or diminished tears, sunken fontanel, dark-colored urine, rapid thready pulse, rapid breathing, lethargy, weakness<br><br>Child takes adequate amounts of fluids and shows no signs of dehydration<br><br>**The Following NOC Concepts Apply to These Outcomes:**<br>Fluid Balance<br>Electrolyte and Acid/Base Balance | Calculate recommended daily fluid intake (1600 ml/m²/day), and base child's fluid requirements on this amount.<br>Increase fluid intake above minimum requirements during physical exercise and emotional stress and during a crisis.<br>Give parents written instructions regarding specific quantity of fluid required daily.<br>Encourage child to drink fluids (set a realistic fluid intake with combination of different fluids which are palatable and healthy for child).<br>Stress importance of avoiding overheating.<br>Teach family signs of dehydration and interventions in case signs are noted (e.g., oral hydration with small amounts, practitioner notification if child is unable to take in fluids or is vomiting).<br><br>**The Following NIC Concepts Apply to These Interventions:**<br>Fluid Monitoring<br>Fluid/Electrolyte Management | To ensure adequate hydration<br><br>To compensate for additional fluid needs<br><br>To encourage compliance with fluid intake<br><br>To encourage compliance with fluid intake<br><br>To avoid excessive fluid loss<br>To avoid delay in hydration therapy |
| **Acute Pain** related to tissue anoxia and clumping of sickled cells (vasoocclusive crisis)<br><br>**Child's/Family's Defining Characteristics**<br>*Subjective and Objective Data*<br>Pain can occur in any location in the body, can be acute in onset and severe, and can be localized or generalized; low-grade fever may be present; localized swelling can occur over joints with arthralgias.<br><br>Child will experience no or minimal pain<br><br>**The Following NOC Concepts Apply to These Outcomes:**<br>Comfort Status<br>Pain Control<br>Risk control | Discuss preventive schedule of medication administration around the clock (ATC) with parents.<br>Encourage high level of fluid intake.<br>Recognize that various analgesics, including opioids and medication schedules, may need to be tried.<br>Reassure child and family that analgesics including opioids are medically indicated, and that a though high doses may be needed, children rarely become addicted.<br>Apply heat, or massage affected area.<br>Avoid applying cold compresses.<br><br>Administer antipyretic medication for fever.<br>Instruct parents to seek medical attention immediately for sudden, persistent headache, weakness on one side of the body, sudden gait or speech problems, or altered mental status.<br><br>**The Following NIC Concepts Apply to These Interventions:**<br>Medication Management<br>Pain Management<br>Patient-Controlled Analgesia (PCA) Assistance | To prevent pain<br><br>To promote hydration<br>To achieve satisfactory pain relief<br><br>To prevent suffering that may result from their unfounded fears about addiction to pain medications<br>To sooth painful tissues<br>To prevent vasoconstriction that may enhance sickling<br>To reduce fever and provide comfort<br>To recognize acute central nervous system (CNS) events to prevent progressive CNS damage |

*Continued*

# NURSING CARE PLAN

## The Child with Sickle Cell Disease—cont'd

| Nursing Diagnosis | Expected Patient Outcomes | Nursing Interventions | Rationale |
|---|---|---|---|
| Risk for Infection related to compromised immune status | Child will remain free of infection | Observe for and report to practitioner any signs of infection immediately. | To ensure preventive measures that decrease risk for infection exposure |
| **Child's/Family's Defining Characteristics** | **The Following NOC Concepts Apply to These Outcomes:** | Promote compliance with prophylactic antibiotic therapy. | To prevent and to treat infection |
| *Subjective and Objective Data* | Infection Severity | Stress importance of adequate nutrition; routine immunizations, including pneumococcal and meningococcal vaccines; protection from known sources of infection; and frequent health evaluation, with regularly scheduled comprehensive evaluation. | To prevent infection and provide adequate calories for tissue growth and function |
| • Fever | Knowledge: Infection Management Control | | |
| • Chills | Risk Detection | Instruct parents regarding signs and symptoms of splenic sequestration including palpating the spleen regularly. | To provide early recognition of splenic sequestration crisis |
| • Pain | | | |
| • Redness | | | |
| • Lethargy | | | |
| • Increased pallor | | **The Following NIC Concepts Apply to These Interventions:** | |
| • Listlessness | | Environmental Management | |
| • Irritability | | Communicable Disease Management | |
| • Increased pulse and respiration | | Medication Prescribing | |
| • History of prior sepsis | | Medication Administration | |
| | | Medication Management | |
| Deficient Knowledge related to understanding of sickle cell disease and its management | Child and family demonstrate understanding of the disease, its cause, and its treatment | Teach family and children characteristics of basic genetic defect (in SCD) and measures to minimize complications. | To minimize complications of sickling |
| | | Stress importance of informing significant health personnel of child's disease. | To ensure prompt and appropriate treatment |
| **Child's/Family's Defining Characteristics** | **The Following NOC Concepts Apply to These Outcomes:** | Explain (to child and family) signs of developing complications such as fever, pallor, respiratory distress, persistent headaches, and pain. | To avoid delay in seeking appropriate treatment |
| *Subjective and Objective Data* | Family Coping | Reinforce basic information regarding trait transmission, and refer to genetic counseling services. | To allow for informed decision making |
| • Lack of understanding | Knowledge: Illness Care | Discuss with family child's condition and treatment requirements, including need for frequent medical attention when child is ill. | To promote family involvement in child's care |
| • Inability to identify signs and symptoms of painful crises | | Encourage and teach parents to be advocates for their child. | To provide support |
| • Inability to follow disease management guidelines | | Educate the school and teachers regarding etiology of sickle cell disease and measures to avoid complications at school. | To provide support and prevent complications |
| • Difficulty describing treatment plan | | Stress with educators the need to provide tutoring and to allow time to make up schoolwork during medically related absences. | To provide support and prevent setbacks in child's education |
| • Improper medication administration | | **The Following NIC Concepts Apply to These Interventions:** | |
| | | Teaching: Disease Process | |
| | | Teaching: Prescribed Medication | |

Patient and Family Education, Spanish Translations—Preventing Spread of HIV and Hepatitis B Virus Infections

# NURSING CARE PLAN

## The Child or Adolescent with Human Immunodeficiency Virus (HIV) Infection

| Nursing Diagnosis | Expected Patient Outcomes | Nursing Interventions | Rationale |
|---|---|---|---|
| Risk for Infection related to impaired body defenses, presence of infective organisms | Infant will not become infected with HIV-1 virus. | Institute measures to prevent newborn exposure to virus from HIV-positive or HIV–unknown-status mother. | To prevent newborn exposure to HIV virus |
| | Child will experience minimized risk of secondary opportunistic infection. | • Administer maternal antiviral medication to HIV-positive woman in labor (Collaborative). | |
| Child's/Family's Defining Characteristics | The Following NOC Concepts Apply to These Outcomes: | • Assist with cesarean section delivery. | |
| *Subjective and Objective Data* | Immune Status | • Bathe infant as soon as body temperature is stable. | |
| • Exposure *in utero* or at birth to HIV-infected mother | Infection Severity | • Avoid maternal breast-feeding until maternal HIV status is known or negative. | |
| • Recipients of blood products, especially children with hemophilia (before testing began in 1985) | Risk Control: Sexually Transmitted Diseases (STD) | • If maternal HIV status is positive, administer antiviral medications to newborn. | |
| | Risk Control: Infectious processes | • Assist with collection of diagnostic laboratory studies (newborn infant). | |
| • Adolescents engaging in high-risk behaviors | Knowledge: Infection Control | Teach HIV-positive mother about ways to prevent spread of virus to newborn (hand washing, avoiding breast-feeding, personal hygiene). | To prevent spread of virus to infant |
| • Recurrent bacterial infections | | Educate mother regarding infant infections and necessity for close medical follow-up. | To identify opportunistic infections in infancy and treat them before immune system is overwhelmed |
| • Pulmonary diseases (especially *Pneumocystis carinii* pneumonia, lymphocytic interstitial pneumonitis, and pulmonary lymphoid hyperplasia) | | Use thorough hand-washing technique when caring for child. | To minimize exposure to infective organisms |
| | | Advise visitors to use good hand-washing technique. | To minimize exposure to infective organisms |
| | | Assist with diagnostic laboratory collection. | To determine optimum treatment |
| | | Administer antiviral medications as prescribed (Collaborative). | To decrease viral replication and symptoms |
| | | Obtain an immunization history. | To assess risk for infectious diseases |
| | | Restrict contact with persons who have infections, including family members, other children, friends, and members of staff; explain that child is highly susceptible to infection. | To encourage cooperation and understanding |
| | | Observe medical asepsis as appropriate. | To decrease risk of infection |
| | | Encourage optimum nutrition and adequate rest. | To promote the body's remaining natural defenses |
| | | Explain to family and older child importance of contacting health professional if exposed to childhood illnesses (e.g., chickenpox, measles). | To ensure that appropriate immunizations can be given |
| | | Administer appropriate childhood immunizations. | To prevent infectious diseases |
| | | Administer antibiotics as prescribed. | To treat infections |
| | | Implement and carry out Standard Precautions. | To prevent spread of virus |

*Continued*

# NURSING CARE PLAN

## The Child or Adolescent with Human Immunodeficiency Virus (HIV) Infection—cont'd

| Nursing Diagnosis | Expected Patient Outcomes | Nursing Interventions | Rationale |
|---|---|---|---|
| | | Instruct others (e.g., family, members of staff) in appropriate precautions; clarify any misconceptions about communicability of virus. | To ensure adequate knowledge |
| | | Teach affected children infection control protective methods (e.g., hand washing, handling genital area, care after using bedpan or toilet). | To prevent spread of infection |
| | | Assess home situation, and implement protective measures as feasible in individual circumstances. | To prevent spread of infection |
| | | **The Following NIC Concepts Apply to These Interventions:**<br>Infection Control<br>Infection Prevention<br>Communicable Disease Management<br>Health Education<br>Medication Management<br>Medication Prescribing<br>Health Screening<br>Immunization/Vaccination Management<br>Infection Protection<br>Medication Administration | |
| Impaired Nutrition: Less Than Body Requirements related to recurrent illness, diarrheal losses, loss of appetite, and oral candidiasis | Child will receive optimum nourishment.<br><br>**The Following NOC Concepts Apply to These Outcomes:**<br>Nutritional Status<br>Nutritional Status: Food and Fluid Intake<br>Sensory Function: Taste and Smell<br>Symptom Control | Provide high-calorie, high-protein meals and snacks. | To meet the body's requirements for metabolism and growth |
| | | Provide foods child prefers. | To encourage eating |
| | | Fortify foods with nutritional supplements (e.g., commercial supplements). | To maximize quality of intake |
| | | Provide meals when child is most likely to eat well. Use creativity to encourage child to eat. | To promote oral intake |
| Child's/Family's Defining Characteristics<br>*Subjective and Objective Data*<br>Observe for manifestations of acquired immunodeficiency syndrome (AIDS) in children:<br>• Growth failure (Failure to thrive)<br>• Lymphadenopathy<br>• Hepatosplenomegaly<br>• Oral candidiasis<br>• Recurrent bacterial infections<br>• Chronic or recurrent diarrhea | | Monitor child's weight and growth. | To promote additional nutritional interventions that can be implemented if growth begins to slow or weight drops |
| | | Administer antifungal medication as prescribed. | To treat oral candidiasis |
| | | **The Following NIC Concepts Apply to These Interventions:**<br>Nutritional Counseling<br>Nutritional Monitoring<br>Nutrition Management<br>Fluid Monitoring<br>Self-Care Assistance: Feeding<br>Teaching: Prescribed Diet<br>Medication Administration | |

| Nursing Diagnosis / Patient Outcomes | Nursing Interventions | Rationale |
|---|---|---|
| **Social isolation** related to physical limitations, hospitalizations, social stigma toward HIV<br><br>Child will participate in peer-group and family activities<br><br>**The Following NOC Concepts Apply to These Outcomes:**<br>Social Interaction Skills<br>Play Participation<br>Social support | Assist child in identifying personal strengths.<br>Educate school personnel and classmates about HIV (while protecting child's personal illness history).<br>Encourage child to participate in activities with other children and family.<br>Encourage child to maintain phone contact with friends during illness or hospitalization.<br><br>**The Following NIC Concepts Apply to These Interventions:**<br>Behavior Modification: Social Skills<br>Recreation Therapy<br>Socialization Enhancement<br>Family Integrity Promotion | To facilitate coping<br>To ensure child is not unnecessarily isolated<br><br>To decrease social isolation |
| **Child's/Family's Defining Characteristics**<br>*Subjective and Objective Data*<br>Neurologic features:<br>• Developmental delay<br>• Loss of previously achieved motor milestones<br>• Possible microcephaly<br>• Abnormal neurologic examination | | |
| **Ineffective Sexuality Patterns** related to risk of disease transmission<br><br>Adolescent exhibits healthy sexual behavior<br><br>**The Following NOC Concepts Apply to These Outcomes:**<br>Personal Well-Being<br>Risk Control: Sexually Transmitted Diseases (STD)<br>Child Development: Adolescence | Educate adolescent about the following:<br>• Sexual transmission of HIV<br>• Risks of perinatal infection<br>• Dangers of promiscuous sexual behaviors<br>• Abstinence, use of condoms<br>• Avoidance of high-risk behaviors<br>Encourage adolescent to talk about feelings and concerns related to sexuality.<br><br>**The Following NIC Concepts Apply to These Interventions:**<br>Behavior Management: Sexual<br>Sexual Counseling<br>Infection Protection<br>Teaching: Safe Sex | To ensure that adolescent has adequate information to identify safe, healthy expressions of sexuality<br><br>To facilitate coping |
| **Child's/Family's Defining Characteristics**<br>*Subjective and Objective Data*<br>• Perinatal infection<br>• Promiscuity<br>• High-risk sexual behaviors | | |
| **Chronic Pain** related to disease process (e.g., encephalopathy, treatments)<br><br>Child will exhibit minimal or no evidence of pain or irritability<br><br>**The Following NOC Concepts Apply to These Outcomes:**<br>Comfort Level<br>Pain Control<br>Pain: Disruptive Effects | Assess pain.<br>Use nonpharmacologic strategies such as distraction, hypnosis, guided imagery.<br>For infants, may try general comfort measures (e.g., rocking, holding, swaddling, reducing environmental stimuli [may or may not be effective because of encephalopathy]).<br>Use pharmacologic strategies (analgesics, NSAIDS).<br>Plan preventive schedule if analgesics are effective in relieving continuous pain.<br>Encourage use of premedication for painful procedures (e.g., use of EMLA, LMX, analgesics).<br>Child may benefit from use of adjunct analgesics (e.g., antidepressants, anticonvulsants) that are effective against neuropathic pain.<br>Use pain assessment record.<br><br>**The Following NIC Concepts Apply to These Interventions:**<br>Analgesic Administration<br>Pain Management | To ensure adequate intervention<br>To help child to manage pain<br><br>To minimize pain<br><br>To treat pain<br>To prevent pain<br><br>To minimize discomfort<br><br>To treat neuropathic pain<br><br>To evaluate the effectiveness of pharmacologic and nonpharmacologic interventions |
| **Child's/Family's Defining Characteristics**<br>*Subjective and Objective Data*<br>• Irritability<br>• Moaning<br>• Rigid position<br>• Refusal to eat or drink<br>• Abnormal neurologic examination | | |

*Continued*

# NURSING CARE PLAN

## The Child or Adolescent with Human Immunodeficiency Virus (HIV) Infection—cont'd

| Nursing Diagnosis | Expected Patient Outcomes | Nursing Interventions | Rationale |
|---|---|---|---|
| Interrupted Family Processes related to having a child with a life-threatening disease | Family will receive adequate support and will be able to meet needs of child. | Recognize family's concerns and need for information. Assess family's understanding of diagnosis and plan of care. Reinforce and clarify explanation of child's condition, procedures, and therapies, as well as the prognosis. Use every opportunity to increase family's understanding of the disease and therapy. Repeat information as often as necessary. Help family interpret infant's or child's behaviors and responses. Set up an appointment time for patient/family education and discussion of concerns. | To increase understanding To increase adherence to treatment schedule |
| **Child's/Family's Defining Characteristics** *Subjective and Objective Data* Family members verbalize: | **The Following NOC Concepts Apply to These Outcomes:** Family Coping Family Normalization Caregiver Emotional Health Parenting Performance Family Functioning Hope Fear Self-Control Knowledge: Treatment Regimen | **The Following NIC Concepts Apply to These Interventions:** Family Support Counseling Family Involvement Promotion Coping Enhancement Family Process Maintenance Caregiver Support Emotional Support Spiritual Support | |
| • Fear of child's death • Lack of understanding of disease • Inability to understand treatment plan | | | |
| Grieving related to having a child with a potentially fatal illness | Family will receive adequate support and will be able to meet needs of child. | **The Following NIC Concepts Apply to These Interventions:** Family Support Counseling Family Integrity Promotion Emotional Support Grief Work Facilitation | |
| **Child's/Family's Defining Characteristics** *Subjective and Objective Data* • Unstable emotions • Depression • Withdrawn behavior • Aggressiveness | **The Following NOC Concepts Apply to These Outcomes:** Family Coping Family Normalization Caregiver Emotional Health Parenting Performance Family Functioning Grief Resolution Dignified Life Closure | | |

*Continued*

Risk for Impaired Parenting
OR
Risk for Impaired Attachment

**Child's/Family's Defining Characteristics**
*Subjective and Objective Data*
• Birth of child with possible chronic illness
• Inadequate child care arrangements
• Prolonged separation
• Potential parent substance use
• Anxiety associated with caring for a newborn
• Lack of financial and social support

Mother of newborn will demonstrate interest in and ability to provide primary care for her newborn.

**The Following NOC Concepts Apply to These Outcomes:**
Caregiver role support
Caregiver Lifestyle disruption
Coping
Parent-infant attachment

Assess mother's perception of newborn and her parental role.
Assess mother's social and financial support systems.
Assist with feeding, diapering, skin care, cord care, and other newborn care as necessary.
Encourage mother in her maternal role (as assessment above warrants) and in abilities to provide basic care for newborn.
Assess strengths of mother in providing parenting activities.
Mobilize maternal financial and supportive resources per above assessment.
Discuss plans for infant care and medical follow-up with mother.
Encourage mother to become involved in newborn care in early postpartum period.

**The Following NIC Concepts Apply to These Interventions:**
Emotional Support
Bottle feeding
Case Management
Family support
Parent Education: Infant

To evaluate mother's caretaking concept
To mutually plan for support system enhancement
To provide emotional support and encouragement
To provide an environment conducive to childrearing
To ensure that adequate medical care is obtained in newborn and infant period to care for infant's medical needs
To foster involvement in care

# Nursing Care of the Child with Neurologic Dysfunction

## NURSING CARE PLAN

### The Child with Bacterial Meningitis

| Nursing Diagnosis | Expected Patient Outcomes | Nursing Interventions | Rationale |
|---|---|---|---|
| Risk for Injury related to presence of harmful bacteria | Child does not experience injury | Assist with diagnostic procedures and tests. | To identify source of infection |
| | | Administer antibiotics as soon as lumbar puncture and blood cultures are obtained. | To implement bactericidal therapy |
| **Child's/Family's Defining Characteristics** | **The Following NOC Concepts Apply to These Outcomes:** Risk Control: Infectious process | Initiate and maintain isolation precautions—private room, standard and droplet-mask, gown, gloves (droplet for at least 24 hours after initiation of antibiotics). | To prevent spread of infection |
| *Subjective and Objective Data* Risk Factors | Risk Control | Maintain IV access for administration of fluids and medications. | To maintain adequate tissue hydration and increase effectiveness of medications |
| • External: Chemical | Risk Detection | Explain all procedures to child at age-appropriate level. | To decrease child's fear of the unknown |
| • Internal: Immune-autoimmune dysfunction | Physical Injury Severity | Monitor child closely for signs of complications such as increased intracranial pressure (ICP), shock, seizure activity, or respiratory distress. | To implement therapy and prevent life-threatening complications |
| • Physical: Abnormal blood (and cerebrospinal fluid [CSF]) profile | | | |

# NURSING CARE PLAN

## The Child with Bacterial Meningitis—cont'd

| Nursing Diagnosis | Expected Patient Outcomes | Nursing Interventions | Rationale |
|---|---|---|---|
| | | Observe child for signs such as change in level of consciousness (LOC), appearance of petechiae, or spontaneous bleeding. | To evaluate tissue hydration status |
| | | Monitor and record fluid intake and output. | |
| | | Implement seizure precautions. | To prevent bodily harm in the event of seizure activity |
| | | Help child achieve position of comfort and reduce environmental stimuli as necessary. | To decrease stimuli that may be irritating to the child's neurologic system |
| | | **The Following NIC Concepts Apply to These Interventions:** | |
| | | Risk Identification | |
| | | Support System Enhancement | |
| | | Environmental Management: Safety | |
| | | Infection Protection | |
| | | Medication Administration | |
| | | Seizure Precautions | |
| | | Vital Signs Monitoring | |
| Acute Pain related to inflammatory process | Child exhibits no or minimum signs of pain. | Allow child to assume position of comfort. | To reduce discomfort |
| | | Elevate head of bed 15 to 30 degrees. | To reduce ICP |
| **Child's/Family's Defining Characteristics** | **The Following NOC Concept Applies to These Outcomes:** | Administer analgesic or other pain reliever. | To manage pain by reduction or removal of pain |
| *Subjective and Objective Data* | Pain Control | Use nonpharmacologic pain management such as distraction. | To manage pain |
| Verbal report | Sensory Function | Allow child's parent to stay with child at all times. | To reduce fear and provide support |
| Guarding behavior | | Allow child to keep favorite stuffed animal, doll, or pillow from home. | To promote comfort and emotional security |
| Observed evidence | | Monitor for indications of increased ICP, meningeal irritation. | To institute therapies to reduce ICP (as necessary) or meningeal irritation and prevent further pain |
| Sleep disturbance | | | |
| *Related Factors* | | | |
| Changes in appetite and eating | | | |
| Autonomic responses (diaphoresis, changes in blood pressure, respiration, pulse) | | | |

Monitor IV site and lumbar puncture site for pain or discomfort. Monitor child's response to analgesic, and encourage child to request pain medication when pain begins; use objective pain scale such as FLACC or FACES Pain Scale (as developmentally appropriate). — To implement pain management strategies and reduce chance of physical trauma

**The Following NIC Concepts Apply to These Interventions:**
Analgesic Administration
Positioning
Environmental Management: Comfort
Teaching: Individual
Pain Management
Distraction

Educate parent(s) about child's illness. — To decrease fear of unknown

Educate parent(s)/family regarding isolation precautions, and encourage frequent hand washing by child and family members. — To keep family informed of child's condition and prevent spread of infection

Provide information about child's condition, progress during hospitalization, and treatment and procedures required. — To reduce anxiety

Allow parent(s) to remain with child as much as possible.

Encourage parent(s) to participate in the child's care as much as feasible. — To promote sense of control and decrease sense of helplessness of child; To promote normalization of family and family functioning

Identify close contacts who may require prophylactic antibiotic therapy. — To prevent spread of infection in close contacts

Initiate discharge planning for home care.

Encourage health maintenance activities such as routine childhood immunizations, including meningococcal vaccine for susceptible individuals. — To involve family in child's care; To prevent childhood illness and promote wellness

**The Following NIC Concepts Apply to These Interventions:**
Family Involvement Promotion
Family Support
Family Process Maintenance
Normalization Promotion
Family Integrity Promotion

---

**Interrupted Family Processes** related to child's serious illness, hospitalization, unfamiliar environment, and change in pattern of routines

**Child's/Family's Defining Characteristics**
*Subjective and Objective Data*
• Changes in patterns and rituals

*Related Factor*
• Shift in health status of a family member

Family function is maintained, and family assumes supportive role of child

**The Following NOC Concepts Apply to These Outcomes:**
Family Coping
Family Functioning
Family Normalization

# Nursing Care of the Child with Cancer

## NURSING CARE PLAN

### The Child with Cancer

| Nursing Diagnosis | Expected Patient Outcomes | Nursing Interventions | Rationale |
|---|---|---|---|
| Risk for Injury related to chemotherapy treatment | Child exhibits no complications of chemotherapy | Administer chemotherapeutic agents using established guidelines. | To prevent inappropriate administration techniques |
| **Child's/Family's Defining Characteristics** | Child will receive prompt, appropriate treatment of complications | Assist with procedures for administration of chemotherapeutic agents. | To promote safer cancer treatment |
| *Subjective and Objective Data* | | Administer medications around the clock to prevent nausea and vomiting before chemotherapy. | To minimize side effects of nausea and vomiting |
| • Anaphylaxis: wheezing, hypotension, urticaria, cyanosis | **The Following NOC Concept Applies to These Outcomes:** | Administer IV fluids as prescribed. | To maintain hydration |
| • Nausea, vomiting | Risk Control | Encourage frequent intake of fluids in small amounts. | To promote hydration |
| • IV infiltration: pain, redness, swelling at IV infusion site | Hydration | Observe for signs of infiltration of intravenous site: pain, stinging, swelling, redness. | To prevent drug infiltration |
| | | Institute policies to treat infiltration if it occurs. | To prevent complications |
| | | Observe child for 20 minutes after infusion of drugs that are associated with risk of anaphylaxis. | To observe for signs of anaphylaxis |
| | | Stop infusion of drug and flush IV line with normal saline if drug reaction is suspected. | To prevent physical harm (anaphylaxis, extravasation, or other localized reaction to drug) |
| | | Have emergency equipment and emergency drugs readily available. | To prevent delay in treatment |
| | | **The Following NIC Concepts Apply to These Interventions:**<br>Chemotherapy Management<br>Nausea Management | |
| Risk for Infection related to depressed body defenses | Child does not exhibit signs of infection. | Use rigorous hand-washing technique. | To minimize exposure to infective organisms |
| **Child's/Family's Defining Characteristics** | Child does not come in contact with infected persons. | Screen all visitors and staff for signs of infection. | To decrease exposure to possible infective organisms |
| *Subjective and Objective Data* | | Use aseptic technique for all invasive procedures. | To decrease chance of infection spread |
| • Fever, altered vital signs, lethargy, change in behavior, septic shock | **The Following NOC Concepts Apply to These Outcomes:** | Monitor temperature. | To detect possible infection |
| | Risk Control | | To evaluate needle puncture sites, mucosa for ulceration, minor abrasions for possible infection |
| | Immune Status | Evaluate child for any potential sites of infection. | |
| | Infection Severity | | |
| | | Provide nutritionally complete diet. | To support body's natural defenses |
| | | Avoid giving live attenuated virus vaccines (e.g., varicella). | To prevent overwhelming infection |
| | | Give inactivated virus vaccines. | To prevent specific infections and to avoid placing the child at risk for acquiring the illness |

| Child's/Family's Defining Characteristics | The Following NOC Concepts Apply to These Outcomes | Interventions | Rationale |
|---|---|---|---|
| | | Administer antibiotics as prescribed.<br>Administer granulocyte colony-stimulating factor (G-CSF) as prescribed.<br><br>**The Following NIC Concepts Apply to These Interventions:**<br>Infection Protection<br>Infection Control<br>Immunization/Vaccination Management | To treat a specific infection<br>To promote production of infection-fighting cells |
| **Imbalanced Nutrition: Less Than Body Requirements** related to loss of appetite<br><br>**Child's/Family's Defining Characteristics**<br>*Subjective and Objective Data*<br>• Weight loss, lack of appetite, nausea | Child's nutritional intake is adequate for growth and development.<br><br>**The Following NOC Concepts Apply to These Outcomes:**<br>Nutritional Status: Food and Fluid Intake<br>Nutritional Status: Nutrient Intake | Encourage parents to relax pressure placed on eating.<br>Allow child any food tolerated.<br>Explain expected increase in appetite if child will be taking steroids.<br>Fortify foods with nutritious supplements.<br>Allow child to be involved in food preparation and selection.<br>Make food appealing to child.<br>Monitor child's weight.<br><br>**The Following NIC Concepts Apply to These Interventions:**<br>Nutrition Management<br>Nutrition Therapy | To educate that loss of appetite is a consequence of chemotherapy<br>To provide food; selections can improve once appetite increases<br>To prepare child and family for this change<br>To maximize quality of intake<br>To encourage eating<br>To encourage eating<br>To monitor child's status |
| **Pain** (Specify: Acute, Chronic) related to diagnosis, treatment, physiologic effects of cancer<br><br>**Child's/Family's Defining Characteristics**<br>*Subjective and Objective Data*<br>• Crying<br>• Withdrawal<br>• Fear of procedures<br>• Reluctance to move<br>• Change in vital signs | Child will experience no pain or reduction of pain to level acceptable to the child.<br><br>**The Following NOC Concepts Apply to These Outcomes:**<br>Pain Level<br>Pain: Disruptive Effects<br>Pain Control | Use pharmacologic and nonpharmacologic interventions before painful procedures.<br>Assess pain with each vital sign measurement.<br>Assess for oral stomatitis and treat with local anesthetics, mouth rinses, or prescribed drugs as necessary.<br>Evaluate effectiveness of pain relief.<br>Administer analgesics as prescribed on preventive schedule (around the clock) when needed.<br><br>**The Following NIC Concept Applies to These Interventions:**<br>Pain Management | To minimize discomfort and minimize or prevent pain<br>To determine level of pain<br>To decrease pain and encourage oral intake of food/fluids<br>To determine effectiveness<br>To prevent pain from recurring |
| **Fear** related to diagnostic tests, procedures, treatment<br><br>**Child's/Family's Defining Characteristics**<br>*Subjective and Objective Data*<br>• Worry and anxiety before procedures<br>• Withdrawal<br>• Lack of control<br>• Outbursts<br>• Anger<br>• Lack of cooperation | Child has reduced fear related to diagnostic procedures and treatment.<br><br>**The Following NOC Concepts Apply to These Outcomes:**<br>Fear Self-Control<br>Pain Control | Explain procedures carefully at child's level of understanding.<br>Explain what will take place and what child will feel, see, and hear.<br>Listen to special requests of child when possible.<br>Provide child with some means of involvement with procedures (e.g., holding a piece of equipment, helping put on bandage, or counting).<br>Implement distraction techniques and pain-reduction interventions.<br><br>**The Following NIC Concepts Apply to These Interventions:**<br>Pain Management | To reduce fear of unknown<br>To provide sense of control<br>To encourage cooperation<br>To provide sense of control, encourage cooperation, and support child's coping skills<br>To reduce pain |

*Continued*

5 - NURSING CARE PLANS

# NURSING CARE PLAN

## The Child with Cancer—cont'd

| Nursing Diagnosis | Expected Patient Outcomes | Nursing Interventions | Rationale |
|---|---|---|---|
| Disturbed Body Image, related to changes caused by cancer and treatment | Child will exhibit positive coping skills. | Encourage child to decide how he or she will cope with hair loss (e.g., wig, cap, or scarf). | To promote early adjustment and preparation for hair loss |
| | | Provide adequate covering during exposure to sunlight, wind, or cold. | To prevent exposure |
| **Child's/Family's Defining Characteristics** | **The Following NOC Concept Applies to These Outcomes:** | Explain that hair begins to regrow in 3 to 6 months and may be a different color and texture. | |
| *Subjective and Objective Data* | Body Image | Encourage good hygiene and grooming. | To reduce risk of infection |
| • Sadness | | Encourage rapid return to peer group and friends. | To prepare child for reactions of others |
| • Depression | | Encourage visits from friends before discharge. | To prepare child for reactions of others |
| • Withdrawal | | | |
| • Anger | | **The Following NIC Concepts Apply to These Interventions:** | |
| | | Counseling | |
| | | Body Image Enhancement | |
| Interrupted Family Processes related to having a child with a life-threatening disease | Child and family demonstrate understanding of the disease and treatment. | Teach parents and child about the disease, and explain all procedures. | To promote understanding |
| | | Advise family of expected side effects and toxicities; clarify which demand medical evaluation. | To prevent delay in treatment |
| **Child's/Family's Defining Characteristics** | **The Following NOC Concepts Apply to These Outcomes:** | Reassure family that reactions are complications of treatment. | To provide support |
| *Subjective and Objective Data* | Family Functioning | Prepare family for what to do when side effects occur. | To prevent delay in treatment |
| • Lack of understanding of disease and treatment | Family Coping | Interpret prognostic statistics carefully, realizing family's level of understanding. | To promote understanding |
| • Inability to identify side effects of treatment | Family Normalization | Schedule time for family to be together without interruptions. | To encourage communication and expression of feelings |
| • Inability to understand child's treatment plan | Knowledge: Illness Care | Help family plan for future. | To promote child's development |
| • Lack of family support | | Encourage family to discuss feelings regarding child's disease. | To encourage expression of feelings |
| | | **The Following NIC Concepts Apply to These Interventions:** | |
| | | Counseling | |
| | | Family Support | |

# Reference Data

## Common Laboratory Tests

| Test, Specimen | Age, Gender, Reference | NORMAL RANGES | |
|---|---|---|---|
| | | Conventional Units | International Units (SI) |
| Acetaminophen | | | |
| Serum or plasma | Therap conc | 10-30 mcg/ml | 66-200 μmol/L |
| | Toxic conc | >200 mcg/ml | >1300 μmol/L |
| Alkaline phosphatase | Infant | 150-420 U/L | 150-420 U/L |
| | 2-10 yr | 100-320 U/L | 100-320 U/L |
| | Adolescent male | 100-390 U/L | 100-390 U/L |
| | Adolescent female | 100-320 U/L | 100-320 U/L |
| Ammonia | | | |
| Plasma or serum | <30 days | 21-95 μmol/L | 21-95 μmol/L |
| | 1-12 mo | 18-74 μmol/L | 18-74 μmol/L |
| | 1-14 yr | 17-68 μmol/L | 17-68 μmol/L |
| | >14 yr | 19-71 μmol/L | 19-71 μmol/L |
| Amylase (serum) | 1-19 yr | 30-100 U/L | 30-100 U/L |
| Anion gap (sodium-[chloride + bicarbonate]) | | 7-16 mEq/L | 7-16 mEq/L |
| Antistreptolysin O Titer (ASO) | | | |
| Serum | 2-5 yr | <160 Todd units | |
| | 6-9 yr | 240 Todd units | |
| | 10-12 yr | 320 Todd units | |
| Alanine | Neonate/infant | 13-45 U/L | 13-45 U/L |
| Aminotransferase | Adult male | 10-40 U/L | 10-40 U/L |
| (ALT) | Adult female | 7-35 U/L | 7-35 U/L |
| Amylase (serum) | Newborn | 5-65 U/L | 5-65 U/L |
| | Adult | 27-131 U/L | 27-131 U/L |
| Antinuclear antibody | Not significant | <1:80 | |
| (ANA) | Likely significant | >1:320 | |
| Base Excess | | | |
| Whole blood | Newborn | (−10)-(−2) mEq/L | (−10)-(−2) mmol/L |
| | Infant | (−7)-(−1) mEq/L | (−7)-(−1) mmol/L |
| | Child | (−4)-(+2) mEq/L | (−4)-(+2) mmol/L |
| | Thereafter | (−3)-(+3) mEq/L | (−3)-(+3) mmol/L |

Modified from Kliegman RM, Behrman RE, Jenson HB, Stanton BF, editors: *Nelson textbook of pediatrics*, ed 18, Philadelphia, 2007; Custer JW, Rau RE, editors: *The Harriet Lane Handbook: A manual for pediatric house officers,* ed 18, Philadelphia, 2009, Elsevier Mosby. *Continued*

| | | NORMAL RANGES | | | |
|---|---|---|---|---|---|
| **Test, Specimen** | **Age, Gender, Reference** | **Conventional Units** | | **International Units (SI)** | |
| Bicarbonate (HCO₃) | | | | | |
| Serum | Arterial | 21-28 mmol/L | | 21-28 mmol/L | |
| | Venous | 22-29 mmol/L | | 22-29 mmol/L | |
| **Bilirubin**, total | | Premature (mg/dl) | Full-term (mg/dl) | Premature (μmol/L) | Full-term (μmol/L) |
| Serum | Cord | <2 | <2 | <34 | <34 |
| | 0-1 d | <8 | <8.7 | <137 | <149 |
| | 1-2 d | <12 | <11.5 | <205 | <197 |
| | 3-5 d | <16 | <12 | <274 | <205 |
| | Older infant | <2 | <1.2 | <34 | <21 |
| Bilirubin, Direct (Conjugated) | | | | | |
| Serum | Neonate | <0.6 mg/dl | | <10 μmol/L | |
| | Infant/child | <0.2 mg/dl | | <3.4 μmol/L | |
| Bleeding Time | | | | | |
| | 1-5 yr | 6 min (2.5-10) | | | |
| | 6-10 yr | 7 min (2.5-13) | | | |
| | 11-16 yr | 5 min (3-8) | | | |
| Estimated Blood Volume | | | | | |
| Whole blood | Term newborn | 78-86 ml/kg | | | |
| | 1-12 mo | 73-78 ml/kg | | | |
| | 1-3 yr | 74-82 ml/kg | | | |
| | 4-6 yr | 80-86 ml/kg | | | |
| | 7-18 yr | 83-90 ml/kg | | | |
| C-reactive Protein (CRP) | | | | | |
| Serum (values given are for males; there is slight difference for females) | 0-90 days | 0.08-1.58 mg/dl | | 0.8-15.8 mg/L | |
| | 91 d-12 mo | 0.08-1.12 mg/dl | | 0.8-11.2 mg/L | |
| | 13 mo-3 yr | 0.08-1.12 mg/dl | | 0.8-11.2 mg/L | |
| | 4-10 yr | 0.06-0.79 mg/dl | | 0.6-7.9 mg/L | |
| | 11-14 yr | 0.08-0.76 mg/dl | | 0.8-7.6 mg/L | |
| | 15-18 yr | 0.04-0.79 mg/dl | | 0.4-7.9 mg/L | |
| Calcium, Ionized | | | | | |
| Serum, plasma, or whole blood | Cord | 5.0-6.0 mg/dl | | 1.25-1.50 mmol/L | |
| | Newborn, 3-24 hr | 4.3-5.1 mg/dl | | 1.07-1.27 mmol/L | |
| | 24-48 hr | 4.0-4.7 mg/dl | | 1.00-1.17 mmol/L | |
| | Thereafter | 4.8-4.92 mg/dl or 2.24-2.46 mEq/L | | 1.12-1.23 mmol/L | |
| Calcium, Total | | | | | |
| Serum | Cord | 9.0-11.5 mg/dl | | 2.25-2.88 mmol/L | |
| | Newborn, 3-24 hr | 9.0-10.6 mg/dl | | 2.3-2.65 mmol/L | |
| | 24-48 hr | 7.0-12.0 mg/dl | | 1.75-3.0 mmol/L | |
| | 4-7 d | 9.0-10.9 mg/dl | | 2.25-2.73 mmol/L | |
| | Child | 8.8-10.8 mg/dl | | 2.2-2.70 mmol/L | |
| | Thereafter | 8.4-10.2 mg/dl | | 2.1-2.55 mmol/L | |
| Carbon Dioxide, Partial Pressure (PCO₂) | | | | | |
| Whole blood, arterial | Newborn | 27-40 mm Hg | | 3.6-5.3 kPa | |
| | Infant | 27-41 mm Hg | | 3.6-5.5 kPa | |
| | Thereafter: Male | 35-48 mm Hg | | 4.7-6.4 kPa | |
| | Female | 32-45 mm Hg | | 4.3-6.0 kPa | |

| | | NORMAL RANGES | |
|---|---|---|---|
| **Test, Specimen** | **Age, Gender, Reference** | **Conventional Units** | **International Units (SI)** |
| Carbon Dioxide, Total (CO$_2$ Content) | | | |
| Serum or plasma | Cord | 14-22 mEq/L | 14-22 mmol/L |
| | Premature (1 wk) | 14-27 mEq/L | 14-27 mmol/L |
| | Newborn | 13-22 mEq/L | 13-22 mmol/L |
| | Infant, child | 20-28 mEq/L | 20-28 mmol/L |
| | Thereafter | 23-30 mEq/L | 23-30 mmol/L |
| Cerebrospinal Fluid (CSF) | | | |
| Opening Pressure (lateral recumbent) | Newborn | 8-11 cm H$_2$O | |
| | Infant/child | <29 cm H$_2$O | |
| **Chloride** | | | |
| Serum or plasma | Cord | 96-104 mEq/L | 96-104 mmol/L |
| | Newborn | 97-110 mEq/L | 97-110 mmol/L |
| | Thereafter | 98-106 mEq/L | 98-106 mmol/L |
| Sweat | Normal (homozygote) | <40 mEq/L | <40 mmol/L |
| | Marginal (e.g., asthma, Addison disease, malnutrition) | 45-60 mEq/L | 45-60 mmol/L |
| | Cystic fibrosis | >60 mEq/L | >60 mmol/L |
| Cholesterol, Total (Lipids) | | | |
| Serum or plasma | Acceptable | <170 mg/dl (LDL <110 mg/dl) HDL 45 (desirable) | <4.4 mmol/L (LDL <2.85 mmol/L) |
| | Borderline | 170-199 mg/dl (LDL 110-129 mg/dl) | 4.4-5.1 mmol/L (LDL 2.85-3.35 mmol/L) |
| | High | ≥200 mg/dl (LDL ≥130 mg/dl) | ≥5.2 mmol/L (LDL ≥3.35 mmol/L) |
| Creatine Kinase (CK) | | | |
| Serum | Cord | 70-380 U/L | 70-380 U/L |
| | 5-8 hr | 214-1175 U/L | 214-1175 U/L |
| | 24-33 hr | 130-1200 U/L | 130-1200 U/L |
| | 72-100 hr | 87-725 U/L | 87-725 U/L |
| | Adult | 5-130 U/L | 5-130 U/L |
| Creatinine | | | |
| Serum | Cord | 0.6-1.2 mg/dl | 53-106 μmol/L |
| | Newborn | 0.3-1.0 mg/dl | 27-88 μmol/L |
| | Infant | 0.2-0.4 mg/d | 18-35 μmol/L |
| | Child | 0.3-0.7 mg/dl | 27-62 μmol/L |
| | Adolescent | 0.5-1.0 mg/dl | 44-88 μmol/L |
| Urine, 24 hr | Premature | 8.1-15.0 mg/kg/24 hr | 72-133 μmol/kg/24 hr |
| | Full-term | 10.4-19.7 mg/kg/24 hr | 92-174 μmol/kg/24 hr |
| | 1.5-7 yr | 10-15 mg/kg/24 hr | 88-133 μmol/kg/24 hr |
| | 7-15 yr | 5.2-41 mg/kg/24 hr | 46-362 μmol/kg/24 hr |
| Creatinine Clearance (Endogenous) | | | |
| Serum or plasma and urine | Newborn | 40-65 ml/min/1.73 m$^2$ | |
| | <40 yr:    Male | 97-137 ml/min/1.73 m$^2$ | |
| | Female | 88-128 ml/min/1.73 m$^2$ | |
| Digoxin | | | |
| Serum, plasma; collect at least 12 hr after dose | Therap conc | 0.8-2.0 ng/ml | |
| | Toxic conc | >2.0-2.5 ng/ml | |

*Continued*

| Test, Specimen | Age, Gender, Reference | NORMAL RANGES | |
|---|---|---|---|
| | | **Conventional Units** | **International Units (SI)** |
| Eosinophil Count | | | |
| Whole blood, capillary blood | | 50-250 cells/mm³ (µl) 50-250 × 10⁶ cells/L | |
| Erythrocyte (RBC) Count | | | |
| Whole blood | Cord | 3.9-5.5 million/mm³ | 3.9-5.5 × 10¹² cells/L |
| | 1-3 d | 4.0-6.6 million/mm³ | 4.0-6.6 × 10¹² cells/L |
| | 1 wk | 3.9-6.3 million/mm³ | 3.9-6.3 × 10¹² cells/L |
| | 2 wk | 3.6-6.2 million/mm³ | 3.6-6.2 × 10¹² cells/L |
| | 1 mo | 3.0-5.4 million/mm³ | 3.0-5.4 × 10¹² cells/L |
| | 2 mo | 2.7-4.9 million/mm³ | 2.7-4.9 × 10¹² cells/L |
| | 3-6 mo | 3.1-4.5 million/mm³ | 3.1-4.5 × 10¹² cells/L |
| | 0.5-2 yr | 3.7-5.3 million/mm³ | 3.7-5.3 × 10¹² cells/L |
| | 2-6 yr | 3.9-5.3 million/mm³ | 3.9-5.3 × 10¹² cells/L |
| | 6-12 yr | 4.0-5.2 million/mm³ | 4.0-5.2 × 10¹² cells/L |
| | 12-18 yr: Male | 4.5-5.3 million/mm³ | 4.5-5.3 × 10¹² cells/L |
| | Female | 4.1-5.1 million/mm³ | 4.1-5.1 × 10¹² cells/L |
| Erythrocyte Sedimentation Rate (ESR) | | | |
| | Term neonate | 0-4 mm/hr | |
| | Child | 4-20 mm/hr | |
| **D-Dimer**, plasma | Adults (positive titer) | ≥1:8 | |
| **Fibrin degradation products** | Adults | Positive titer <1:50 | |
| Fibrinogen | | | |
| Plasma | Term Newborn Day 1 | 283 mg/dl (167-309) | 2.83 g/L |
| | 1-5 yr | 276 mg/dl (170-405) | 2.76 g/L |
| | 6-10 yr | 279 mg/dl (157-400) | 2.79 g/L |
| | 11-16 yr | 300 mg/dl (154-448) | 3.0 g/L |
| Galactose | | | |
| Serum | Newborn | 0-20 mg/dl | 0-1.11 mmol/L |
| | Thereafter | <5 mg/dl | <0.28 mmol/L |
| Urine | Newborn | ≤60 mg/dl | ≤3.33 mmol/L |
| | Thereafter | <14 mg/24 hr | <0.08 mmol/d |
| Glucose | | | |
| Serum | Cord | 45-96 mg/dl | 2.5-5.3 mmol/L |
| | Newborn, 1 d | 40-60 mg/dl | 2.2-3.3 mmol/L |
| | Newborn, >1 d | 50-90 mg/dl | 2.8-5.0 mmol/L |
| | Child | 60-100 mg/dl | 3.3-5.5 mmol/L |
| | Thereafter | 70-105 mg/dl | 3.9-5.8 mmol/L |
| Whole blood | Adult | 65-95 mg/dl | 3.6-5.3 mmol/L |
| CSF | Adult | 40-70 mg/dl | 2.2-3.9 mmol/L |
| Urine (quantitative) | | <0.5 g/d | <2.8 mmol/d |
| Urine (qualitative) | | Negative | Negative |

Glucose Tolerance Test (GTT), Oral
Serum

| | | Normal | Diabetic | Normal | Diabetic |
|---|---|---|---|---|---|
| Dosages | | | | | |
| Adult: 75 g | Fasting | 70-105 mg/dl | ≥126 mg/dl | 3.9-5.8 mmol/L | ≥7 mmol/L |
| Child: 1.75 g/kg of | 60 min | 120-170 mg/dl | ≥200 mg/dl | 6.7-9.4 mmol/L | ≥11 mmol/L |
| ideal weight up to | 90 min | 100-140 mg/dl | ≥200 mg/dl | 5.6-7.8 mmol/L | ≥11 mmol/L |
| maximum of 75 g | 120 min | 70-120 mg/dl | ≥200 mg/dl | 3.9-6.7 mmol/L | ≥11 mmol/L |

| Test, Specimen | Age, Gender, Reference | NORMAL RANGES | |
|---|---|---|---|
| | | **Conventional Units** | **International Units (SI)** |
| Glucose Tolerance Test (GTT), Oral—cont'd | | | |
| **Glycosylated hemoglobin Hb A1c** ** desired goal for type 1 diabetic children | 0-6 yrs | <8.5% but >7.5% | |
| | 6-12 yrs | <8% | |
| | 13-19 yrs | <7.5% | |
| | Target goal for nonpregnant adults | ≤6.5% | |
| Hematocrit (HCT, Hct) Whole blood | 1 d (capillary) | 48%-69% | 0.48-0.69 vol fraction |
| | 2 d | 48%-75% | 0.48-0.75 vol fraction |
| | 3 d | 44%-72% | 0.44-0.72 vol fraction |
| | 2 mo | 28%-42% | 0.28-0.42 vol fraction |
| | 6-12 yr | 35%-45% | 0.35-0.45 vol fraction |
| | 12-18 yr: Male | 37%-49% | 0.37-0.49 vol fraction |
| | Female | 36%-46% | 0.36-0.46 vol fraction |
| Hemoglobin (Hb) Whole blood | 1-3 d (capillary) | 14.5-22.5 g/dl | 2.25-3.49 mmol/L |
| | 2 mo | 9.0-14.0 g/dl | 1.40-2.17 mmol/L |
| | 6-12 yr | 11.5-15.5 g/dl | 1.78-2.40 mmol/L |
| | 12-18 yr: Male | 13.0-16.0 g/dl | 2.02-2.48 mmol/L |
| | Female | 12.0-16.0 g/dl | 1.86-2.48 mmol/L |
| Hemoglobin A Whole blood | | >95% of total | >0.95 fraction of Hb |
| Hemoglobin F Whole blood | 1 d | 77% total Hb | |
| | 5 d | 76.88% total Hb | |
| | 3 wk | 70% total Hb | |
| | 6-9 wk | 52.9 % total Hb | |
| | 3-4 mo | 23.2% total Hb | |
| | 6 mo | 4.7% total Hb | |
| | 8-11 mo | 1.6% total Hb | |
| Immunoglobulin A (IgA) Serum | Cord | 1.4-3.6 mg/dl | 14-36 mg/L |
| | 1-3 mo | 1.3-53 mg/dl | 13-530 mg/L |
| | 4-6 mo | 4.4-84 mg/dl | 44-840 mg/L |
| | 7-12 mo | 11-106 mg/dl | 110-1060 mg/L |
| | 2-5 yr | 14-159 mg/dl | 140-1590 mg/L |
| | 6-10 yr | 33-236 mg/dl | 330-2360 mg/L |
| | Adult | 70-312 mg/dl | 700-3120 mg/L |
| Immunoglobulin D (IgD) Serum | Newborn | None detected | None detected |
| | Thereafter | 0-8 mg/dl | 0-80 mg/L |
| Immunoglobulin E (IgE) Serum | Male | 0-230 IU/ml | 0-230 kIU/L |
| | Female | 0-170 IU/ml | 0-170 kIU/L |

**American Diabetes Association: Standards of medical care in diabetes—2010, *Diabetes Care* 33(Suppl 1):S11-S61, 2010.    *Continued*

| | | NORMAL RANGES | |
|---|---|---|---|
| **Test, Specimen** | **Age, Gender, Reference** | **Conventional Units** | **International Units (SI)** |
| Immunoglobulin G (IgG) | | | |
| Serum | Cord | 636-1606 mg/dl | 6.36-16.06 g/L |
| | 1 mo | 251-906 mg/dl | 2.51-9.06 g/L |
| | 2-4 mo | 176-601 mg/dl | 1.76-6.01 g/L |
| | 5-12 mo | 172-1069 mg/dl | 1.72-10.69 g/L |
| | 1-5 yr | 345-1236 mg/dl | 3.45-12.36 g/L |
| | 6-10 yr | 608-1572 mg/dl | 6.08-15.72 g/L |
| | Adult | 639-1349 mg/dl | 6.39-13.49 g/L |
| Immunoglobulin M (IgM) | | | |
| Serum | Cord | 6.3-25 mg/dl | 63-250 mg/L |
| | 1-4 mo | 17-105 mg/dl | 170-1050 mg/L |
| | 5-9 mo | 33-126 mg/dl | 330-1260 mg/L |
| | 10-12 mo | 41-173 mg/dl | 410-1730 mg/L |
| | 2-8 yr | 43-207 mg/dl | 430-2070 mg/L |
| | 9-10 yr | 52-242 mg/dl | 520-2420 mg/L |
| | Adult | 56-352 mg/dl | 560-3520 mg/L |
| **International Normalized Ratio (INR)**—only for patients on coumarin | DVT target INR | 2-3 sec | |
| | Prosthetic heart valve | 3-4 sec | |
| Iron | | | |
| Serum | Newborn | 100-250 mcg/dl | 18-45 μmol/L |
| | Infant | 40-100 mcg/dl | 7-18 μmol/L |
| | Child | 50-120 mcg/dl | 9-22 μmol/L |
| | Thereafter:   Male | 65-170 mcg/dl | 12-30 μmol/L |
| | Female | 50-170 mcg/dl | 9-30 μmol/L |
| | Intoxicated child | 280-2550 mcg/dl | 50.12-456.5 μmol/L |
| | Fatally poisoned child | >1800 mcg/dl | >322.2 μmol/L |
| Iron-binding capacity, total (TIBC) | | | |
| Serum | Infant | 100-400 mcg/dl | 17.90-71.60 μmol/L |
| | Thereafter | 250-400 mcg/dl | 44.75-71.60 μmol/L |
| Lead | | | |
| Whole blood | Child | <10 mcg/dl | <0.48 μmol/L |
| | Toxic | ≥70 mcg/dl | ≥3.38 μmol/L |
| **Leukocyte count** (WBC count) | | ×1000 cells/mm³ (μl) | ×10⁹ cells/L |
| Whole blood | Birth | 9.0-30.0 | 9.0-30.0 |
| | 24 hr | 9.4-34.0 | 9.4-34.0 |
| | 1 mo | 5.0-19.5 | 5.0-19.5 |
| | 1-3 yr | 6.0-17.5 | 6.0-17.5 |
| | 4-7 yr | 5.5-15.5 | 5.5-15.5 |
| | 8-13 yr | 4.5-13.5 | 4.5-13.5 |
| | Adult | 4.5-11.0 | 4.5-11.0 |
| CSF (cell count) | | ×1000 cells/mm³ (μl) | ×10⁶ cells/L |
| | Preterm | 0-25 mononuclear | 0-25 |
| | | 0-10 polymorphonuclear | 0-10 |
| | | 0-1000 RBCs | 0-1000 |
| | Newborn | 0-20 mononuclear | 0-20 |
| | | 0-10 polymorphonuclear | 0-10 |
| | | 0-800 RBCs | 0-800 |
| | Neonate | 0-5 mononuclear | 0-5 |
| | | 0-10 polymorphonuclear | 0-10 |
| | | 0-50 RBCs | 0-50 |
| | Thereafter | 0-5 mononuclear | 0-5 |

| Test, Specimen | Age, Gender, Reference | NORMAL RANGES | | International Units (SI) |
|---|---|---|---|---|
| | | Conventional Units | | |
| Leukocyte Differential Count | | | | |
| Whole blood | Myelocytes | 0% | 0 cells/mm$^3$ ($\mu$l) | Number fraction 0 |
| | Neutrophils—"bands" | 3%-5% | 150-400 cells/mm$^3$ ($\mu$l) | Number fraction 0.03-0.05 |
| | Neutrophils—"segs" | 54%-62% | 3000-5800 cells/mm$^3$ ($\mu$l) | Number fraction 0.54-0.62 |
| | Lymphocytes | 25%-33% | 1500-3000 cells/mm$^3$ ($\mu$l) | Number fraction 0.25-0.33 |
| | Monocytes | 3%-7% | 285-500 cells/mm$^3$ ($\mu$l) | Number fraction 0.03-0.07 |
| | Eosinophils | 1%-3% | 50-250 cells/mm$^3$ ($\mu$l) | Number fraction 0.01-0.03 |
| | Basophils | 0%-0.75% | 15-50 cells/mm$^3$ ($\mu$l) | Number fraction 0-0.0075 |
| Lipase (serum) | 0-90 days | 10-85 U/L | | 10-85 U/L |
| | 3-12 mo | 9-128 U/L | | 9-128 U/L |
| | 1-11 yr old | 10-150 U/L | | 10-150 U/L |
| | >11 yr | 10-220 U/L | | 10-220 U/L |
| Mean Corpuscular Hemoglobin (MCH) | | | | |
| Whole blood | Birth | 31-37 pg/cell | | 0.48-0.57 fmol/cell |
| | 1-3 d (cap) | 31-37 pg/cell | | 0.48-0.57 fmol/cell |
| | 1 wk-1 mo | 28-40 pg/cell | | 0.43-0.62 fmol/cell |
| | 2 mo | 26-34 pg/cell | | 0.40-0.53 fmol/cell |
| | 3-6 mo | 25-35 pg/cell | | 0.39-0.54 fmol/cell |
| | 0.5-2 yr | 23-31 pg/cell | | 0.36-0.48 fmol/cell |
| | 2-6 yr | 24-30 pg/cell | | 0.37-0.47 fmol/cell |
| | 6-12 yr | 25-33 pg/cell | | 0.39-0.51 fmol/cell |
| | 12-18 yr | 25-35 pg/cell | | 0.39-0.54 fmol/cell |
| | 18-49 yr | 26-34 pg/cell | | 0.40-0.53 fmol/cell |
| Mean Corpuscular Hemoglobin Concentration (MCHC) | | | | |
| Whole blood | Birth | 30%-36% Hb/cell or g Hb/dl RBCs | | 4.65-5.58 mmol Hb/L RBCs |
| | 1-3 d (cap) | 29%-37% Hb/cell or g Hb/dl RBCs | | 4.50-5.74 mmol Hb/L RBCs |
| | 1-2 wk | 28%-38% Hb/cell or g Hb/dl RBCs | | 4.34-5.89 mmol Hb/L RBCs |
| | 1-2 mo | 29%-37% Hb/cell or g Hb/dl RBCs | | 4.50-5.74 mmol Hb/L RBCs |
| | 3 mo-2 yr | 30%-36% Hb/cell or g Hb/dl RBCs | | 4.65-5.58 mmol Hb/L RBCs |
| | 2-18 yr | 31%-37% Hb/cell or g Hb/dl RBCs | | 4.81-5.74 mmol Hb/L RBCs |
| | >18 yr | 31%-37% Hb/cell or g Hb/dl RBCs | | 4.81-5.74 mmol Hb/L RBCs |
| Mean Corpuscular Volume (MCV) | | | | |
| Whole blood | 1-3 d (cap) | 95-121 $\mu$m$^3$ | | 95-121 fl |
| | 0.5-2 yr | 70-86 $\mu$m$^3$ | | 70-86 fl |
| | 6-12 yr | 77-95 $\mu$m$^3$ | | 77-95 fl |
| | 12-18 yr: Male | 78-98 $\mu$m$^3$ | | 78-98 fl |
| | Female | 78-102 $\mu$m$^3$ | | 78-102 fl |
| Activated Partial Thromboplastin Time (aPTT) | | | | |
| | Term infant | 42.9 sec (31.3-54.3) | | |
| | 1-5 yr | 30 sec (24-36) | | |
| | 6-10 yr | 31 sec (26-36) | | |
| | 11-18 yr | 32 sec (26-37) | | |

*Continued*

| Test, Specimen | Age, Gender, Reference | NORMAL RANGES | |
|---|---|---|---|
| | | Conventional Units | International Units (SI) |
| Phenylalanine | | | |
| Serum | Preterm | 2.0-7.5 mg/dl | 120-450 µmol/L |
| | Newborn | 1.2-3.4 mg/dl | 70-210 µmol/L |
| | Thereafter | 0.8-1.8 mg/dl | 50-110 µmol/L |
| Platelet Count (Thrombocyte Count) | | | |
| | Newborn (after 1 wk, same as adult) | $84\text{-}478 \times 10^3/mm^3$ (µl) | $84\text{-}478 \times 10^9$/L |
| | Adult | $150\text{-}400 \times 10^3/mm^3$ (µl) | $150\text{-}400 \times 10^9$/L |
| Potassium | | | |
| Serum | Newborn | 3.0-6.0 mEq/L | 3.0-6.0 mmol/L |
| | Thereafter | 3.5-5.0 mEq/L | 3.5-5.0 mmol/L |
| Plasma (heparin) | | 3.4-4.5 mEq/L | 3.4-4.5 mmol/L |
| Urine, 24 hr | | 2.5-125 mEq/d (varies with diet) | 2.5-125 mmol/L |
| Protein, Total (Serum) | | | |
| | Preterm | 4.3-7.6 g/dl | 43-76 g/L |
| | Newborn | 4.6-7.4 g/dl | 46-74 g/L |
| | 1-7 yr | 6.1-7.9 g/dl | 61-79 g/L |
| | 8-12 yr | 6.4-8.1 g/dl | 64-81 g/L |
| | 13-19 yr | 6.6-8.2 g/dl | 66-82 g/L |
| CSF | | Lumbar: 8-32 mg/dl | 80-320 mg/L |
| Prothrombin Time (PT) | | | |
| Whole blood (Na citrate) | In general | 11-15 sec (varies with type of thromboplastin) | 11-15 sec |
| | Newborn | Prolonged by 2-3 sec | Prolonged by 2-3 sec |
| Reticulocyte Count | | | |
| Whole blood | Adults | 0.5%-1.5% of erythrocytes or 25,000-75,000/mm$^3$ (µl) | 0.005-0.015 (number fraction) or $25,000\text{-}75,000 \times 10^6$/L |
| Capillary | 1 d | 0.4%-6.0% | 0.004-0.060 (number fraction) |
| | 7 d | <0.1%-1.3% | <0.001-0.013 (number fraction) |
| | 1-4 wk | <0.1%-1.2% | <0.001-0.012 (number fraction) |
| | 5-6 wk | <0.1%-2.4% | <0.001-0.024 (number fraction) |
| | 7-8 wk | 0.1%-2.9% | 0.001-0.029 (number fraction) |
| | 9-10 wk | <0.1%-2.6% | <0.001-0.026 (number fraction) |
| | 11-12 wk | 0.1%-1.3% | 0.001-0.013 (number fraction) |
| **Rheumatoid Factor** | <30 U/ml | | |
| Salicylates | | | |
| Serum, plasma | Therap conc | 15-30 mg/dl | 1.1-2.2 mmol/L |
| | Toxic conc | >30 mg/dl | >18.5 mmol/L |
| Sodium | | | |
| Serum or plasma | Newborn | 134-146 mEq/L | 134-146 mmol/L |
| | Infant | 139-146 mEq/L | 139-146 mmol/L |
| | Child | 138-145 mEq/L | 138-145 mmol/L |
| | Thereafter | 136-146 mEq/L | 136-146 mmol/L |
| Urine, 24 hr | | 40-220 mEq/L (diet dependent) | 40-220 mmol/L |
| Sweat | Normal | <40 mEq/L | <40 mmol/L |
| | Indeterminate | 45-60 mEq/L | 45-60 mmol/L |
| | Cystic fibrosis | >60 mEq/L | >60 mmol/L |

| Test, Specimen | Age, Gender, Reference | NORMAL RANGES | | | |
| --- | --- | --- | --- | --- | --- |
| | | **Conventional Units** | | **International Units (SI)** | |
| Specific gravity | | | | | |
| Urine, random | Adult | 1.002-1.030 | | 1.002-1.030 | |
| | After 12-hr fluid restriction | >1.025 | | >1.025 | |
| Urine, 24 hr | | 1.015-1.025 | | | |
| Thrombin time | | | | | |
| Whole blood (Na citrate) | | Control time ±2 s when control is 9-13 s | | Control time ±2 s when control is 9-13 s | |
| Thyroxine, Total ($T_4$) | | | | | |
| Serum | 1-3 day term | 8.2-19.9 mcg/dl | | 106-256 nmol/L | |
| | 1 week | 6-15.9 mcg/dl | | 77-205 nmol/L | |
| | 1-12 mo | 6.1-14.9 mcg/dl | | 79-192 nmol/L | |
| | 1-3 yr | 6.8-13.5 mcg/dl | | 88-174 nmol/L | |
| | 3-10 yr | 5.5-12.8 mcg/dl | | 71-165 nmol/L | |
| | Thereafter | 4.2-13 mcg/dl | | 54-167 nmol/L | |
| Triglycerides (TG), Total | | Male (mg/dl) MEAN | Female (mg/dl) | Male (g/L) 90th percentile | Female (g/L) |
| | Cord | 34 | | | |
| | 1-4 yr | 56 | 64 | 85 | 95 |
| | 5-9 yr | 52 | 64 | 70 | 103 |
| | 10-14 yr | 63 | 72 | 94 | 104 |
| | 15-19 yr | 78 | 73 | 125 | 112 |
| Triiodothyronine ($T_3$), Free | | | | | |
| Serum | Cord | 20-240 pg/dl | | 0.3-3.7 pmol/L | |
| | 1-3 d | 200-610 pg/dl | | 3.1-9.4 pmol/L | |
| | 6 wk | 240-560 pg/dl | | 3.7-8.6 pmol/L | |
| | Adults (20-50 yr) | 230-660 pg/dl | | 3.5-10.0 pmol/L | |
| Triiodothyronine, Total ($T_3$-RIA) | | | | | |
| Serum | Cord | 30-70 ng/dl | | 0.46-1.08 nmol/L | |
| | Newborn | 72-260 ng/dl | | 1.16-4 nmol/L | |
| | 1-5 yr | 100-260 ng/dl | | 1.54-4 nmol/L | |
| | 5-10 yr | 90-240 ng/dl | | 1.39-3.70 nmol/L | |
| | 10-15 yr | 80-210 ng/dl | | 1.23-3.23 nmol/L | |
| | Thereafter | 115-190 ng/dl | | 1.77-2.93 nmol/L | |
| Urea Nitrogen | | | | | |
| Serum or plasma | Cord | 21-40 mg/dl | | 7.5-14.3 mmol/L | |
| | Premature (1 wk) | 3-25 mg/dl | | 1.1-9 mmol/L | |
| | Newborn | 3-12 mg/dl | | 1.1-4.3 mmol/L | |
| | Infant or child | 5-18 mg/dl | | 1.8-6.4 mmol/L | |
| | Thereafter | 7-18 mg/dl | | 2.5-6.4 mmol/L | |

# Index

Page numbers followed by *f* indicate figures; *t*, tables; *b*, text in boxes.

337